KV-732-636

FIGHTING FIT

FIGHTING FIT

HEALTH, MEDICINE
AND WAR IN THE
TWENTIETH CENTURY

KEVIN BROWN

In memory of Harry and Ethel Lazenby, Rob and Jennie Brown

When you see millions of the mouthless dead across your dreams in pale battalions go, say not soft things as other men have said, that you'll remember. For you need not so.

Charles Hamilton Sorley, 1915.

NEWCASTLE LIBRARIES

C447405700

Bertrams	27/11/2008
616.98	£20.00

First published 2008

The History Press Ltd
The Mill, Brimscombe Port
Stroud, Gloucestershire, GL5 2QG
www.thehistorypress.co.uk

© Kevin Brown, 2008

The right of Kevin Brown to be identified as the Author
of this work has been asserted in accordance with the
Copyrights, Designs and Patents Act 1988.

All rights reserved. No part of this book may be reprinted
or reproduced or utilised in any form or by any electronic,
mechanical or other means, now known or hereafter invented,
including photocopying and recording, or in any information
storage or retrieval system, without the permission in writing
from the Publishers.

British Library Cataloguing in Publication Data.
A catalogue record for this book is available from the British Library.

ISBN 978 0 7509 4649 0

Typesetting and origination by The History Press Ltd
Printed in Great Britain

Contents

List of Illustrations   6

Preface   8

1. National Inefficiency   13

2. Medicine in Khaki   37

3. Business not as Usual   66

4. Spanish Rehearsal   88

5. Healing for Victory   110

6. Road to Utopia   139

7. Behind the Wire   164

8. Trauma and Terror   191

Notes   215

Bibliography   258

Index   284

List of Illustrations

1   Boer War casualties.
2   Young doctors and students of St Mary's Hospital Medical School.
3   Sir Almroth Wright.
4   Medical inspection.
5   No. 14 General Hospital.
6   Advanced Dressing Station near Ypres, 20 September 1917.
7   Wounded soldiers fill the wards.
8   Troops blinded by tear gas during the Battle of Estaires, 10 April 1918.
9   A makeshift laboratory.
10 The welfare of children was a concern on the Home Front in the First World War.
11 Rehabilitation: limbless First World War soldiers learn to walk with artificial legs.
12 Blood transfusion pioneer Frederic Duran i Jordà, 1936.
13 VAD (Voluntary Aid Detachment) take on the duties of nurses during the Second World War.
14 A reflection of the strategic importance of penicillin during the Second World War.
15 A nurse and infant with their gas masks, 1940.
16 Nurses and babies leave Great Ormond Street Children's Hospital during the great evacuation of 1939.
17 Soldiers are exhorted to stay clean and avoid the temptations that might reduce their fighting capacities.
18 A wartime cookery demonstration.
19 Archibald McIndoe encourages members of the Guinea Pig Club to enjoy themselves, Christmas 1944.
20 Civilian doctors and nurses.

21 The emergency hospital set up after the liberation of Buchenwald Concentration Camp, 1945.
22 Weary Dunlop and Jacob Markowitz are depicted amputating a thigh.
23 Evacuation by Sikorski S-51 Dragonfly helicopter, Korea, 26 June 1953.
24 Wounded Vietnamese soldiers are winched to safety.

Preface

War and medicine make strange bedfellows. The main purpose of war is to injure, maim and kill. Medicine, by contrast, is dedicated to healing and maintaining good health. Opposing as they may seem, these aims are not totally incompatible. If a nation is to maintain its fighting capability, it requires a healthy citizenry. It also needs to have the means of repairing the ravages inflicted by war on the human body in order to return its servicemen to action as quickly as possible, since, in the words of the great medical humanist Sir William Osler, it is 'strange that man who dominates Nature has so far departed from Nature as to be the only animal to wage relentless war on his own species'.[1] In a modern democracy, a state must be prepared to patch up the damage done to its soldiers by warfare in return for its citizens being ready to risk life and limb; as the Home Front has become as much a battlefield as the theatres of war, medical services for civilian casualties have become part of that implicit pact between state and combatant.

The twentieth century has been marked by wars of great savagery in which technological advances have made the killing machine ever more efficient and deadly. That rapid pace of technological advance in medicine has generally kept pace with the developments in the sinews of war. Indeed in many ways, warfare has accelerated changes in medical practice, though not without opposition from diehard conservative practitioners of military medicine, and has encouraged new ways of looking at things that have been beneficial to patients in general. Both war and medicine in the last century have been impelled by a drive to modernity.[2] Osler believed that the monster of war had brought the blessings of 'the enormous number spared the misery of sickness, the unspeakable tortures saved by anaesthesia, the more prompt care of the wounded, the better surgical technique, the lessened time to convalesce, the whole organization of nursing' and judged that 'the wounded soldier would throw his sword into the scale for science – and he is right'.[3] Yet the picture is not entirely positive. War can impede progress because limited resources are used on the means of waging warfare rather than on drugs or medical care.[4] War has also unleashed callousness towards injury and has perverted medicine from its nobler ethics, not only under authoritarian regimes but wherever it may be accepted that the ends justify the means. Medicine is not a noble calling above the society in which it operates: it is conditioned by, and an integral part of, that society.

The intimacy in the relationship between health, medicine and war is reflected in the language used to describe medicine. We speak of the battle against infection, we wage war on bacteria and patients fight for life. At the same time metaphors for illness can be used in a military context. Military planners talk of 'surgical strikes'. British serviceman liberating France in 1944 were urged to understand that 'when anyone has been living for a long time suffering from privation or in a concentration camp, and is suddenly let out, it takes him time to recuperate. And France had developed under the German occupation much of the physical depression of a huge sick-room, and much of the mental stress of a huge concentration camp'.[5] The Italian futurist artist Virgilio Retrosi depicted the First World War as a giant abscess covering the world with the sores of misery, sickness and taxation.[6] Such terminology reinforces the idea of the heroism of medical pioneers and military doctors. It also suggests that in modern warfare, two battles are ongoing simultaneously, the military one of the armed servicemen and the medical one of the doctors, nurses, stretcher-bearers and medical scientists.

This book tells the story of the interrelationship of these two wars over the course of the twentieth century, a subject surprisingly up to now lacking an overview, such as this one, for the whole century. There are tales of heroism and the ideal of the noble warrior, but there are also accounts of the misery caused by warfare and of inhumanity. Yet, there remains in the popular imagination a romantic tinge of heroism attached to the image of the tending of the sick in the heat of battle. Most war films or dramas would be incomplete without a background of ambulances, first aid posts and Red Cross armbands or the heroic figure of the doctor or nurse. Such imagery is often irresistible because so striking. When the opera director Emilio Sagi updated Donizetti's *La Fille du Régiment* to a Second World War setting for a 2005 production at the Teatro Carlo Felice in Genoa, he had Patrizia Ciofi's Marie don a nurse's headdress to tend the wounded leg of Juan Diego Flórez's Tonio to make him into a soldier fit to fight and ready for the tenor's effortless achievement of his successive nine high Cs.[7] The nurse always remains the beautiful 'Rose of No Man's Land' and the sick and wounded are similarly handsomely idealised. War is never like that and the casualties rarely suffer as picturesquely as in art. Warfare by its very nature is nasty and brutish even when it is justified. Medicine is often very messy.

Yet even out of the chaos and confusion of war can emerge unexpected benefits. It is outside the scope of this book to investigate the ways in which military technology and hardware devised for one purpose subsequently can have entirely pacific benefits in a different context for which they were never envisaged, but we ought to be aware of these possibilities. A classic case of this is ultrasound scanning, which had its origins in a sound-wave device to detect icebergs invented by the American Lewis Nixon in 1906 and subsequently developed to detect the presence of enemy U-boats. By the Second World War, sonograms were being used to detect gallstones, brain tumours, breast cancer and rectal obstructions. Then in the late 1950s the Scottish gynaecologist and obstetrician Ian Donald, a veteran of the First World War, moved on from using ultrasound scanning to detect ovarian cysts to producing clear echoes of babies in the mother's womb to check for foetal abnormalities.[8]

While this book was being written, the newspapers were full of stories of casualties from the fighting in Iraq and Afghanistan, the deplorable closure of specialist military hospitals, the resultant problems in treating wounded service personnel in the general wards and clinics of the National Health Service, and the psychological problems faced by people returning from an unpopular war that their country perhaps should never have got involved in. It seemed as if the pact promising the soldier that he and his dependents would be looked after medically and financially if wounded or killed, in return for risking his life in his country's service, had been breeched.[9] Yet, with military forces stretched, the role of the army doctor in maintaining the health and physical fitness of the soldiers in his unit remains as important as ever.[10] Sometimes it seems as if nothing has been learned from the experience of the last century. It does give immediacy to the themes running through this book and, as always, the past informs the present and the present helps us towards an understanding of history. Yet, however much there might seem to be similarities, it is as well to remember that society a hundred years ago was different from how it is now. What happened in the past was conditioned by a world that is remote from our own and must be understood in its own setting. Medicine, war and society are interrelated and not separate areas of study: to understand one, we need to know something about all and in the context of the times, not by projecting the concerns of 2007–8 back to the 1900s. At the same time, it is by looking at the subject over a long period of time that we can better see the development of war and medicine over a century that has known few periods of true peace.

As ever, many people were very helpful while I was researching this book. I am grateful to Bill Frankland, who has relived the ordeal of his experiences as a prisoner of war of the Japanese in Singapore during the Second World War. Michael Wolach has spoken of the absence of any medical aid during his time in a Soviet camp. Barbara Gammon and Betty Ashton have described their experiences of nursing during the Second World War. Andrew Bamji has kindly given me access to the records of Harold Gillies's First World War work on plastic surgery at Queen Mary's Hospital Sidcup and has liberally given his time in discussing the subject with me, displaying his great enthusiasm for the topic. At the Queen Victoria Hospital, East Grinstead, Bob Marchant very generously gave me access to the collections of the Queen Victoria Hospital Museum, showed me around the hospital as it is today and pointed out buildings surviving from when Archibald McIndoe was treating burnt airmen there in the 1940s, as well as sharing his memories of working with McIndoe in the post-war years. Nicholas Baldwin, Archivist at Great Ormond Street Children's Hospital, has supplied references to child welfare during the First World War. From Ellen Reace, I have learned of the experiences of Londoners evacuated to safer areas to have their babies, and their desire to return to the heavily bombed capital during the Second World War. I have happy memories of discussing the First World War influx of female medical students with James Garner when he was doing his history of medicine dissertation on that very topic. Myer Salamon, Richard Keeler, Neil Handley, Bernard Dixon, Maria Lorentzon, Elise Younger, John Grabenstein and João Carlos Boléo-Tomé, secretary-general of the Fundação Casa de Bragança, have suggested some useful references. Robin Touquet has recommended some leads on more recent military medicine and reminded me of the similarities between military field medicine and the work of modern Accident and Emergency departments. I wish to thank too everyone at The History Press concerned with the commissioning and editing of this, my third book for them.

I must especially mention the assistance of Lluis Martinez, sub-editor of *Avui* in Barcelona, who has proved himself the most helpful of friends over the last five years, and that of his son Guillem whose native Catalan and Spanish tongues and ability in English has facilitated communication between us. Without Lluis's guidance about sources and contacts, the chapter on medicine in the Spanish Civil War would have been infinitely poorer. I also wish to thank Miguel Lozano of the Hospital Clinic, University of Barcelona, the family of Dr Frederic Duran, and Montserrat Mira, daughter of Dr Emili Mira.

Without the resources of countless libraries and archives, the research for this book would have been impossible. Even with the benefits of desktop access through the Internet to many journals, which allow references in them to be consulted without leaving one's seat, there is no substitute for visits to archives and libraries that contain material that is often unique and will never be available online. Such visits may involve more effort and be harder work, but they are so much more rewarding. I wish to thank the staff of the National Archives at Kew; the Wellcome Library; the National Archives and Records Service of the United States; the National Academy of Sciences in Washington DC; the Imperial War Museum; the Royal Society Library; the Musée International de la Croix Rouge et du Croissant Rouge; the Deutsches Hygiene Museum; the National Center for Agricultural Utilization Research in Peoria, Illinois; the Pfizer Records Centre at Sandwich; the Pfizer Information Center in New York; the Rockefeller Archives Center; the Paul Ehrlich Institut; the British Library; the Bodleian Library and the Library of Congress. Long may we all continue to have such unfettered access to such banks of knowledge that are the mainspring of knowledge and scholarship. I have also taken inspiration from visits to medical and military museums throughout the world, too innumerable for all to be mentioned. Their collections of artefacts and interpretative displays can provide that imaginative spark needed to bring the past alive or suggest an otherwise elusive insight.

London, 11 November 2007.

I

National Inefficiency

It started off as a *Boys' Own* adventure both for the troops and for the young doctors seeing active service in the early days of the Boer War that broke out in October 1899. The young newly qualified medic was urged to seize his 'chance of seeing actual fighting, and, maybe, of proving himself to be something more than a non-combatant' and was reminded that 'a chance such as this does not often come of widening one's view of life, of foreign travel, of active service and of good pay into the bargain.'[1] What no one at the time could know was that the new century so soon to dawn was to be a century of total war in which health and medicine were to assume great importance for good and ill, nor that this colonial adventure straddling the 'Century's corpse outleant'[2] was to prefigure the relationship between medicine and warfare in the years to come. For the time being though, a recruit could happily claim that 'we live in tents, comfortable enough, though everything is covered with dust' and complacently boast of 'what a brotherhood our profession is! Although I know none of the men here, almost all of us have mutual acquaintances'.[3] This spirit of supreme confidence of a quick victory by an efficient modern army against a weak force of Boer farmers shared by army doctors and soldiers alike was soon to meet its nemesis in the form of three British defeats in the aptly christened 'Black Week' of December 1899. Few could have foreseen that it would be another two and a half years before the might of the British Empire, represented by over 400,000 British troops, could prevail over a seemingly insignificant enemy.[4] Wars in the coming twentieth century were rarely to go according to predictions either in duration or outcome.

Despite initial appearances to the contrary, the Boer commandos were actually better armed in many ways than the British Army at first. They could call upon an impressive arsenal of modern Mauser 0.276 rifles,

Krupp cannons and French Creusot siege-guns, not to mention a stock of more ammunition than they could hope to use. Moreover, 'these hard-bitten farmers with their ancient theology and their inconveniently modern rifles' turned out to be unsurpassed as horsemen and even more superb as marksmen, easily able to pick off British officers at 1200yds.[5] The resultant gunshot wounds were clean and it was soon found best to leave them to heal themselves as far as possible. Vincent Warren Low, tending over 300 wounded in a small field hospital in one week from the Battles of Paardeburg and Driefontein in February 1900, noted that 'the most striking feature of the ordinary modern bullet wound is its asepticity' and that 'assuming no complication existed, both [entrance and exit wounds] healed in the course of a few days under a scab, and, as a rule, gave rise to no inconvenience, though occasionally a little pain and stiffness existed in the course of the track of the bullet'.[6] A Canadian Scout had been wounded by a Mauser bullet a week before reporting sick and this 'had not prevented him riding some 20–30 miles daily'. Low ascribed this to the shape, structure and size of the bullet, although many of his fellow surgeons were more inclined to put it down to 'the dryness and asepticity of the South African atmosphere' despite the fact that shell wounds invariably suppurated and shrapnel wounds tended to drive small pieces of shirt or khaki uniform into the wound which also caused infection whereas 'the wedge-like modern bullet made as clean a perforation of the clothes as it did the skin'.[7]

That it was possible to wait for a wound to be treated by a doctor for sometimes considerable periods was partly owing to the fact that each soldier now carried a 'first field dressing' for immediate use at the height of battle. These packages contained a couple of sterile dressings in waterproof covers, comprising gauze pads stitched to a bandage, together with a safety pin. The Prussian Army had been the first to use such dressings and they were an item of standard issue to British troops from 1884.[8] Soldiers in the Boer War and subsequent wars of the twentieth century were able to apply the dressings to themselves if they were not too badly wounded or to their comrades to stave off infection. Yet many soldiers would be seen 'with their dressings a long way from their wounds'.[9] Nevertheless the field dressing also allowed regimental medical officers in the midst of battle to collect 'their wounded in the nearest sheltered positions they could find, which owing to the hilly nature of the ground was usually close to the fighting line; here they were dressed and attended to, and no attempt was, or could be, made to move them further to the rear until the fighting had ceased'.[10]

It was perhaps just as well that the majority of the wounds could be left undressed for some time as the rapid pace of many of the battles on the veldt meant that the sudden evacuation of a casualty clearing station or field hospital might become necessary at short notice. Lieutenant Wingate was giving chloroform to a wounded officer being operated upon during the Battle of Paardeburg when the Boers began to shell the hospital tents and 'two bullets whistled through the operating tent over our heads'. With barely time to finish operating upon their patient, the doctors had to abandon their tented hospital, load their wagons with the wounded under fire and travel two miles before it was safe to stop and 'dead beat, with all our wounded except two poor fellows who died en route, we camped or rather laid down on the veldt and slept'. For the exhausted and wounded soldiers there lay ahead a night of intense thirst since the enemy had control of the nearby river and had captured the hospital's water carts.[11]

Frederick Treves, surgeon to Queen Victoria and now in charge of the No. 4 Field Hospital, was shocked by the sight of the casualties from the Battle of Colenso on 15 December 1899, men whom a few hours earlier he had witnessed marching off with a devil-may-care attitude only to return 'burnt a brown red by the sun, their faces ... covered with dust and sweat ... blistered by the heat' and their 'blue army shirts ... stiff with blood.' All of them 'seemed dazed, weary and depressed'.[12] Although he was an experienced surgeon, the horrors of war still turned his stomach as he surveyed the men lying on stretchers covered with tarpaulin as slight protection against the rain that had now started to pour down; one man paralysed by a bullet in his spine was trying vainly to move his limbs, other men were kicking around deliriously on the wet grass to which they had fallen from their stretchers, and the piles of discarded bullet-riddled helmets and blood-soaked uniforms littered the ground. For him, there lay a ceaseless round of amputation ahead.

There was not even time to remove the dead and, during one hectic operating session, Treves noticed what seemed to be a corpse lying below the operating table. The man had been shot through the face and his 'features were obliterated by dust and blood', leaving only his blood-clotted moustache visible. Treves was taken aback to see 'this apparently inanimate figure' raise his head and open his eyes to see what was happening when an amputated limb fell onto him. For most of the casualties there was not to be such a happy ending even if they actually reached the operating theatre in good time.[13]

Transport was a major problem bedevilling the British Army during the war in South Africa, but it was perhaps at its most grievous in its effects on the care of the sick and wounded. Liaison between stretcher-bearer companies and the field hospitals was often poor, with bearer companies simply dumping the wounded at the short-staffed field hospitals where they might be left waiting a long time for treatment. There was no simple line of command to link these two units responsible for battlefield medicine. Moreover, many of the stretcher-bearers were not specially trained orderlies but were 'the outlaws, who are useless for regimental work, and handed over to the M[edical] O[fficer] to carry his bags about'. Such 'useless ignorant fellows' could kill their patients 'by the clumsy jerky way' they carried the stretcher. One medical officer who saw a soldier who had been wounded in the abdomen die on a stretcher lamented that he 'could not make the men, who were untrained, understand the stretcher was to be carried absolutely level and not jerked'.[14] It was felt throughout the army and even into the corridors of the War Office that 'probably nothing has come more prominently under the notice of army medical officers in this campaign than the necessity of combining the field hospital and the bearer company into one unit under one commanding officer'.[15] A model for this was the New South Wales Ambulance, which comprised a unified field hospital and bearer company, 'everything necessary for the performance of its special duties', and had proved itself to be efficient.

However, little could be done to make the ox-drawn ambulance wagons without springs comfortable for the men travelling in them. William Burdett-Coutts, war correspondent for *The Times*, complained in April 1900 that 'many of the wounded were sent back to Kimberley in bullock wagons, and we can well imagine the excruciating suffering caused by such a method of conveyance'.[16] It was remarkable that there were very few accidents involving them on the march from the Modder River to Pretoria following the British reverses of the aptly named 'Black Week' of December 1899, although there were doubts about their true value when their weight and the number of animals they required to pull them was compared with the relatively few sick and wounded they could carry.[17] Indeed General Buller considered them so unsuitable for the stony terrain of the veldt that he recruited a team of some 2000 volunteer stretcher-bearers as a substitute for them, mainly from British-born Uitlander refugees from the Boer Republics.[18] With them were 800 volunteers from the Indian community of Natal led by a twenty-eight-year-old barrister Mohandras K. Gandhi, keen to show loyalty to the British Empire in the non-belligerent role of stretcher-bearer.[19] The medical horrors of war and seemingly needless death were to reinforce Gandhi's innate pacifism.

Altogether some 22,000 British troops were to die during the war and more than five times that number were to be wounded or incapacitated by disease. However, of those soldiers who died, two thirds of them were the victims not of wounds inflicted in battle but of infectious disease.[20] Above all, it was typhoid that proved the greatest killer in this war rather than the armed warrior. War and typhoid, often known as enteric fever, were old companions. In the Spanish American War of 1898, one fifth of the United States armed forces had contracted it and six times the number of soldiers who died in combat died from the fever. Out of 107,973 soldiers, there were 20,738 cases of typhoid with 1,580 deaths. In the majority of the volunteer regiments involved, the disease tended to break out within two months of the men going into camp and was the result of poor sanitation, flies carrying the contagion and dusty conditions.[21] This pattern was to be all too familiar during the war in South Africa where the disease also struck standing camps rather than troops constantly on the move. The infection was also spread by the 'plagues of flies' so common on the veldt 'for it was a most difficult task to prevent them from settling on the sore lips and gums of men, and then inoculating any food or drink they might come into contact with'.[22] Of the 557,653 officers and men serving, 57,684 caught enteric fever. There were 8,225 deaths from it compared with the 7,582 men who died of wounds.[23]

Typhoid victims are often infected by eating food or drinking water contaminated by the bacillus *Salmonella typhi*, which had only been identified as recently as 1880 by Carl Eberth and Edwin Klebs. Once the bacillus reaches the small intestine, it multiplies and enters the bloodstream. After some ten to fourteen days the symptoms begin to manifest themselves, often starting off with a fever, headaches and pains in the muscles and joints that make rest difficult if not impossible. Constipation in the early stages of the illness may be followed by watery green or bloody diarrhoea. By the second week of the infection, the patient is often too weak and dizzy to get out of bed when stricken with diarrhoea, with the result that the bedclothes are frequently soiled. Meanwhile, the fever, accompanied by fits of shivering, increases until it reaches 104°F or even higher. The skin is hot and dry, the lips scab-encrusted and the tongue blackened. Not surprisingly, the patient often begins to ramble mentally. In many cases the intestine wall is perforated and there is massive gastrointestinal haemorrhaging, the major causes of death from typhoid. In 1896 Ferdinand Widal had devised a blood test for the diagnosis of typhoid fever but there was to be no effective treatment for the dreaded disease until the discovery of the antibiotic chloramphenicol in 1948. For the late nineteenth-century patient the infection meant great suffering with no hope of any effective treatment; for the doctor of the age it represented a failure in the therapeutic tools at his command.[24] William Osler, the great doyen of medical humanism, was in no doubt that 'typhoid fever has been one of the great scourges of armies, and kills and maims more than powder and shot'. Writing in 1914, on the eve of a conflict in which this was to change, he despaired that 'the story of recent wars forms a sad chapter in human inefficiency'.[25]

The Hospital Field Service in South Africa soon found it impossible to cope with the horrors of an outbreak of typhoid that shocked the public at home already reeling from news of military setbacks and heavy battlefield casualties. An epidemic spread through besieged Ladysmith, the hot, dusty railway junction walled in by a ridge of hills in which around 13,500 British troops were trapped. Three field hospitals were set up within the town and an isolation hospital for typhoid cases set up in a no man's land at Intombi, beyond the perimeters of the town to which typhoid cases were sent. Out of a garrison of 13,500 these hospitals treated 10,688 cases of sickness between November 1899 and February 1900, during which four months 393 people died of the disease. At first, when Sir George White and his men had flocked into Ladysmith at the end of October, the hospitals had seen mainly battle casualties. One nurse, Miss Charleson found those early days heady ones as 'trembling from want of rest, strangely excited at the thought of seeing – for the first time – the wounded from a field of battle ... by the dim light of many lanterns, I traced a moving mass of ambulances carrying the wounded and the dead' from the Battle of Modderspruit. An improvised hospital was set up in the town hall and the nurses handed out warming cups of hot Bovril to the wounded. Meanwhile in the operating theatre, surgeons operated on hopeless case after hopeless case: 'alas for the brave Gordons, many of them with their heads shattered by shells, or with hair matted with gore, and faces grey with suffering'.[26] Such horrific injuries did not stop this nursing sister from taking a romantic view of the dying wounded hero, the death of Commander Egerton of HMS *Powerful*, prompting her to write in her diary on 2 November 1899 that 'his face was pale and peaceful, a tender heroic smile was on his lips, and his eyes had no pain in them, only a look of satisfaction for having done his duty, and a glory in dying for his country'.[27] She had a more realistic view of wounded privates, noting that 'always Tommy was very anxious to get his bullet for the missus'.[28] As the siege went on and typhoid raged, her romanticised view of war was to be greatly modified.

The hospital at Intombi Sprut had been established for the isolation of typhoid and dysentery sufferers. By agreement with the Boer General Piet Joubert, hospital trains bearing a white flag were allowed to transport patients there each day. Once there, they were forbidden to return to Ladysmith. Intombi was a 'dismal spot' and when it rained the camp became a swamp. Nurse Charleson was 'obliged to wade from one marquee to another in a very short dress, shod with long gun boots and with a waterproof bag on my head' when tending her patients.[29] It was no better in dry conditions when the heat of the sun made conditions in the tents unbearable. The patients were deliberately deprived of what medicines and comforts were available in Ladysmith by the military authorities in charge in order to save them for the defenders within the besieged town. Nurse Charleson's diary recorded her despair about being 'shut up in that hollow with so many sick and wounded, surrounded by high mountains in which our enemies were seated with their long-reaching guns; we were indeed to be pitied'. She noted that 'daily the camp was becoming more unhealthy, and the food rationings decreasing. Nothing but a good, sound constitution could have possibly overcome these obstacles'.[30]

It was little wonder that sick men tried to stay in one of the hospitals in Ladysmith rather than be sent to such a hellhole. In order to prevent journalists from seeing what was happening out there, any press correspondent stricken with enteric fever was allowed to stay in the town though it was compulsory for all other sufferers to be sent to the isolation of Intombi.[31] George Steevens, the dashing war correspondent for the *Daily Mail*, had complained soon after the beginning of the siege that there was nothing to do other than eat, drink and sleep and that unless Ladysmith were to be relieved soon, 'we die of dullness', but was destined himself to die a horrible death from typhoid shortly before Christmas 1899 in one of the insalubrious Ladysmith hospitals.[32]

Conditions in the hospitals were bad enough at the height of the typhoid epidemic but were made worse by the actions of Colonel Exham, the Principal Medical Officer who, desirous of being able to present a neat list of supplies at the end of the siege, had forbidden the issue of such meagre comforts as sago, arrowroot and brandy to the sick whilst ensuring that these were diverted for the use of journalists, civilians and senior officers.[33] At the same time Exham was obsessed with the tidiness of the field hospitals, prompting Major Donegan, who was in charge of the 18th Field Hospital, to complain 'God almighty! We have four doctors for 120 patients scattered over three churches and thirty-six tents, and the P[rincipal] M[edical] O[fficer] only worries whether the men's clothes are neatly folded, or if their boots are in line.'[34]

Bad as the ravage of typhoid was at Ladysmith with its grim average of ten deaths a day, it was to be far worse at Bloemfontein after its occupation by General Roberts in March 1900. Almost 1,000 troops were to die in the epidemic which had been partly caused by many of Roberts's troops drinking water from the Modder River, heavily polluted by the corpses of men and horses killed in the recent Battle of Paardeburg fought there. Neglect of elementary hygiene compounded the problem. Where attention was paid to adequate sanitation, it was possible to control typhoid. At 6th General Hospital, Naauwpoort, a simple and effective sewage system had been devised by the Royal Engineers who had also provided pumps for an adequate water supply. Moreover, the hospital staff had incinerated all soiled dressings and the excreta of typhoid patients, thereby ensuring that 'up to date we have passed over 2000 patients through No. 6 General Hospital, and there is not a case of enteric fever to be traced to the surroundings of the hospital'.[35] Less care was taken at Bloemfontein. Soon there were funeral processions through the dusty streets of the town every afternoon mocking the recent triumphal entry of the army that was now burying its dead with the minimum of ceremony.

Arthur Conan Doyle working in a voluntary hospital at Bloemfontein saw the outbreak of enteric fever at Bloemfontein as 'a calamity the magnitude of which had not been foreseen and which even now is not fully appreciated'. In one month alone, 10–12,000 men had gone down with 'the most debilitating and lingering of continued fevers' and over half of the doctors, nurses and medical orderlies attending the sick had themselves caught the disease.[36] William Burdett-Coutts, a journalist and Unionist MP, denounced in the columns of *The Times* the scandal of the failure of the Hospital Field Service:

> hundreds of men to my knowledge were lying in the worst stages of typhoid, with only a blanket and a thin waterproof sheet … between their aching bodies and the hard ground, with no milk and hardly any medicines, without

beds, stretchers or mattresses, without linen of any kind, without a single nurse amongst them, with only a few soldiers to act as orderlies and with only three doctors to attend on 350 patients.[37]

Yet despite it being 'obvious that for many years the department of healing has not advanced *pari passu* with the department of maiming',[38] the Army Medical Department was unwilling to co-operate with civilian volunteer hospitals notwithstanding it being recognised that such hospitals as the Portland Hospital offered superior standards of care and accommodation to anything provided by the Royal Army Medical Corps.[39] Perhaps co-operation was not as great as it may have been because of a feeling that the private hospitals were getting in the way of the army organisation and that 'they should not be allowed to force themselves up towards the Front in the place of organised military hospitals'.[40] Jurisdictional rivalries only worsened the lot of the sick and dying.

All these deaths from typhoid could so easily have been prevented had the troops been vaccinated. Only a few years before the outbreak of the war a vaccine against typhoid fever had been developed by Almroth Wright, professor of pathology at the Army Medical School at the Royal Victoria Hospital at Netley overlooking Southampton Water. Yet, despite it coming from an army medical establishment that was gaining a reputation for its research, the military authorities were suspicious of the new vaccine and even more so of the man who had produced it. Wright was an abrasive, acrimonious figure made for controversy who made no concessions to his critics however much he may have antagonised them and biased them against his ideas. There had been resentment against his appointment to the post at Netley in 1892 when this relatively unknown thirty-one-year-old civilian with as yet little experience in the field of pathology had been given the job in preference to older, more experienced army officers.[41] By this time, despite having followed an erratic career path that had veered from the humanities to the sciences and from law to medicine before he finally chose to concentrate on medical research, he was already acutely conscious of his own ability and impatient of anyone who disagreed with him. It was an attitude that was later to earn him the nicknames of 'Sir Almost Right' and 'Sir Always Wrong' from his many opponents who did not share his own extremely high opinion of himself.[42] He was not averse to telling the president of one military tribunal to which he was giving evidence that 'I have given you the facts, I can't give you the brains.'[43]

At Netley, he had developed a diagnostic test for Malta Fever and a vaccine against this prolonged, relapsing illness. So confident was he that this vaccine would work that he tried it out on himself and then injected himself with live organisms only to find that the vaccine did not work after all.[44] When he had recovered from a long and distressing bout of Malta Fever, he turned his attention in 1896 to the problem of producing a vaccine against the much more serious typhoid fever. It had taken great personal courage for Wright to test his vaccine against Malta Fever on himself, yet there were even greater dangers in injecting a human being with this virulent organism, the typhoid bacillus, in however attenuated a form. Still firm in his belief in the principle of vaccination and encouraged by the success of Waldemar Haffkine in using heat-killed bacteria in an anti-cholera vaccine, he developed a heat-killed vaccine which he tested on himself, his colleague David Semple and sixteen trainee medical officers. These young officers were accustomed to military discipline and to obeying orders but were also inspired by their charismatic chief's confidence in what he was asking them to do. The initial effects were alarming. The officers concerned soon felt faint and suffered from vomiting and a loss of appetite. The worst affected of them remained weak and 'looked somewhat shaken in health for some three weeks after'.[45] Wright, having learned his lesson with Malta Fever, decided against infecting himself with typhoid to see whether the vaccine did actually work, but injected one intrepid young man with live typhoid bacilli with no ill effects. More extended clinical trials following a typhoid outbreak at Maidstone Insane Asylum in 1897 and with the Indian Army in 1898 also gave encouraging results but were too sketchy and incomplete to confirm Wright's faith in his vaccine.[46] The outbreak of the Boer War offered just the opportunity he needed to try out his vaccine in wartime conditions and give him the chance he craved to make a difference to the health of the troops.

Unfortunately, the new vaccine was not received by serving military medical officers with the same enthusiasm Wright had shown for it. Only 14,628 soldiers actually volunteered to be inoculated, which amounted to no more than four per cent of the total. There was little support and much suspicion from the army doctors. There was a general history of popular hostility to compulsory vaccination, which had raged ever since Edward Jenner had first developed his smallpox vaccine at the end of the eighteenth century with many doctors opposed to the very idea of inoculation.[47] Moreover many of them actually believed that anti-typhoid inoculation caused the fever in the first place; and the severity of the reactions to it, which could leave a man unfit for duty for several days, only reinforced military hostility to inoculation.[48] Wright explained such adverse reactions as representing a 'negative phase' in the treatment, a period immediately after inoculation when immunity was diminished before it could be enhanced. Since this made men more vulnerable to infection in the short term, it meant that inoculation must take place before they were exposed to infection and made it potentially dangerous during an epidemic. Wright also recommended a second booster injection to increase protection, but this advice made it even more of a deterrent to the adoption of the vaccine. Some wooden cases containing supplies of the vaccine were even dumped over the sides of troopships leaving Southampton Water within sight of Wright at Netley to be returned to him by the coastguards.[49]

Those doctors who actually inoculated soldiers during the voyage out to South Africa were to report adverse reactions made worse in some cases by seasickness. One civilian surgeon was able to round up 200 volunteers aboard SS *Sicilian*, but two of them fainted 'with fright' immediately after the needle was injected. Within ninety minutes, nearly all the men injected began to feel ill, some with cramp in the abdomen, others with nausea and violent vomiting or diarrhoea, and all with a rise in temperature. It was to be three days before any of them began to recover. The surgeon concerned was also inoculated and was soon 'unable to move hand or foot without assistance' while the 'two glands in my groin were swollen to the size of pigeon's eggs'.[50] Such strong reactions, though actually very common, were put down by some doctors to the sera being too strong.[51] It was no wonder that many men did not volunteer, even if their regimental medical officers recommended the injections, when they saw the effects on their comrades.

As a result of the low number of troops inoculated, it was impossible to perform any accurate statistical analysis of the results of using the vaccine. Wright, who was sceptical about statistics at the best of times, had no doubt about its value and advocated the compulsory vaccination of troops against typhoid. His many enemies in the military hierarchy, headed by David Bruce, discoverer of the cause of Malta Fever and one of the disappointed candidates for Wright's chair in pathology, were hostile to any form of inoculation let alone any involving compulsion. As a result, the army board advising the War Office on scientific issues recommended that voluntary inoculation be suspended and that it should only be resumed if Wright prepared a detailed proposal 'showing exactly on what lines and with what precautions he would propose that the system should be carried out'.[52]

An Army Medical Services committee on anti-typhoid inoculation was established in 1904 after Wright had mobilised medical and scientific support against this decision; it concluded that 'the practice of anti-typhoid inoculations in the army has resulted in a substantial reduction in the incidence and death rate from enteric fever among the inoculated' and recommended resumption of voluntary vaccination for troops.[53] However, the critics of vaccination enlisted the support of the statistician Karl Pearson, who attacked the rigour of Wright's methods of analysis.[54] Wright, who had left the Army Medical Service in 1902, was to spend the next decade fighting for official recognition of the value of vaccination that he believed could have saved so many lives in South Africa.[55] It was only once William Leishman, Wright's successor at the Royal Army Medical School now based at Millbank, London, had undertaken further research into the effects of anti-typhoid sera that vaccination was reintroduced on a voluntary basis in 1912.[56]

However, it was not only among the British armed forces that the inadequate response to the treatment of infectious disease was to provoke a scandal.[57] Boer women and children incarcerated in the first concentration camps of the twentieth century were to suffer from the ravages of epidemics just as much as the men who were fighting, although measles rather than typhoid was to be the bigger killer. These camps were General Kitchener's response to the Boer guerrilla warfare that characterised the last phases of the conflict. They were established as refuges for Boer women and children made homeless by the burning of farms thought to be harbouring the commandos. It was a policy which freed the Boer men from the distraction of looking after their families and added to the determination of the 'bitter enders' to carry on what was by now a hopeless struggle. Those families who tried to stay in their farms seemed to be 'very badly off' and were short of sugar, salt and matches. If they left home to seek refuge in a camp, their homesteads were burned in line with the policy 'to destroy everything likely to be of material use to the enemy' if it had not been purloined by British soldiers, with 'a most brilliant reputation for looting', first. Even many an army doctor 'became somewhat of an adept at fowl-snatching'.[58] For some Boer families the camps were at first refuges as much as prisons, but not for long.

Soon death from malnutrition and disease swept through these badly sited, unhygienic camps. At the camp at Mafeking women were washing clothes in excrement-fouled water, the latrines were not properly disinfected and slop water was just emptied next to the tents. There was no mortuary despite a rising death rate. Fresh meat and vegetables were not available as part of the rations, even though they could easily have been bought from the nearby town. However, it was not just the negligence of the British Army that was to blame for creating such unsanitary conditions.[59] The Boer women were also blamed by observers for having 'a horror of ventilation' which directly caused 'the pestilential atmosphere of the tents' which could best be described as 'stinking'.[60] Farming families accustomed to leading healthy if isolated lives had not built up resistance to infectious diseases. By the end of the war, well over 20,000 women and children had died in the camps, a quarter of all women and children from the Boer Republics.[61]

Conditions at Heilbron were made even worse when the army interned a group of Boer families infected with measles in a camp unable to cope with the influx of the sick, many of whom were housed in 'miserable sheds or stables, and one hovel was one surely meant for a pig or some poor native and yet a young girl, dangerously ill lay in it'.[62] Such a policy outraged the suffragette Millicent Fawcett, the leader of an all-women committee appointed by the British government to enquire into conditions in the camps: 'There is barely language too strong to express our opinion of the sending of a mass of disease to a healthy camp; but the cemetery at Heilbron tells the price paid in lives for the terrible mistake.'[63]

Conditions in the camps had first been exposed by the Quaker Emily Hobhouse who had been horrified at what she had witnessed during her visit to them between December 1900 and May 1901:

> I began to compare a parish I had known at home of 2,000 people where a funeral was an event – and usually of an old person. Here some twenty to twenty-five were carried away daily ... it was a death rate that had not been known except in the times of the Great Plagues ... the whole talk was of deaths – who died yesterday, who lay dying today, who would be dead tomorrow.[64]

Alfred Milner, British High Commissioner for South Africa, although privately blaming the scandal on military mismanagement, was so angered by Hobhouse's rhetorical mission to publicise the scandal, that he arranged for her to be arrested and deported when she attempted to return to South Africa in October 1901.[65]

However, by that time Mrs Fawcett's Ladies' Committee had been sent out by the War Office to investigate the conditions in the camps. Unlike Hobhouse, who was often dismissed as hysterical in her response to the camps, all of these practical and down-to-earth women, including two doctors and a nurse, believed that the war was just and that in wartime unpleasant measures might have to be taken against enemy civilians. Yet, they were appalled by what they saw and recommended relief measures including the provision of trained nurses in the camps, improved rations and proper equipment for the sterilization of the linen used by typhoid patients, though their interest did not extend to the native Africans who had also been interned.[66]

Just as Hobhouse and the Fawcett Commission's reports had galvanised action to improve conditions in the camps, it was Burdett-Coutts's revelations of 'the growing scenes of neglect and inhumanity, of suffering and death, which have been the lot of the British soldier in the closing chapter of this war'[67] that provoked the usual governmental response to any official scandal, the appointment of a royal commission 'to consider and report upon the care and treatment of the sick and wounded during the South African Campaign' under the chairmanship of Sir Robert Romer. Evidence was taken from officers of the Royal Army Medical Corps (RAMC), civilian surgeons and the sick and wounded themselves. The commission found that the scale of the war had taken the authorities by surprise and that the RAMC had come under great pressure and had neglected sanitation in the field, but its conclusion that in general the Corps had generally overcome its own very considerable shortcomings was certainly a whitewash that bore little relationship to the reality of what had actually happened.[68] The evidence pointed towards a breakdown of the army medical organisation especially with regard to sanitation, transport, the response to infectious diseases, and manpower, however brave and dedicated individual officers may have been. The whole question of the failure to introduce inoculation against typhoid was ignored.

Yet the outcome of this commission should have come as no surprise to anyone, for there was a feeling within the RAMC that 'this war is the first occasion on which the existing medical organisation has been tested, and in spite of the reduced scale, it has stood the test remarkably well'.[69]

E.W. Herrington, a doctor at Bloemfontein, had no doubts after a visit from the Hospital Commission that:

> I do not think that the RAMC will come badly out of the enquiry but will, in the future, have their hands greatly strengthened. They were not able to do impossibilities and did their best with what material they could seize upon, whilst no one could foresee that there would be such a terrible outbreak of enteric after Paardeburg, or that the disease would be of such virulent a type.[70]

Nonetheless, the RAMC had come very close to breaking down under the pressure of war. When the war broke out, the Corps was only one year old, having been formed as recently as June 1898 from an amalgamation of the Medical Staff Corps, made up of medically trained soldiers, and the doctors of the Medical Staff. Up to this time the Staff Corps, men of 'regular, steady habits and good temper … possessed of a kindly disposition', had had no officers while the Medical Staff of the Army Medical Department were all officers without any men to command.[71] Only with the formation of the RAMC were medical officers given the same status and rank as other officers within the British Army but they still continued to be looked down upon as inferior by both the army and their fellow civilian doctors to whom medical military service was seen as a last resort for medical men unable to afford a footing in general practice or even to find a paid appointment with the poor law authorities. Recruitment to the Corps was also deterred by the inferior terms of service offered to army doctors within the armed forces even if they enjoyed officer status. Whereas an eighteen-year-old cavalry subaltern was paid £400 a year in allowances to enable him to maintain two servants, two horses and stabling, the £200 salary and £70 allowances paid to an older, medically qualified RAMC subaltern was not enough for him 'to keep up a smart civilian and military kit and subscribe freely to everything that is going on'.[72] If better doctors were to be recruited, the army had to offer them more attractive conditions of service and more authority in enforcing health and sanitary regulations. It was little wonder that on the outbreak of the Boer War the new Corps was still undermanned and its inadequacies had been only too visible, but the experience had offered salutary lessons which were to be heeded over the next few years.

The years between the end of the Boer War and the outbreak of war in 1914 were ones of reform for the army medical services just as they marked a period of army reform in general under the War Secretary Lord Haldane. The status of the military doctor was regularised and it was suggested that candidates for the RAMC should be 'British subjects of unmixed European blood, not more than 28 years of age, and shall possess a recognizable qualification to practice'. The medical officers were given responsibility for all medical and sanitary services in their area. Salaries and the status of army medical officers were raised and provision made for study leave.[73] In 1904 the director-general of the Army Medical Department was raised to a rank immediately below that of an adjutant-general, which ensured that his voice would be heard when it came to military planning. The Royal Army Medical College was transferred from Netley to London in 1907 ensuring that it was more in touch with wider developments in the medical world of the capital and was no longer regarded as a seaside holiday for men taking courses there. The veteran bacteriologist Alexander Ogston was very concerned that there was no provision 'for the formation of a Sanitary Corps, consisting of officers specially charged with the duty of carrying out proper sanitary measures in peace and war, and a staff of men trained to ensure the requisite measures being carried into effect'.[74] In 1906 a school of sanitation was opened at Aldershot for the training of regimental officers and non commissioned officers that could form the nucleus of hygiene detachments. Military hygiene courses also became a regular part of the syllabus for army doctors. Field ambulances replaced the old stretcher-bearer companies. Research was commissioned into water filters and water sterilizing carts.[75] The need for a medical reserve to cope with greater needs in the event of war was met by the formation of a territorial army unit modelled on the RAMC. This reorganisation under the aegis of the director-general Alfred Keogh was to shape the RAMC into a much more effective medical service, one that was at last prepared to fight the Boer War so recently over. Sir Frederick Treves gave his approval to the removal of 'the grave defects brought to light in the Report of the South African Hospital Committee' and predicted that 'it will be the finest service in the world in time'.[76]

Army nursing did not escape rationalization in the rush to repair the deficiencies revealed by the war. An Army Nursing Service had been formed in 1881 and this had been supplemented by Princess Christian's Army Nursing Service Reserve from 1887, but women still lacked any status as regular members of the armed forces and were not supposed to nurse close to the battle zones. The Boer War demonstrated the need for the employment 'of nurses in fixed hospitals for the care of the wounded and of fever and dysenteric patients, and such others as can properly be nursed by females'.[77] A committee under the chairmanship of St John Broderick recommended the amalgamation of the army and Indian Nursing Services to form Queen Alexandra's Imperial Military Nursing Service 'under the immediate control of Her Majesty Queen Alexandra as President'.[78] However, Queen Alexandra was determined to be consulted and have her way on everything, from the size of buttons on the uniform to the role of the Lady Superintendent or Matron-in-Chief.[79] The Queen's interest was often counter-productive and a trial to any one who opposed her well-meaning but always regal interference. Lord Haldane as Secretary of State for War was not the only person to consider her a nuisance when he came up against her in replacing Princess Christian's Army Nursing Reserve with the rationalized Queen Alexandra's Imperial Military Nursing Service Reserve and establishing the Territorial Army Nursing Service in 1908. Exasperated by his dealings with the Queen, Haldane complained that 'she is about the stupidest woman in England'.[80] However, there was nothing he could do to counter royal influence in army nursing.[81]

Military medical and nursing reform was part of a wider obsession with 'National Efficiency' which reverses in the Boer War had brought to the fore, though their origins lay in an underlying unease that economically and militarily Britain was being overtaken by an armed, vigorous and prosperous German Empire. The fear was that if the mighty British forces could be brought to the verge of defeat by simple South African farmers, they would stand no chance against a well-disciplined, well-equipped and well-trained German Army. If Britain was to survive it had to modernise itself. Linked in with such fears of national decline were the revelations of the deplorable physical condition of many of the men volunteering for service in South Africa. Over a quarter of volunteers at some recruiting depots were rejected as unfit for military service. The journalist Arnold White revealed that at Manchester three out of five recruits failed to meet the low physical standards of a minimum height of 5ft 3in, a chest measurement of 33in and a weight of 115lb. At York, Leeds and Sheffield, forty-seven per cent of recruits failed to meet these standards and twenty-six per cent were additionally rejected on account of defective vision or hearing, decayed teeth, ill-health or 'dull intellect'.[82] Major-General Sir John Frederick Maurice argued that such statistics suggested that the environmental conditions in which the working classes lived were seriously depleting the reserve of fit men from which the soldiers were recruited.[83] All of this was to influence debate on social policy for many years to come.[84]

In the short term, an interdepartmental committee of enquiry into physical deterioration was set up to consider the important question of whether the British race was in terminal decline and unable to bear the Imperial burden. As the Boer War was the first time since the Crimean War that large numbers of the adult male population had been weighed, measured and tested for physical weakness, no one could be sure whether the conditions that had been reported were the result of progressive racial degeneracy or merely of an unhealthy urban environment. The report, as would be expected from a commission made up exclusively of civil servants, was reassuring in its findings that there was no clear evidence of inherited physical degeneracy. However, evidence given to it confirmed White's charge about the physical condition of recruits and suggested that dirt, ill-nourishment and neglect were responsible for much of the ill-health uncovered, but that this could be remedied if the conditions producing it were improved. A clear connection was made between the evils of the slums and national security: an unhealthy citizenry meant a declining national power and physical weakness directly corresponded to military weakness. Yet, these evils could be overcome since 'those inferior bodily characters which are the result of poverty (and not vice, such as syphilis and alcoholism), and are therefore acquired during the lifetime of the individual, are not transmissible from one generation to another. To restore, therefore, the classes in which this inferiority exists to the mean standard of national physique, all that is required is to improve the conditions of living, and in one or two generations all the ground that has been lost will be recovered'.[85] The recommendations of the report were conventional ones that social reformers had been urging for about twenty years, including the medical inspection of school children, school meals for the needy, physical education in schools, the education of girls about child care and cookery, and more rigorous enforcement of the existing sanitary regulations. They were given more cogency by their importance for the future of Britain as a world power and Sir William Taylor, Director-General of the Army Medical Services expressed the hope that 'the inquiry might end in suggestions that will lead to the institution of measures which will result in bringing about a marked improvement of the physique of the classes from which our recruits are at present drawn'.[86]

Although the medical profession and many social reformers welcomed the report, others were less convinced that physical deterioration was not a reality and were concerned about the differential birth rate, whereby the unhealthiest stock among the poorest working classes were having more children than the healthier middle classes. The statistician Karl Pearson was concerned that a quarter of the population would produce half of the next generation and that as the best stocks, as he considered the professional classes to be, were dying out, the worst stocks, the dysgenic poor, were multiplying. The racial fitness of the population would determine its survival chances and Britain's differential birth rate could be seen as foreshadowing the collapse of the British Empire.[87] This war-induced panic created an atmosphere congenial to the launch of the eugenics movement with its schemes of race improvement through encouraging breeding among the better classes and discouraging it among the unfit.

The quality of future good citizens mattered as much as the quantity, a concern which encouraged eugenicists to ally with social reformers, unconvinced of there being any evidence of hereditary racial degeneration, in order to improve conditions for the next generation upon whom national survival might depend. Infant welfare was at the heart of public health concerns. Even before the war, there had been concern about the dangers to mothers and babies from untrained midwives, but, despite attempts to regulate the profession through unsuccessful bills in 1890 and 1899, it was not until 1902 that the Midwives' Act banned unregistered midwives from practising. One midwife instructor, Emilia Kanthack, linked training in midwifery with the creation of little imperial assets and the fight against race-deterioration in 1907, stating that 'we want not only to keep babies alive, but we want them to be healthy young animals'.[88] Mothers were urged to breastfeed their babies because of a belief among medical experts that the use of dirty feeding bottles, contaminated milk or tinned, sweetened, skimmed milk was causing a high infant mortality rate from diarrhoea. Maternity and child welfare clinics were also established all over the country, following the opening of the St Pancras School for Mothers in 1907, where mothers could be given advice on feeding, and the babies could be weighed. Health visitors were also employed by many of the more progressive local authorities.[89] Meanwhile, mothercraft and domestic science lessons for girls became more prominent in schools, a preparation for their future responsibilities and roles in the home.[90] The Fabian Society called for 'the endowment of motherhood', which involved a combination of family allowances and publicly financed infant welfare centres, in order to encourage 'fit parenthood'.[91]

It was not just the role of the mother that was being emphasised as a solution to the problems exposed by wartime recruitment. If Britain was to maintain the Empire, it was important to ensure the physical health and nourishment of a new generation of schoolchildren who would represent the future imperial army. Imperial rivals were already making such provision. Japan made provision for the medical inspection of schoolchildren and Germany provided baths, food and medical services in its schools, both nations being very much in advance of Britain in welfare matters. In 1905 free school meals were introduced for needy schoolchildren. School medical inspections followed in 1907, primarily to provide an accurate anthropometrical survey of school-age children that would help to establish whether physical deterioration was indeed a reality, and also reveal the true extent of preventable disease. Once these inspections had revealed a picture of widespread ill health, the way was open for the establishment of a school medical service staffed by nurses.

School clinics were set up when it proved too costly and difficult to refer cases to local hospitals. The first clinic was established by Margaret McMillan in London in 1908, and by the end of 1913 there were 260 school clinics in 139 local education authorities around the country. Dental treatment was offered, though in the days of foot-operated drills it was often distressing for the child. By 1914 free eye-tests were widely available although the parents had to pay towards the costs of the spectacle frames. Perhaps the most visible results of the service were the reduction in the number of children carrying lice or ringworm.[92] Nevertheless in 1913 more than fifty per cent of schoolchildren still had bad teeth, ten per cent were carrying vermin, ten per cent had seriously defective vision and five per cent had defective hearing.[93] A healthier people could not be created overnight, especially without more investment from the State and less continued reliance on voluntary action, but the aftermath of the Boer War had been a great impetus to social advance by focusing on already existing concerns as matters of urgency.

Physical training and sport were more immediate ways of improving the fitness of young people. It was a matter of contemporary concern that by the age of seventeen many young working class men had passed their peak of fitness and their bodies were taking the toll of a passion for gambling and stimulants such as alcohol and tobacco, varied with a poor diet of bread, tea and salt fish. As a result, 'the lack of self-improvement which they have exhibited is bound up with their physical condition.

At seventeen they become street loafers – practically the only available source of recruiting for the army'.[94] The Majority Report of the 1909 Royal Commission on the Poor Laws recommended that 'with a view to the improvement of physique, a continuous system of physical training should be instituted, which might be commenced during school life and be continued afterwards'.[95] It was widely accepted that the armed forces were effective in improving the bodily fitness of their men and that through army drill the bodies of these recruits were 're-formed into more manly shapes'.[96] Military drill for boys had been introduced in elementary schools from 1871 and was supplemented by a Swedish drill for girls from 1881. The whole question of physical education in schools was brought into focus by the Boer War and forced the War Office and Board of Education to take concerted action. In 1901 the Physical Training Committee made provision for regular inspection of physical classes in schools to ensure that drill was being correctly taught and in line with military thought on the subject.[97]

Both the army and Board of Education adopted the gymnastic exercises of Swedish drill, with its emphasis on the toning of the stomach, ensuring that physical training in elementary schools mirrored that of army training camps. This represented a move away from German drill, which used Indian clubs, dumb-bells, horizontal and parallel bars, rings and vaulting horses for muscular development of the biceps and shoulders. However, there was less emphasis on organised games such as football, rugby or cricket except as supplements to drill, despite the emphasis on sports in promoting manliness in public schools. It was left to such organisations as cadet forces, university settlements, the Church Lads' Brigade, the Boys' Brigade and the Boy Scouts to use sports to improve the physique of working-class boys by physical exercise in the open air, and to improve their character through imbuing them with the code of the gentleman.[98] The influence of the young middle-class men who introduced the working-class boys to sports in this way was often immense when it came to encouraging them to keep fit and healthy. Arthur Bullock, a young London medical student, was an inspiration to the boys of the Pauline Mission at King's Cross, established by St Paul's School, and 'attracted them by his skill in athletics' and the lessons he gave them in gymnastics so that 'many of them still practice the exercises he taught them in order to increase their chest measurements and thus pass the test and get into Khaki'.[99] It was one answer to the question of how to raise the standards of recruits.

Whereas the Boer War had brought into the spotlight the inadequacies of the British army preparedness for the medical aspects of modern warfare, the Russo-Japanese War of 1904–5 offered a model of how it should be done. No less an authority than Sir William Osler approved of the efficiency of the Japanese medical services and noted that 'no great war has ever been conducted with such forethought for the preservation of the fighting unit, and in consequence the mortality from typhoid fever and dysentery was exceptionally low'.[100] Part of the success of the Japanese forces in preventing disease was owing to their medical officers having status within the army. Not only were their roles well defined but they had the same status as other officers of similar rank and the authority to issue instructions on sanitary matters. Moreover, the Japanese medical officer 'is proud of his profession which is considered by the whole army to be a highly honourable one'.[101]

The medical organisation of the Japanese forces was based on that of the German Army but lines of command were 'much shorter, less detailed and less cumbersome' and had 'proved as perfect a machinery for the purposes of this war, at any rate, as can well be devised'.[102] There were clear lines of responsibility from the principal medical officer of the field forces down to the principal medical officers of depot divisions and the regiments, and thence to the medical services with the military units. Each battalion had two medical officers attached to it who would set up regimental 'sick rooms' or infirmaries in standing camps, and aid stations and temporary dressing stations in the field. Crucially, these medical officers had complete control over sanitary matters in the area in which they were stationed.[103] This emphasis on sanitation as the province of the army doctor was seen as essential for the control of infectious diseases.

There was also a separate department dealing with the transport of the sick and wounded which had no counterpart in European medical regiments of the time but which proved extraordinarily efficient in evacuating the wounded from field hospitals down the line to trains and ships.[104] Yet, the Japanese stretcher-bearers did not have an easy time of it. After the Battle of Sha Ho in October 1904 they had to go backwards and forwards over a distance of ten miles to transport 342 wounded soldiers from the battlefield to a dressing station. Chinese coolies and carts were employed to supplement the work of the stretcher-bearers and also 'one might see a long straggling line of wounded marching from the dressing station to field hospital'.[105] The operating tables were improvised from solid Chinese cupboards salvaged from houses and operations were performed by the light of sperm candles since the Japanese were reluctant to use 'any lights that would indicate any of their positions to the enemy'.[106]

Western observers especially praised the fact that not only did the Japanese medical service work efficiently in conditions of modern warfare but 'there is an entire absence of that sentiment, which, in Western nations, is apt to exaggerate those defects into so-called medical scandals' because 'the Japanese soldier who is wounded considers his sufferings as nothing compared with the hardships and dangers of his comrades who are left in the fighting'.[107] It was a cultural difference which was even more marked, though less appealing to Europeans, in the Japanese practice of not treating wounded soldiers on the battlefields, especially in cases of 'severe wounds of the brain, in which the skull was shattered and the brain substance protruding', because of the Japanese belief that it was 'a special honour to be killed outright in battle ... and not considered inhumane to leave on the field a case so hopelessly injured that death is likely to occur within an hour or two'.[108] Despite the apparent modernity of Japan, older cultural traditions made its people act differently from what would be considered humane in Europe.

The Russian medical response to the war with Japan was less efficient. The Army Medical Department was supposed to make provision for all the sick and wounded but in practice depended heavily on back-up from the Red Cross, which provided most of the necessary drugs and modern appliances like X-rays. Many wealthy Russians vied with each other to provide Red Cross units and 'the hope of social reward was sometimes partly the reason for their liberality'. One success was the work of the surgeon Princess Vera Gedroitz, who performed successful abdominal surgery from a well-equipped hospital train that she was able to bring close to the Front. Otherwise, the resultant medical arrangements were 'on much too small a scale for modern great battles' and suffered from poor co-operation between the Red Cross and army services.[109]

Within the Russian Army responsibilities were divided, doctors had no disciplinary or administrative powers and 'the man who is responsible for the supply of medicines is not responsible for their use'.[110] At Port Arthur, this administrative inefficiency resulted in some hospitals being oversupplied with drugs and equipment while others were in dire need.[111] With doctors unable to enforce sanitary regulations it is little wonder that there was an outbreak of typhoid because the troops disliked the taste of boiled water.[112] Yet, despite all this neglect, the Russian soldier remained in remarkably good health, better perhaps than that of his Japanese counterpart, which was put down to his being 'of such good physique, and as a rule so inured to privation in his own home that he can … stand campaigning better than any other European soldier'.[113]

For western observers the lessons of the Russo-Japanese War were that scientific medicine was the key to military efficiency, with clear lines of command and sufficient attention paid to the important matters of sanitation and military hygiene. Japan, which seemed to have modernised its services and improved upon its Western models, was widely admired and offered a way forward in modern military medicine.[114] Certainly, the conflict between Russia and Japan offered a contrast to British experience during the Boer War, but these first wars of the twentieth century were to seem like nothing when a much greater struggle broke out just when the lessons of the earlier wars seemed to have been learned, but were to prove less useful than anyone might have expected.

2

Medicine in Khaki

One of the very first casualties of the First World War was the hospital at Belgrade. The Austro-Hungarian Empire began its war of revenge for the assassination of the Archduke Franz Ferdinand and his morganatic wife by shelling the Serbian capital on 28 July 1914. There the hospital windows were shattered, broken glass littered the ward floors and patients screamed with terror. Some of them tried to get out of their beds to escape the nightmare, but there was nowhere for them to go. No one was in any doubt that war had broken out as shocked silence punctuated the explosions.[1]

Somehow the shelling of a hospital was prophetic of the horrors of the next four years when medicine would be challenged in new ways and some of the old gentleman-like attitudes lost in the face of modern, mechanised warfare. A new, more brutal way of waging war was to cause confusion and uncertainty but out of the wreckage came innovations that changed the very practice of medicine.

At first, just like in the Boer War at the beginning of the century, it was all a great adventure. The conflict was not expected to last long, enthusiastic crowds thronged the streets of the capitals of Europe and once again doctors and nurses were no more immune to war fever than any one else in that generation of 1914. Soon like their contemporaries, they were to learn what warfare really meant, but to begin with they joined up in droves for fear of missing their chance of a lifetime of taking part in what was seen as 'the great game'. Many doctors in khaki regretted that their role was non-combatant and eagerly sought out the accoutrements of war, though more mature doctors ridiculed the 'mild-looking surgeons arriv[ing] at the front armed to the teeth, with swords, revolvers and ammunition, clanking spurs, map cases, field glasses and compasses strung all round them, and on their left arm the brassard with the Red Cross. We called them "Christmas Trees".'[2]

Some of them chaffed at not being allowed to fight. Henry Souttar, serving as a surgeon in Flanders, was shown around a chateau vandalised by the occupying Germans and he 'itched to pull the lever and to scatter withering death' among the enemy in revenge.[3] German doctors, subject to universal conscription, were already more militarised in their practices and way of thought from their period of compulsory military service, than the volunteer civilian doctors in Britain, but were equally gung-ho. The likelihood of their being wounded or killed was not at the forefront of the thoughts of the young men flocking to the colours as war fever gripped Europe. Nor was the illusion of war as something of a 'lark' immediately dispelled. In the early months of the war, a medical officer attached to the Middlesex Regiment was able to write home that he was 'very fit, very brown, eat like a lion, have congenial work and companions, sleep well and have little to complain of', though he did admit that 'it seems extraordinary that we should be desolating everything, and except for very violent and forcible reminders, at times it is difficult to realize that the war is really in progress'. What struck him most of all was that 'the birds sing just the same, though heavy firing and bursting shells surprise them continually'.[4] What he did not comment on were the human casualties from the fighting that disturbed the birdsong. Instead he depicted warfare as positive and life enhancing compared with the monotony of civilian life, a view shared by his counterparts on the opposing side in this war. Benno Ziegler, a German medical student from Freiburg, declared in September 1914, only a month before his own death in battle, that 'it shall not be my fault if I am not a Man when I come home'.[5]

In the rush to join up in the heady patriotic days of August, the ill health of the population was once again revealed as a cause of national shame. The medical inspection of recruits at the recruiting depots revealed the raw material from which Kitchener's New Army was to be created and 'compelled us to take stock of the health and physique of our manhood; this stocktaking has brought us face to face with ugly facts'.[6] At Aldershot, 300 'first footers … of the most variegated texture' lined up at the depot door, 'some lean, some fat, some smart, some unkempt, but all looking very cheerful and hopeful'. Ten men at a time were marched into the depot and ordered to strip before the two doctors waiting to give them a cursory examination of their general physique, chest, tongue, mouth and teeth and to question them as to their state of health, age and occupation. Only the most obviously unfit were turned down entirely, including a lame tramp who was also blind in one eye, a London draper's assistant with a twisted spine and a veteran soldier with syphilitic ulcers on his legs. Less obvious disabilities got through. The doctors were instructed not to turn anyone down who could be usefully employed by the state. Even many of 'the weeds among the young men, the cigarette victims, the pasty-faced, flat-chested youths, those who had lived down dark alleys and in unhygienic surroundings all their lives' were considered redeemable and 'capable of being made into better men' through marching, drilling, gymnastics, decent food, good quarters, baths and cleanliness. Men who were not healthy enough to be turned into good soldiers through the efforts of the drill sergeant might be fit for home defence or roles as batmen or mess servants.[7] It was believed that all could be made more manly by military service.

New recruits were placed into three categories. Class A was fit for general service overseas, B for service abroad in a support capacity and C for home service only. In 1917, by which time conscription was the norm, the system was changed and four grades were introduced. Grade One soldiers were those men fit for service who would formerly have been in Class A. Men in Grade Two were deemed capable of walking six miles 'with ease', while Grade Three recruits were unsuitable for combat but could be given ancillary roles. Men placed in Grade Four were rejected as utterly unfit.[8] D.H. Lawrence was called up in 1916 and immediately rejected on account of having suffered from tuberculosis after he had been examined by two doctors 'who knew the sacredness of another naked man'.[9] Yet, as the war went on and more soldiers were needed, conscription was introduced, standards were lowered and men could be reclassified from C to A without further medical inspection.[10]

While some doctors were only too ready to pass men as fit for service, others were more concerned about the effects of their colleagues being so 'careless about the attestation of recruits' since it meant that many men who should never have undertaken military service because of hernias, varicose veins, defective teeth, chronic heart disease, poor eyesight and chronic bronchitis had later to be discharged; 300 such men enlisted in the Seaforth and Gordon Highlanders and 'were clothed, fed and paid for 6–8 weeks, sent the length of Great Britain, sent home again with a suit of clothes and 20 to 30 shillings in pocket'.[11] It was a waste of scarce resources in a period when 'one of the greatest problems of a nation at war is the proper use of manpower so that maximum results can be obtained at minimum expenditure'.[12]

When the United States entered the war in 1917, the American Psychological Association advocated that the United States War Department use intelligence tests to screen mental incompetents from the army in the same way that the physically unfit could be identified by medical inspections. At first the army authorities were sceptical but by the beginning of 1918 psychological examiners were at work in all the training camps administering the Stanford–Binet test. This had first been developed by the French psychologist Alfred Binet and then refined by Lewis Terman of Stanford University. More difficult 'alpha tests' were given to the literate and 'beta tests' to the illiterate recruits in an attempt to identify superior, average and inferior intelligence and select potential officer material. Critics pointed out that the tests were culturally biased towards white Anglo-Saxon protestants, and the American armed forces, never entirely convinced of the value of the tests, rejected the testing system in January 1919. However, intelligence testing was widely adopted in the American school system after the war.[13]

For those men not returned home as mentally or physically unfit but sent out to France and Belgium, casualties were soon to be a commonplace, many of them sustained when men had left the trenches and were crossing the shell-pocked wastes of no man's land. During daylight it was often impossible to do anything to help these wounded men, though their comrades felt frustrated at having to leave them in agony lying in the 'wet mud of manured fields until their torn trousers and their wounds were so soaked in a mixture of blood and dirt that it was impossible to get the torn muscles mechanically clean let alone aseptic'.[14] It was four hours before anyone noticed one of Benno Ziegler's comrades in the German Army almost bleeding to death after a shell-splinter had carried away the lower part of his thigh, but only Ziegler and another soldier had the courage to try to rescue him while 'the enemy's rifle-bullets were still whizzing from the edge of wood' and then had to carry him six miles to a field hospital.[15]

Many army doctors seized the opportunity for the heroics and action that their non-combatant status denied them and risked their own lives to tend to the wounded. For one medical officer it was 'a most exciting journey' as he crawled along ditches to rescue a badly wounded officer in a trench and returned with him under 'a shower of bullets … if the smallest piece of one's body was to be seen' to his temporary field hospital set up in an abandoned farmhouse. Unfortunately, one of the stretcher-bearers showed his foot while crawling along and was wounded so 'I had to take him on my back for the rest of the journey'.[16] Rescuing the wounded from No Man's Land was indeed something dreaded by many soldiers. The poet Charles Sorley, who was himself to be killed in action at Loos in 1915 aged only twenty, was only too aware of the horrors of 'carrying a piece of living pulp' and the 'curious inarticulate cry' of a man close to death.[17] Despite being a sensitive youth, he confessed that he felt a 'horrible thankfulness' when faced by the dead rather than a living casualty since 'we won't have to carry him in under fire, thank God, dragging will do: hauling in of the great resistless body in the dark, the smashed head rattling: the relief that the thing has ceased to groan'.[18] The heroics of doctors in bringing in the wounded, by contrast, provided 'a magnificent example of courage, cheerfulness and determination to the fighting men' and were morale boosting.[19] Noel Chavasse, a former Olympic athlete, became the supreme war hero for the Royal Army Medical Corps after earning the Victoria Cross in 1916 for having saved the wounded under heavy fire. He had not always been so popular with his superiors: his insistence on wearing the Glengarry of the Liverpool Scottish Regiment to which he was attached rather than correct RAMC uniform almost led to his arrest as a German spy, and he had once hidden the evidence of a self-inflicted wound and sent the malingerer back down the line. He was killed by a shell as he worked in a dressing station during the 1917 Battle of Passchendaele, having earned a bar to his VC by continuing to treat the wounded despite twice having been wounded in the head himself.[20]

It was not only extroverts like Chavasse who risked their lives as army doctors to save their patients. Arthur Bullock was 'quiet and reserved in manner' with 'a sincere consciousness of his own limitations and abilities' but that did not stop him from being killed while doing his duty in attending to the wounded under shellfire on the battlefield.[21] The 'quiet, unassuming' Reginald Wooster, considered by his commanding officer to be 'a most pleasant member of our Mess', was killed with his medical orderly while going forward with an attack on the enemy in order to attend the wounded.[22] A few war memorials were to commemorate in marble such heroics. On the Croydon War memorial, a wound is being bandaged while on the Port Sunlight memorial two fit men prepare to defend a wounded soldier.[23] However, such self-sacrificing heroics were not universally appreciated and it was felt by many that it was 'impossible to be of much use in the trenches' and that a doctor was of more value if he remained at his first aid post where he could offer treatment than risking his life in the heat of battle.[24] The 'gallant but fatal efforts to succour one wounded man' could deprive a whole unit of medical aid, leading to calls for medical officers to be forbidden to expose themselves too recklessly, but heroes continued to be heroes.[25]

For most wounded men, though, it was only after dark that stretcher parties could bring them back to the regimental aid post. The stretcher-bearers were taught how to apply the Thomas Splint for compound fractures of the femur to immobilise the legs of the wounded while blindfolded as preparation for the conditions in which they would have to rescue the men before bringing them to the first-aid post. Here they received immediate medical attention from a regimental medical officer, often consisting of little more than a rough dressing, a hot drink, a cigarette and liberal doses of morphia to deaden the pain.[26] Often less welcome were the religious ministrations of the padre, who was frequently perceived as being partial to members of his own denomination, though Salvation Army officers were generally more respected since they were seen as helpful to all the wounded in practical rather than preachy ways.[27] Then the wounded would be sent on the slow, agonizing journey by horse-drawn ambulance wagon to an Advanced Dressing Station and finally to a main dressing station or to a casualty clearing station several miles from the front line where they could be operated upon. These casualty clearing stations were usually located near to a railway siding so that the wounded could be easily loaded on to ambulance trains that would take them to the base hospitals.[28] It was a system common to all the belligerent armies and designed for a rapid and mobile war but was soon adapted to deal with the static nature of trench warfare. At the beginning of the war, first aid posts had been established in ruined farmhouses or churches,[29] but as trench warfare became more settled they took on a more permanent character in a series of heavily propped and timbered passages in the trenches.[30]

The transport of the wounded was to be a problem throughout the war. There were calls to replace the uncomfortable and slow horse-drawn ambulances with more modern, faster motor ambulances whereby 'many lives would have been saved and much suffering would have been avoided'.[31] However, Colonel Arthur Lee, who was reporting on the medical conditions in France to Lord Kitchener, considered motor ambulances to be best for short runs and dismissed complaints that it was taking too long to transfer the wounded by train with the observation that 'in the interest of the wounded themselves, even 24 hours delay, or even more, in a hospital train would nearly always be preferable to a quick transfer by motor ambulances', especially in the special 'hospitals on wheels' with their doctors, nursing sisters, operating theatres and supply of invalid foods.[32] Yet even Lee admitted that in the early days of the war, the wounded had to compete for space on ordinary trains with civilians and the French government fleeing from Paris, an exodus of panic which meant that 'it is not surprising that our wounded should have taken a long time in getting down from the front, or that they had to travel in trains that were crowded and were certainly none too comfortable'.[33] Almost two years later back in Britain, hospital and leave trains from France were stopped for five days at Easter 1916 so as not to interfere with holiday traffic.[34] Nevertheless, British arrangements were superior to French arrangements for evacuating the wounded from the Front. At Dunkirk, 600 wounded *poilus* were left lying on dirty straw with very little medical attention for over five days. The only French hospital trains were model trains built for universal exhibitions and the French medical director general admitted that the evacuation system did not work well.[35] Corporal Robson of the London Scottish Regiment was appalled by the sight of 'the wounded all jumbled together ... plastered with dried mud and blood' in ordinary trucks rather than the 'swagger shows with beds, nurses and red crosses'.[36]

The casualty clearing stations had originally been intended as mobile units serving as a link between the field ambulances and the base hospitals where casualties could be assessed and given immediate basic treatment before being passed down the line. However, it was soon realised that, in order to avoid potentially fatal delays in the treatment of war wounds, many of them abdominal or head injuries, surgery would have to take place closer to the Front. Sir Arthur Bowlby, consultant surgeon for surgery, argued for more casualty clearing stations, effectively forward hospitals, to be established closer to the fighting line where this much needed surgery could take place.[37] Here, much of the emergency surgery of the war took place in conditions that would have horrified many of the surgeons if they had had to operate in them in their own hospitals at home. They were faced with rows of 'virile bodies brought to nothing but a slug on the ground'.[38] It surprised them to find that 'with surgery on rather bold lines it was extraordinary how much could be done, especially in the way of saving limbs', although it was an advantage to be 'dealing with healthy and vigorous men, and once they got over the shock of injury they had wonderful powers of recovery'.[39] The lesson of the Boer War had been that complex abdominal surgery could be safely left until the patient had been evacuated to a base hospital. The effects of high explosive missiles on the abdomen now suggested that early surgical intervention offered the best hope of survival. Experience also soon taught that the French surgical practice of *débridement*, or the complete excision of foreign objects and the damaged wound tissue, at the earliest possible opportunity was the most effective approach if gas gangrene were to be avoided. After this surgical preparation, the wound was treated with antiseptics using a system devised by Alexis Carrel and Henry Dakin. This Carrel-Dakin method involved the constant cleansing of the wounds using a solution of sodium hypochlorite administered by a series of tubes, but was not always practicable in the face of an inrush of fresh casualties. When it was adopted, there was a reduction in the number of amputations.[40]

Another life-saving innovation to be tested on the battlefields was blood transfusion. The French surgeon Alexis Carrel had developed a new technique, known as anastomosis, for sewing together arteries and veins in 1902. The American surgeon George Crile had built on this to develop a procedure for attaching a donor's artery directly to a recipient's vein so as to avoid blood clotting in transferring blood, which he first used in 1905. Other transfusion methods were also developed for this person-to-person transfusion using syringe-needles, a Y-shaped cannula and syringe, and a temporary glass storage tube coated with paraffin to stop coagulation of the blood. However, there remained a problem that had doomed many transfusions ever since the first attempts at blood transfusion in the seventeenth century, the incompatibility of a lot of the blood transferred between many donors and recipients. Karl Landsteiner in Vienna noticed, when investigating failed transfusions in 1900, that in some cases fusing the blood of two individuals together caused the red cells to clump together and that the patient died. Since this did not occur in all cases, he concluded that clumping depended on the presence, or absence, of two antigens, substances that produce antibodies, on the surface of the red blood cells. He named these two antigens type 'A' and type 'B'. When blood containing the two different antigens was mixed together, clumping occurred, but nothing happened when antigens of the same type were mixed together or with blood containing no antigens. Blood cells lacking in antigens were named 'O'; a fourth type of blood, 'AB', containing both antigens was later identified. People with blood type 'O' could be universal donors. This discovery of blood groups was to have immense implications for safe blood transfusion, but Landsteiner's discovery was to be ignored for many years. It was too difficult and time-consuming to match blood types and often impossible in emergency conditions. Moreover, the transfusion technique based on Carrel and Crile's methods was difficult to perform under wartime conditions since it needed experienced staff, specialised instruments and a calm setting, impossibilities on the battlefield. It was also an inexact method and sometimes the recipient received too little blood, or else the donor was bled until he looked ashen or fainted from lack of blood. In response to the rushed conditions at casualty clearing stations, indirect methods of transfusion using syringes and transfer tubes were introduced, based on procedures already used in some American hospitals. The French surgeon and urologist Emile Jeanbreau advocated the use of sodium citrate to prevent clotting, but there was some prejudice against using any additives in the blood.[41]

New techniques were less than useless at the height of the bloodiest of battles if the equipment was not there to use them. Harvey Cushing, a surgeon with the American Expeditionary Force, lost track of the days during heavy operating sessions in an evacuation hospital on the Marne in July 1918 in primitive conditions compared with those he was accustomed to at Harvard Medical School where he was professor of surgery. Such basics as X-ray equipment,[42] Dakin's fluid and even dressings were not to be found. He was forced to use 'little compressed bundles of ancient gauze and tabloid finger bandages ... to dress the stinking ruins of these poor lads'. The scene was one of utter confusion and chaos as he dealt ceaselessly one after another with 'amputations of the thigh – sucking chest wounds – mutilations – German wounded ... stinking'. Exhausted, he lay down on an empty operating table, went to sleep and fell off the table.[43]

Cushing's own expertise was with head wounds, having built up a reputation for operating on brain tumours before the war, and he was to impress observers with his use of a magnet to extract metal fragments from the brains of the injured after X-rays had located them. The introduction of steel helmets in 1915 had reduced the incidence of head wounds but there still remained plenty of work for a brain surgeon. On one occasion a piece of a missile proved difficult to extract when Cushing magnetised a six-inch nail which he used to make contact with the metal fragment before withdrawing the nail from the brain in the hope that the foreign body would come out too. A large audience had gathered to watch this but was disappointed when nothing happened and Cushing began to grumble like a golfer might 'scold his golf ball'. On the third attempt, with his magnetised nail, he was successful.[44] His precision and meticulousness so essential for neurosurgery were considered a handicap in battlefield operating.[45] In an attempt to speed things up, he began to use a catheter to suck out depressed bone fragments just as he used a magnet to remove the shrapnel from the brain and operated using a local anaesthetic, talking to the conscious soldier as he performed brain surgery on him.[46] The German surgeon Professor Bier, a pioneer of spinal anaesthesia, used similar methods of extracting shell splinters from brains by using an electric current to magnetise specially shaped pieces of metal attached to special metallic blocks, weighing up to 500lb, lowered by pulleys and then yanked up to remove the shrapnel. However, his success rate was not high and many of his patients later died of meningitis or were paralysed as a result of the brain damage they had suffered from their wounds and treatment.[47]

The unfortunate patient was often understandably wary of the medical treatment he received. Otto Heinebach, a German conscript, was distressed when his 'best comrade', his abdomen torn open by a shell, tried to prevent the stretcher-bearers and doctor from dressing his wound and begged in vain to be given a drug to relieve the pain, refusing to be reassured or comforted by the doctor.[48] When ether was used as an anaesthetic, it caused a 'chestiness' that was particularly unpleasant for heavy smokers. Nitrous oxide was a better anaesthetic than either ether or chloroform but it was in short supply and reserved for the most severe surgical cases.[49] In many German field hospitals, the wounded lay closely packed together on stone floors with only a little straw to cushion them, 'many of them lying with their brains exposed and the wounds covered with flies', and very few attendants to look after them.[50] When senior medical student Stephen Westman from Freiburg University was injured in 1915 and lying on a straw mattress in a church, he was reprimanded for not lying at attention when a medical officer passed him; he ought to have lain with his arms 'stiffly outstretched over the blankets, as if on their trouser seams, like green recruits on the barrack square', but, 'with every bone in my body aching', he did not care about the correct and uncomfortable military protocol.[51] In Eric Maria Remarque's classic novel of the war *All Quiet on the Western Front*, based on the author's own experiences, Franz Kemmerich lies in a dressing station after having his leg amputated, ignored by the doctors when a selection of fitter patients is made for transport aboard a hospital train. When the narrator Paul asks a doctor to attend to his dying friend, the doctor callously dismisses the request with the comment 'How should

I know anything about it, I've amputated five legs today'.[52] Nineteen-year-old Kemmerich dies in an 'atmosphere of carbolic and gangrene', his watch stolen by an orderly.[53]

Robert Graves had similar views on British medical orderlies when he was wounded, calling the RAMC by their less than complimentary sobriquet of 'the Rob All My Comrades' and accusing them, without any real evidence, of having stolen everything he possessed except for a few papers in his tunic pocket and a ring that was too tight to pull off his finger. His finger was festering 'because nobody could be bothered with a slight thing like that', but he received more sympathetic attention for the more serious haemorrhaging in his lung.[54] Private Alex Moffat of the London Scottish Regiment fumed that 'RAMC men should be shot, our wounded and dying travelling five days in a train from the front and they don't even look after them or give them water to drink'.[55] What such critics were often unaware of was that for many of the men seriously wounded with abdominal injuries a drink of water could have been harmful and RAMC orderlies were forbidden to do more than moisten their lips.

If ordinary servicemen were wary of the care they might receive from their own medical services, they were even more concerned about what would happen if they fell into the hands of the enemy, castigated by opposing sides as brutal and unhygienic in their procedures. German medical officers and even members of the Red Cross were accused, like their RAMC counterparts, of being uncaring and 'stealing from saddle bags and haversacks, but without the slightest move on their part to assist in the heavy work of attending to the wounded'. Wounded prisoners were herded together without regard to sanitation or ventilation and, forbidden to dig sanitary trenches, leaving them with no choice but to foul the ground close to where they were being imprisoned. Captain Middleton of the RAMC regarded such a lack of 'decency in these matters being medieval and to our minds disgusting'.[56] The hospital for prisoners of war in Berlin was infested with bugs, burned out by the attendants with a painter's spirit lamp.[57] By the later stages of the war when the Allied blockade of Germany began to bite, medical supplies were in short supply and doctors had to use bandages made from crepe paper or lace curtains and cellulose paper was used instead of cotton wool, even though it quickly dissolved into a sodden mess when soaked with blood and pus. Surgeons were reduced to scrubbing up with ersatz soap made from sand mixed with soap, whilst rubber gloves were an unknown luxury.[58] No wonder that there were complaints of the primitive standards of the German medical services, though it was a situation forced upon them. The Germans in their turn believed that the English clasp knife for removing stones from horses' hooves was 'used for picking out the eyes of their wounded'.[59] In reality, doctors from both armies had a professional duty towards the wounded, regardless of whether they were their own soldiers or the enemy. For A.A. Martin, there could be 'no nationality amongst the men in a hospital, and English, French and German all had a little bit of floor space and a bit of straw' in his improvised field hospital in a schoolhouse at Bethune.[60] It was an attitude shared by German doctors who similarly made no distinction when treating Allied wounded.[61]

Almroth Wright, consulting physician to the British Expeditionary Force, whose anti-typhoid vaccine was to prove the lifesaver in this war that it ought to have done in South Africa, was appalled at the suffering of the wounded. His abiding memory of the war was of the 'quiet, muffled tramp of the soldiers passing through the night' as he rested in his billet. This made him even more determined to work 'very hard because it makes me unhappy to see these wounded boys lose their limbs or their lives through infection, which could if we had the knowledge be cured'.[62] This brought him once again into the heart of controversy so familiar to him from his attempts to gain recognition for his vaccine during the Boer War. He had left the Army Medical School at Netley in 1902 to work at St Mary's Hospital, Paddington, where he had been able to achieve his ambition of establishing his own semi-autonomous medical research institute, the Inoculation Department, in which the hospital wards could be considered an extension of the laboratory, but on the outbreak of war, he had offered the services of his department to the War Office and had been appointed to the rank of lieutenant-colonel and given the task of establishing a laboratory for the study of wound infections at the Casino at Boulogne, now converted into the Fourteenth General Hospital.[63] Now, from this base, he was determined to make his views on the inadequacies of the army medical services known and was unafraid of clashing with his army superiors and colleagues.

Wright was especially opposed to the official policy of evacuating all casualties back to England at the earliest opportunity, often at the very time when their wounds either needed to be excised or sutured. By the time that they arrived at the military hospitals at home, it might be too late for an operation to be viable. Lives were being lost and treatment hindered and delayed by such inflexibility. Meanwhile, medical officers were kept idle during quiet periods on the Western Front when there was a shortage of doctors and hospital beds on the home front. After the Battle of the Marne in 1914 he denounced this iniquitous situation: 'The surgeons are accumulated in France while the wounded are accumulated in England. It almost looks as if the problem proposed has been to keep the wolf, the sheep and the cabbage of the puzzle from ever finding themselves on the same side of the water'.[64]

With a total disregard for military protocol, Wright appealed directly to the Prime Minister, Lloyd George, and the Minister for War, Lord Derby, and his personal friend the ex-Prime Minister Lord Balfour, as well as submitting a memorandum on his proposals for reform through the usual military channels. Although he was the arch individualist with a disregard for any authority but his own, Wright now found himself arguing for the setting up of a Medical Intelligence and Investigation Department to standardise military medicine. Increasingly, he had become concerned about the lack of co-ordination between erstwhile civilian practitioners now serving in the Royal Army Medical Corps who had continued with their pre-war methods of treatment in the very different conditions of total war in which they were 'untaught and inexperienced'. While praising the administrative successes of the Army Medical Services in organising hospitals, ambulances, medical staff and nurses, he lambasted the failure of anyone to take responsibility for a uniform method of treatment and accused them of being 'hypnotised by the plea of "Military Exigencies"'.[65]

The authorities were antagonised by the violation of military protocol in the way the proposals had been presented as much as by the trenchant opinions expressed. Sir Arthur Sloggett, Director General of Army Medical Services in France, was keen to have Wright recalled from France in disgrace. Only the fact that Wright had many powerful friends able to intervene prevented his recall but his proposals were shelved to his chagrin.[66] The 1917 Howard Commission on Medical Services in France ignored most of his suggestions and praised the RAMC for its flexibility and 'the success with which an organisation, designed for a small Army, has been rapidly expanded to meet the requirements of an Army of millions and has proved itself as adaptable to trench warfare, as to the war of movement for which it was originally intended', including innovations that Wright actually approved of such as the mobile bacteriological laboratories which had first appeared just before the Battle of the Aisne in 1914 and which allowed for swifter identification of, and action to contain, infectious diseases such as enteric and cerebro-spinal fever.[67]

What Wright justifiably could take pride in was his role in preventing a repetition from the Boer War of needless deaths from typhoid. His insistence that British troops be vaccinated with the anti-typhoid vaccine he had developed back in 1897 was perhaps his greatest contribution to medicine during the war. He had been arguing his case since the end of the Boer War for compulsory inoculation of troops and in 1914 he lobbied his acquaintance Lord Kitchener and also took his case before the public using his usual tactic of a letter to *The Times* to appeal for public support for inoculation. He warned that 'an army, going out on active service, goes from the sanitary conditions of modern civilization straight back to those of barbarism' and that typhoid was endemic in northern France.[68] Kitchener was easily persuaded and all regimental medical officers were encouraged to offer inoculation to their men. Although it was still optional, Kitchener gave an added inducement to its take-up by insisting that only men who had been inoculated could be sent overseas to fight. Yet there were still men who avoided inoculation. Many doctors thought it ought to be compulsory. Surgeon Arthur Martin declared that 'soldiers should not be allowed liberty of conscience' but should obey orders and be inoculated 'in spite of the screechings of fanatics suffering from distorted cerebration'.[69] The United States armed forces already had introduced inoculation against typhoid on a voluntary basis in 1909 and had made it compulsory from 1911 onwards with three doses being given to new soldiers at intervals of one week as soon as they enlisted.[70] A commission appointed by the French government had also recommended anti-typhoid inoculation for anyone at risk of infection but the Académie de Médicine had failed to endorse its conclusions, though French colonial troops were all vaccinated.[71] With the acceptance of inoculation for the British Army, Wright mobilised the resources of his own Inoculation Department for the large-scale production of his vaccine; throughout the war some ten million doses were supplied to the British, Belgian, French, Russian and Serbian armed forces, at first free of charge though it was not long before British government grants were sought to fund the project.[72] As a result there were only 1,191 deaths among British soldiers from typhoid during the war, mainly of men who had managed to evade inoculation, rather than the 120,000 deaths that have been estimated as likely without it.[73] Paratyphoid was causing problems on the Eastern Front, so killed cultures of paratyphoid bacilli 'A' and 'B' were added to the anti-typhoid vaccine, which now became known as a T.A.B. vaccine. Tetanus too was reduced to manageable proportions by the introduction of an anti-tetanus serum thanks to the influence of Wright's old adversary David Bruce.[74]

The German Empire, with its generals mindful of the havoc reaped by typhoid during the Franco-Prussian war of 1870, had considered the question of compulsory anti-typhoid inoculation in 1905. Wright had many friends and admirers in the German medical and scientific community, including the eminent bacteriologist Robert Koch who had laid the foundations of the scientific study of infectious disease, and they did not hesitate in recommending Wright's vaccine.[75] Despite this, the German Army only adopted a very limited policy of inoculation although it did screen all conscripts for typhoid and anyone found to be a carrier was invalided out of the service. It was not enough. Following an outbreak of typhoid on the Western Front in 1915, inoculation was made mandatory.[76]

As important as inoculation in preventing disease was attention to the unglamorous but essential field of sanitation. Sanitary units were made responsible for clearing up newly occupied territory, incinerating rubbish, filling in latrines and disposing of excreta, disinfecting clothes and ensuring that the troops had access to clean drinking water. The French were less particular and did not set up sanitary squads until November 1916, much to the disgust of their British allies.[77] In many areas, British officers had to act to improve on Gallic inadequacies. In the absence of French doctors, British military doctors would treat French civilian patients and work with the French authorities to maintain public health, as much to the benefit of their own men as the French, though the motive in giving such humanitarian aid was tied up with ideas of helping an ally whose country was suffering more than one's own: 'the duty is one which the British nation is in honour bound to undertake, when it is remembered that we are not only defending France against the Germans but defending our own country at the same time, with the advantage of fighting our battles on French soil'.[78] In 1915 a serious epidemic of enteric fever broke out among the civilian population near Ypres, threatening the health of the troops billeted in that much bombarded town. Despite 'the diplomatic difficulties attendant upon removing a stricken but ignorant civilian population from its own homes to the care of strangers', an attempt was made to isolate the typhoid sufferers away from the troops but proved impossible.[79] However, even the best of arrangements could break down under pressure and during the rapid movement of divisions during the Battle of the Somme in 1916 there was an outbreak of dysentery as a result of the failure of the sanitary squads to keep up with the action.

The shameful neglect of measures for disease prevention was one of many mistakes made at Gallipoli and in Mesopotamia. Flies spread dysentery, diarrhoea and gastroenteritis among the wounded at the ill-fated Gallipoli assault on Turkey. Latrines were even cruder than those on the Western Front and soiled dressings and other rubbish were left lying around. There was a shortage of stretchers and the very dead went unburied in the heat of battle.[80] Medical officers felt frustrated when 'the evacuation of the wounded, maintenance of water supply and sanitation have required all one's efforts to carry out in a way not satisfactory indeed, but sufficient to save one from a feeling of abject incompetence'.[81] The campaigns in Mesopotamia were no better. There the chief problems were enteric disease, dysentery, malaria and such deficiency diseases as scurvy and beri beri. There were cases of cholera and plague in Basra.[82] Above all 'the conditions of the sick and wounded … left much to be desired and anxiety was felt as to the medical and general arrangements being such that proper care for the sick and wounded soldiers in that trying climate could be ensured'.[83] The enemy was blamed for their poor standards of hygiene and 'most of the epidemics of dysentery in our advancing troops were traceable infection from polluted areas occupied by the Turks'.[84] Lawrence of Arabia, the desert hero, shared this low view of Turkish hygiene when he took command of a Turkish hospital after he had liberated Damascus near the end of the war. Entering the hospital, he was assailed by the 'sickening stench' and the sight of the stone floor 'covered with dead bodies, side by side, some in full uniform, some in underclothing, some stark naked' which were being gnawed away by rats. Those patients still living were in just as bad a condition, 'each man rigid on his stinking pallet, from which liquid muck had dripped down to stiffen on the cemented floor'.[85] Lawrence took charge of this charnel house, saw to the burial of the dead, disinfection of the wards and the clean-up of the patients only for a British major, mistaking him in his Arab dress for a native, to splutter at him, 'Scandalous, disgraceful, outrageous, ought to be shot' before smacking him on the face for his brutality in seemingly neglecting the sick in his charge.[86]

Back in the trenches of the Western Front it was rats, not Turks, that threatened health by contaminating food and spreading disease such as Weil's Disease (infective jaundice) and bubonic plague. The naturalist Philip Gosse was appointed as Rat Officer to draw up schemes for destroying the rats and training officers in vermin control.[87] Among his duties was performing inquests on dead rats to see what they had died from, the most usual cause being a blow from a soldier's stick. One rat had swollen glands, which suggested to Gosse and his colleague Adrian Stokes, a bacteriologist investigating Weil's Disease, the possibility that it might have bubonic plague, which was endemic on the Eastern Front and might have been brought to France by the transfer of a German division. They infected a guinea pig with micro-organisms from the swollen glands of the dead rat and it too died of plague-like symptoms. Under the microscope the bacteria seemed to resemble *bacillus pestis*, responsible for bubonic plague. William Leishman, adviser in pathology to the British Expeditionary Force was called in and declared that the rat had died of 'chicken plague', an obscure disease harmless to humans. However, Leishman was unsure of his diagnosis and ordered 50,000 doses of anti-plague vaccine from the Lister Institute just in case he was wrong. He was not.[88] It was an expensive hesitancy and modesty of which Almroth Wright and many of the generals would never have been guilty.

Lice were an even greater threat than rats to personal hygiene and health in the trenches. Not only were they a source of an unpleasant itch and an affront to the sensibilities of the more fastidious recruit or conscript accustomed to greater standards of cleanliness than were possible in the field, but they also spread disease including relapsing fever, typhus and trench fever, although it was not until 1918 that David Bruce established the causal link between trench fever and the despised louse.[89] In their billets, soldiers using matches to drive the lice from the seams of their uniforms were a common sight, though such efforts were more often than not in vain. The poet Isaac Rosenberg described one soldier tearing off from his throat 'a shirt verminously busy' which was soon 'aflare over the candle he'd lit while we lay' only to be followed by his comrades who all 'sprang up and stript' to hunt their own lice in 'a demons' pantomime'.[90] Much more effective was the all-too welcome and too rare opportunity to have a bath and for the steam disinfection of soiled uniforms. Companies of 'mud-caked, verminous and woe-begone looking scarecrows' entered at one end of the improvised bathhouses only to emerge after forty-five minutes 'rosy-cheeked, bright-eyed, comparatively well-dressed and in wildly hilarious spirits'.[91] Fumigation in delousing stations was also standard for German soldiers, with more luxurious facilities for officers, though at least one general complained because his underwear was so long in returning from fumigation with formalin while he waited with the most junior of officers.[92] On the Eastern Front, delousing pits were developed in Russia and Rumania, dugouts heated by brick stoves to eighty or ninety degrees

Centigrade in which clothing was hung or placed on racks.[93] They were more effective than an attempt to treat uniforms chemically to prevent the growth of gas-forming bacteria, but such chemicals as pyxol merely proved an irritant to the skin, especially when the soldiers trying out such garments sweated profusely following exercise in hot rooms.[94]

Linked with the difficulty for the humble Tommie, Fritz and *poilu* of keeping himself clean was the problem of trench foot, in which the foot went black, ulcerous and rotted away; this new condition first became a matter of major concern in November and December 1914 as a result of cold, water-logged conditions in the trenches.[95] Various ineffective remedies were tried out, including putting rum in the boots of the men, wrapping the feet in cotton wool and placing braziers of hot charcoal in the trenches before it was recognized that the best treatment and preventative was to wash the feet regularly, change socks frequently and wear comfortable, waterproof boots.[96] It was also noticed that 'neither the Indian troops nor the Germans appear to have suffered to anything like the same extent as the British white troops', a fact explained by the habit of Indian and German soldiers of wearing outsize boots and wearing a second pair of socks in cold weather'.[97]

The maintenance of personal hygiene was difficult enough in the trenches of the Western Front but on the Eastern Front was almost impossible with more extreme winters. It was here that epidemics really took their toll. Like the war itself, the typhus epidemic began in Serbia, with 10,000 cases as early as November 1914. Within six months, the number of deaths had reached 150,000, with a sixty per cent death rate. The casualties included thirty per cent of all Serbian physicians. Conditions in Serbian hospitals outside Belgrade were primitive, with sacks of hay serving as mattresses in many of them, and doctors and nurses could not avoid the ubiquitous lice that spread the disease as they went about their work.[98] Even when sanitary precautions were taken, it was impossible to avoid infection. Mabel St Clair Stobart set up a hospital camp, staffed by women doctors under the aegis of the Serbian Relief Fund at Kragujevatz, the Serbian military headquarters, that was 'a model in outdoor sanitation' in which the patients were kept free of infection though the staff went down with typhoid fever rather than typhus.[99] When the German Army invaded Serbia in the autumn of 1915 Mrs St Clair Stobart's unit took part in the retreat across the mountains of Albania, 'a memory of mental and physical suffering, which will cause life henceforth to be seen through darkened spectacles', in which some

150,000 Serbs died.[100] German troops took the infection of typhus home with them and it spread through prisoner of war camps, most notoriously at Wittenberg where many British officers died.[101] Typhus also spread through Russia, Ukraine and eastern Poland. In Russia, one consequence of the 1917 revolution and the ensuing civil war was that typhus rampaged uncontrolled. From 1917 to 1921, there were 25 million cases with almost 3 million deaths in one of the worst typhus outbreaks recorded. Lenin remarked that 'if socialism does not defeat the louse, the louse will defeat socialism'.[102]

Despite the ravages of infectious disease in Eastern Europe, it soon became apparent that wound infections rather than epidemics would pose one of the major medical problems of the war, yet there was little understanding of the subject and little research had been undertaken into it. In South Africa, where most of the injuries had indeed been simple, clean bullet wounds, there had been no need to attempt any bacteriological investigation of wound infections. Now in 1914, multiple wounds from numerous pieces of shrapnel from high explosive shells were more common, sepsis was rife and gas gangrene and tetanus were responsible for ten per cent of all deaths in field hospitals. It was not what the textbooks had led doctors to expect and regimental medical officers commented that they had seen 'great gaping wounds as big as your fist made by rifle bullets, either fired at short range or after ricocheting'. Popular myth told of men whose lives had been saved by pocket Bibles, silver cigarette cases or a threepenny bit carried in a waistcoat pocket, but in fact 'any object of that sort incites a rifle bullet to produce more horrid wounds' which could become badly infected.[103] However, most of the infection came from the soldiers' own clothing, their uniforms having been dirtied by soil fertilised by horse manure, which had been contaminated by the organisms that cause gas gangrene and tetanus.[104] In many cases, the only way of stopping the gas gangrene from spreading was amputation of the affected limb. Lice and maggots, in cases where flies had laid their eggs in open wounds, were often seen crawling from under bandages and plaster of Paris casts, yet it was noticed that maggots, 'these highly unpleasant creatures acted as scavengers, so to speak, and the wounds looked fresh and clean'.[105] In October 1914 Sir Alfred Keogh, Director-General of the Army Medical Service, was not exaggerating when he declared that 'We have in this war gone straight back to all the septic infections of the Middle Ages'.[106]

Almroth Wright was determined to come up with a solution to the problem. It soon became clear that the cause of the problem was actually the liberal use of antiseptics on the wounds by medical officers brought up on the doctrine that the answer to infection was that proposed by Lord Lister in the late nineteenth century, the use of antiseptics to kill off the bacteria. The antiseptics were negating the body's own defences and the bacteria thus were able to flourish unchecked.[107] Wright had long believed that chemical antiseptics were more harmful to the white blood cells than infective bacteria, but his views were not shared by most army surgeons who found it difficult to accept that antiseptics might not only be useless but could be potentially damaging.[108] In order to demonstrate this to sceptical military surgeons, Alexander Fleming, one of Wright's most loyal disciples, with the ingenuity and flair for improvisation that was his hallmark, made an artificial wound from a test tube, which he heated to soften its walls before drawing out spikes from it, using the glass blowing skills that were so useful in the laboratory and which in peacetime he had used to make glass animals for the amusement of children. The spiked tube was then filled with a liquid infected with bacteria, which he then emptied and replaced with an antiseptic. This was incubated for twenty-four hours before being emptied in its turn and replaced with a liquid culture medium in which any bacteria could grow. When he incubated this for one more time, the original bacteria were found to be as virulent as they had been from the beginning. It was obvious that the bacteria had remained in the hollow spikes of the tube untouched by the bacteria. Having established this, Fleming then tested his hypothesis that the antiseptics not only failed to penetrate the crevices of the wound but were also absorbed by the dressings and dead tissue on the surface of the wound. He filled a test tube with the coloured antiseptic gentian violet, pushed a plug of cotton wool through it with a glass rod so that the fluid was forced through the cotton wool and then showed that the fluid on top of it was colourless because the plug had absorbed all of the antiseptic. Thus he demonstrated how antiseptics could not penetrate the jagged edges of the wounds of modern warfare with the result that the bacteria had an open road into the wound and could multiply unchecked in its irregular edges.[109] He then went on to prove that the bacteria were not only useless in the treatment of war wounds, but could be positively harmful by actually encouraging the growth of bacteria in the blood serum.[110]

This in-depth investigation of war wounds suggested to Wright and Fleming the best means of dealing with the infections: diseased and dying tissue should be cut off, the wounds should be cleansed with a mild saline solution and then closed to further sterilise them. The use of clean dressings would then offer protection against further bacterial infection.[111] It was sensible advice but aroused controversy like everything else that Wright was involved in. Sir William Watson Cheyne, the President of the Royal College of Surgeons, mounted a challenge against this salt-water treatment in defence of the use of antiseptics to treat wounds. The debate became acrimonious and almost amounted to a personal duel between the two medical knights, in which Wright dismissed his opponent's views as 'imaginative fiction' and 'blindfolded by prejudice'.[112] Nevertheless, perhaps even in reaction to the intemperance of Wright's criticism of the venerable President of the Royal College of Surgeons, the prevailing view among doctors remained that if the available antiseptics did not work, then the only thing to do was to use a stronger antiseptic. Newer and stronger antiseptics, such as iodine, iodoform, eusol, gentian violet, flavine and acridine were no improvement on carbolic acid. The only antiseptic that proved to be any good was Carrel-Dakin solution containing sodium hypochlorite, which soon lost its antiseptic qualities when poured on a wound and turned into a simple saline solution such as that advocated by Wright and Fleming all along.[113] Yet, sensible though this salt treatment may have been, it was caught in the crossfire of medical and military politics and was not widely adopted until the Second World War; much to Wright's chagrin antiseptics continued in use in field stations throughout this war.[114] It was little consolation when shortly after the end of the war a surgeon who had opposed him admitted in the national press that 'We all said Wright was mistaken about his antiseptics: but it was we who were mistaken'.[115]

The problem of wound infection was perhaps the most serious to come out of the new technology of war and the attempts to overcome it were of major importance, but from 22 April 1915 onwards a new more frightening and sinister development appeared with the first use of poison gas by the Germans in the Ypres Salient. This new resort to chemical warfare, masterminded by Fritz Haber working with the chemical firm of IG Farben, was at first greeted with outrage by the British, but very soon they followed suit and set up their own gas unit, which, led by Major Howard Foulkes, soon developed the more deadly phosgene as an alternative to the chlorine gas used in the initial German attack; in January 1916, they mixed the two gases together to form a deadly new compound called 'White Star'.[116] Such attacks were frightening to the men involved, and could backfire on the perpetrator if the prevailing wind blew the gas back to their own lines. One chlorine gas attack on the night of

23–24 May 1915 'came over as a dense whitish green cloud sufficient even at the Asylum at Ypres to blot out houses and trees from view' and to fill the asylum cellars 'with a fog'. Respirators and helmets with pads of cotton wool soaked in hyposulphite solution had been issued to the men, but, unfortunately, no one had instructed them in the proper use of the new fangled gas masks, though they were improvements on the early advice to 'piss on your handkerchiefs and tie them over your faces' to neutralise the chloride.[117] In German dressing stations, gas casualties were stripped of their uniforms, washed and bandaged. They then lay completely naked with only a blanket to keep them warm for up to two days before ambulances could make it through the intense shelling.[118] Mustard gas in shells was used by the Germans from 1917 and proved particularly deadly as its high boiling point of 223 degrees Centigrade meant that its characteristic garlic or mustard aroma 'could be smelt in Ypres on the day following the bombardment'. The initial effect of a mustard gas attack was an irritation of the nose and throat, but after eighteen hours the eyes of the victim became irritated and he would have fits of vomiting. If the liquid came into contact with his skin, there would be blistering.[119] Mustard gas was responsible for eighty per cent of gas casualties.[120]

One of the most striking images to emerge from the war was John Singer Sargent's painting *Gassed* depicting a line of men, their eyes covered by blindfolds, groping their way along a duckboard towards a medical aid tent through a battlefield of corpses, each man with his hand on the shoulder of the man in front of him and being guided by a medic. In another line, a man vomits. In the distant background, soldiers play football, their physical and visual fitness sadly and eloquently contrasting with the victims of mustard gas who were once as hale and vigorous as them.[121] The painting was inspired by what Sargent had witnessed as a war artist at a dressing station at Le Bac-du-Sud on the road between Arras and Doullens in July 1918, where men who had been gassed were arriving in six-strong parties, their eyes covered by pieces of lint.[122] Sargent's famous picture is echoed in many contemporary photographs.[123] Wilfred Owen provides in his verse an alternative image of 'an ecstasy of fumbling fitting the clumsy helmets' and of a gassed man with 'the white eyes writhing in his face' and 'the blood come gargling from the froth-corrupted lungs'.[124] What no contemporary account could do was depict the long-term broken health, partial blindness and ceaseless coughing suffered by the survivors of gas attacks in the years to come.

Also lasting and even more visible was the horrific mutilation of face wounds. Steel helmets might offer protection against brain injuries, but the face still remained exposed to shell fragments and shrapnel. Close range and low velocity rifles produced big entry wounds and many men had their jaws and noses blown away or were blinded.[125] For the ophthalmologist there was the problem of ensuring that men with eye injuries could see anything at all. Large magnets were used to remove metal fragments from eyes in which the retina had been detached when the eyelids had been lacerated by large pieces of shrapnel.[126] Wood splinters too could cause extensive damage.[127] Many of these ophthalmic injuries were depicted in a remarkable series of drawings by the composer William Wallace, who had briefly returned to his original career as an ophthalmologist for the duration of the war as Eye Specialist for the London District and Inspector of Ophthalmic Centres for the Eastern Command.[128]

It was the need to do something for severely disfigured men that led to the birth of modern plastic surgery. Reconstructive surgery itself was not new and had its origins in classical India and its rebirth in Renaissance Europe, but was given a stimulus by the sickening facial injuries now being seen in military hospitals. The first British jaw and plastic surgery unit was set up by the dentist Charles Valadier at Wimereux in the summer of 1915. The military medical establishment was suspicious of a dentist dabbling in reconstructive surgery and insisted that the ear, nose and throat surgeon Harold Gillies should assist him and keep an eye on him. Inspired by what he saw, Gillies returned to the Cambridge Military Hospital at Aldershot and established his own facial injuries team of surgeons, dentists, anaesthetists, radiologists and medical illustrators. He was one of the first reconstructive surgeons to show an interest in the aesthetics of plastic surgery. At this time, German plastic surgery was more concerned with getting mutilated men back into battle with little concern about their appearance. Even the usually aesthetic French showed slight regard for the final appearance of the men with facial injuries that they worked on. Gillies, though, was of a different mettle and attempted to improve the appearance of the men. Henry Tonks, Professor of Fine Art at the Slade School, drew pastels of the injuries and of the subsequent appearance of the men after surgery. Broken and septic teeth were removed, dentures fitted, broken bones reset and skin–grafting carried out to reconstruct noses and jaws. Gillies showed his patients albums containing photographs of handsome young men and asked them to choose the chin or other feature they would most like. Psychologically it did the patient more good than the use of masks, known as 'Tin Faces', to cover the worst and largest facial injuries. As casualties began to flood in from the Battle of the Somme in July 1916 and Gillies was faced with 2,000 cases of jaw and facial mutilation, 'men maimed to the condition of animals', he found it more difficult to give every man full personal attention. He also needed more facilities than the Cambridge Military Hospital could offer and in 1917 established the new Queen's Hospital at Sidcup specifically for reconstructive surgery. Here, he and his team laid the foundations of modern plastic surgery, though their work has often been forgotten in comparison with later developments during the Second World War, which it prefigured.[129]

The disfigurements so awfully and yet so strangely beautifully depicted by Henry Tonks in pastels and the photographs showing the hideously deformed features of the men being treated by Gillies are horrific, but even the photographs of the men after treatment can shock.[130] All the skill of the plastic surgeon could not restore young men to how they had once looked nor hide entirely the rough and scared ravages of war. Some of the men requested no further surgery, especially if their facial disfigurement was 'slight' and they were afraid that any further action might cause more visible scarring.[131] For others, prolonged and painful surgery was necessary, such as an able seaman aged twenty, who had suffered severe cordite burns to his face, neck and hands on board HMS *Malaya* at the Battle of Jutland in May 1916 and was unable to close his mouth.[132] Not admitted to the Queen's Military Hospital until August 1917, his nose and hands had to be rebuilt and even when he was finally discharged in September 1920 he remained horribly disfigured by scar tissue.[133] Even when the reconstruction of the face was relatively simple and successful, it could be a long-drawn out process. A twenty-year-old soldier who lost his nose from a gunshot wound in 1917 needed five operations in which a new nose was fashioned from a flap of skin on his forehead and four years in hospital before he could present an acceptable face to the world.[134] For some of the men, the treatment was not only long and painful, but could also be ultimately unsuccessful. A twenty-year-old private in the Second Lincolnshire Regiment received gunshot wounds to the nose and left eye on the first day of the Battle of the Somme on 1 July 1916. He underwent six unsuccessful operations to reconstruct his nose and eyelids over the next eighteen months only for the surgeon to discharge him in January 1918 with the comment 'Total result: unsatisfactory. Advised to return for further treatment'. He returned two years later for that further attempt at rhinoplasty, reconstruction of the nose, only for scar tissue to block the nasal airway before he succumbed to a streptococcal infection of his nose. The next series of operations were more successful but when he was finally discharged in October 1921 he was told that he would have to return for further treatment to improve the line of his new nose and left eyebrow.[135] For him the sickening horror of war would always be there in the mirror.

Not all war injuries were visible. The mental scars could be just as debilitating and long lasting as a physical wound. Shell-shock was a new phenomenon recognizing for the first time mental breakdown as a result of the effects of battle. The term, coined by Charles Myers in 1915, was soon applied to a wide variety of wartime mental disorders though its name suggested an erroneous connection between the effects of a shell exploding and the development of neurotic symptoms.[136] In Scott Fitzgerald's 1934 novel *Tender is the Night*, a Swiss psychiatrist tells the doctor hero Dick Diver that 'we have some shell-shocks who merely heard an air raid from a distance. We have a few who merely read newspapers'.[137] Real soldiers traumatised by war regularly complained of palpitations, chest pains, tremors, joint and muscle pains, loss of speech or deafness and often broke down in tears when asked to describe their experiences at the Front. Already by December 1914, large numbers of men with the British Expeditionary Force were being sent back to England suffering from 'nervous and mental shock'. Myers, a forty-one-year-old Cambridge psychologist, was appointed as Specialist in Nervous Shock to investigate the problem and arrange for the dispatch of such cases from France to England. It soon became clear to Myers that the army was making a serious mistake in treating men who had broken down mentally and emotionally under the strains of war as if they were lunatics; such treatment could actually push them into genuine insanity. Instead of sending them back to mental hospitals in Britain, he argued for the treatment of these men in specialist hospitals a few miles from the Front where they could be treated quickly and returned to military service where possible so as to avoid unnecessary wastage of manpower; if their problems were too deep seated for a return to action, rapid treatment of their neuroses would at least allow them to return to normal civilian life rather than become war pensioner burdens on the state. However, there was an entrenched lack of sympathy for mental illness within the army, which linked any such weakness with lack of moral fibre.[138] A distinction was made between 'shell-shock (wound)' resulting from concussion from military action and 'shell-shock (sick)' which was seen as an emotional reaction to the stress of battle and had a stigma attached to it.[139]

Nevertheless, as a reaction to the acute manpower shortages following the Somme, Myers was given the go ahead to set up 'Not Yet Diagnosed Nervous' centres, based on similar centres established by the French neurologist Georges Guillan, near the Front where soldiers could be rested, medicated, fed and put through a programme of graduated exercises and route marches to allow them to be speedily returned to combat. Many of the physicians running these units had little faith in psychiatry or the use of hypnotism to reveal underlying problems, and eventually a demoralised Myers returned to the United Kingdom on sick leave. The major part of his responsibilities passed to the neurologist Gordon Holmes, who believed that psychoanalysis was undermining military efficiency and that the doctor's role was to treat physical symptoms only. Real men would not weaken but would obey the music hall artiste Harry Lauder's exhortation to 'keep right on to the end of the road'. However, Myers's model of 'forward psychiatry' was adopted by the Americans when they arrived in France and set up psychiatric field hospitals run by divisional psychiatrists to whom all shell-shock cases were referred.[140]

Emotional shell-shock was seen as a condition more likely to affect 'people of finer intellects',[141] a type of sensitive young man who is unable to sleep and turns to drink to try to control his fears as exemplified by the figure of Captain Stanhope in R.C. Sherriff's post-war play *Journey's End*.[142] The psychologist W.H.R. Rivers believed that officers suffered a different kind of breakdown from their men because they were better educated, more sensitive and had a greater sense of duty. This meant that they had to repress their instinct for flight from danger and show courage as a good example to their men. Privates, however, had not been brought up to show a stiff upper lip and could express themselves with 'sulphurous language' as 'a safety valve for repressed emotion', though Rivers was perhaps underestimating the ability of all classes to curse and swear. He was on safer ground in arguing that sensitive men were unable to build up strategies for coping with 'strains such as have never previously been known in the history of mankind'.[143] Charles Wilson, a medical officer who was later, ennobled as Lord Moran, to be Winston Churchill's personal physician in the Second World War, thought that blank, unimaginative men fared best while sensitive, imaginative ones were most likely to suffer a breakdown, yet paradoxically it was the imaginative man who made the better leader and whose qualities were most needed in wartime: 'it is not what happens out here but what men think may happen that finds the flaw in them, yet it is the thinking soldier that lasts in modern war.'[144] The intelligent officer was the manly soldier, but he was more sensitive to danger. In John Buchan's popular novel of 1916 *Greenmantle*, the seasoned fighter Peter Pienar, a man 'to whom courage is habitual', finds in the confusion of the trenches that the taste of fear 'seems to wash away his manhood'.[145] Shell-shock was emasculating as much as it was debilitating.

Whereas the ordinary shell-shocked soldier was likely to find himself confined as a morally weak hysteric in a county lunatic asylum[146] or executed for cowardice and desertion,[147] the neurasthenic officer was usually treated more sympathetically in special hospitals for officers such as Craiglockhart Hospital near Edinburgh. Billiards, badminton, bowls, croquet, cricket, golf and water polo filled the days of the patients in a frenzy of forced, communal physical activity. The nights were different as the 'hospital became sepulchral and oppressive with saturations of war experience ... feet padding along passages which smelt of stale cigarette smoke ... an underworld of dreams haunted by submerged memories of warfare and its intolerable shocks and self-lacerating failures to achieve the impossible'.[148] It was to Craiglockhart that Siegfried Sassoon was sent in 1917 after denouncing the war while recovering from war wounds. A hitherto dashing and daring subaltern, his new anti-war position was ascribed to shell-shock, 'the disintegration of those qualities through which they had been so gallant and selfless and uncomplaining', and he was sent for psychiatric treatment rather than the court martial his 'act of wilful defiance' deserved.[149] He was treated by W.H.R. Rivers, a fifty-one-year-old, socially awkward, sexually repressed psychiatrist with a passion for anthropology. The two men bonded, their friendship imbued with the homo-erotic tensions arising from Rivers's repressed homosexuality and Sassoon's increasingly angry admission of his own attraction to men. Rivers too had doubts about 'whether the continuance of the war was justifiable' but was obliged to 'cure [him] of his pacifist errors and persuade him to return to the fight'.[150] Before leaving Craiglockhart, Sassoon had become friendly with another shell-shocked poet, Wilfred Owen, whose therapist Arthur Brock believed that cold baths, swimming, early morning walks and ceaseless activity was the answer to introspection and nightmares of the horrors of the trenches. This treatment honed Owen as a soldier while his friendship with Sassoon sharpened his poetic genius. It was among 'men whose minds the Dead have ravished' that Sassoon found his poetic voice only to be killed on his return to action.[151]

Sassoon and Owen were treated differently from each other by their psychiatrists at Craiglockhart, one being encouraged to discuss his fears and the other to displace them with physical activity, but their therapies were gentler than those experienced by many of their contemporaries. Lewis Yealland, a Canadian neurologist working at the National Hospital for the Paralysed and Epileptic in Queen's Square, London, used faradism, electric shock treatment, on his patients. One man was 'strapped in a chair for twenty minutes at a time while strong electricity was applied to his neck and throat; lighted cigarettes had been applied to the tip of his tongue and hot plates had been placed at the back of his mouth'; this went on for four hours until the man was cured, perhaps from fear as much as anything marvellous about the treatment.[152] Similar methods were used by the Mannheim neurologist D. Kaufmann, an example followed by many other German doctors, but his 'sadistic attack on the patient' was attacked by the British as emblematic of the authoritarian brutality of Teutonic medicine. Max Nonne, a Hamburg neurologist, preferred to use hypnotism and was filmed healing a group of writhing and twitching men, naked except for their underwear, with a few words and clicks of his fingers. However, like battle scenes in many contemporary war documentaries, it was all staged for the camera with patients Nonne had previously cured and then rehypnotized. The German Army looked on these victims of shell-shock as unworthy of the traditions of the German soldier and accepted that they could better serve the Fatherland as farm labourers or factory workers than be returned to the Front for which they were so obviously unfitted.[153]

In many ways the First World War had been a successful one for medicine, whose practitioners had risen to the challenges posed by modern warfare. The physician Sir Thomas Clifford Allbutt claimed in 1919 that the war had transformed medicine from 'an observational and empirical craft to a scientific calling'.[154] Doctors had been exposed to new medical technology and methods that they were to take with them into civilian life. Many of the wartime innovations, though, had had their origins in work carried out before the war, suggesting to the pioneering historian of medicine Fielding Garrison that 'the medical innovations and inventions ... seem clever, respectable but not particularly brilliant' compared with the administrative achievement of organising medical services in a world war.[155] Yet, the demands of war left little time for the considered reflection that might have led to brilliance in peacetime and some of the improvised responses to the new demands of war were bold and imaginative. However, there was some resistance to new ideas and techniques even when introduced more diplomatically than by Almroth Wright, and most doctors continued along their old lines of thought. Above all it was essential to do what was necessary to save lives for 'the primary objects ... are to get the disabled, physically and mentally, fit to fight again'.[156] It was winning the war that mattered and for that soldiers fit for the task were needed.[157] Even if no longer fit to fight, they still had a part to play in national survival. The doctor and writer Georges Duhamel was well aware of this when he wrote that 'the mutilated owed something more to their country: they had given their blood, they would now give up their sons' and put words into the mouth of one of his doctor characters that 'each time I amputate a limb and save a man, I think of the race: this fellow will still be a good stud'; even those men incapacitated for fighting had a part to play if their lives could be saved for the breeding of the next generation of soldiers.[158] Medicine had indeed played an important part in maintaining fighting forces for all the belligerent powers, whether they were to be victors or vanquished in this war and prepared to rear a new generation to fight in the next. As the medical humanist Sir William Osler was well aware, 'Hygeia holds the trump card and gives victory to the nation that can keep a succession of healthily efficient men in the field'.[159]

3

Business not as Usual

Crowds gathered at Charing Cross Station in July 1916 to watch the arrival of casualties from the Battle of the Somme, an event often seen as marking the end of any illusions of chivalry in war and in its horror ushering in the modern age of warfare. The moment was captured by the official war artist J. Hodgson Lobley in an oil painting 'Outside Charing Cross Station, July 1916', which epitomises Britain at this crucial moment during the First World War. The grandiose buildings of the station reflect the grandeur of the British Army in contrast to the pitiable state of the returning soldiers. Newspaper placards headline the war news and posters advertising continental holidays for a more peaceful time ironically make the point that instead of dispatching peaceful tourists abroad the same railways nowadays bring back the wounded and dying. The now redundant American Currency Exchange underlines this, for the exchange effectively has become one of wounded soldiers for fit, healthy young men. The crowds of besuited men and millinered women going about their affairs ostensibly as in peacetime and watching the scene cannot remain unaffected by the consequences of what they see.[1] Civilian health was influenced by the war just as much as that of the injured troops. The mood of the Home Front might have been business as usual but the war had its effect all the same.

Almost from the outbreak of the war, military requirements took priority over the needs of women, children and men not in the armed forces. Winning the war was what mattered, whatever the sacrifice demanded. The care, nursing and rehabilitation of wounded soldiers now mattered more than the already patchy provision of medical services for everyone else. Whereas in Germany plans had been made for the conversion of public buildings and barracks blocks into hospitals in the event of war, Britain was caught unprepared when war came. The War Office had realised that the number of beds in the regular military hospitals would be inadequate and had made arrangements to take over some schools, asylums and voluntary hospitals but that only amounted to about 20,000 beds on mobilisation in August 1914. Fortunately, the public mood was generous and some 5,000 buildings were offered for use as hospitals, including Lambeth Palace, stately homes, schools and colleges.[2] Not all premises offered were suitable nor was their offer always in the best interests of the donor. Louisa Gurney was Lady District Superintendent of the Jesmond Nursing Division of the St John's Ambulance Brigade, as well as headmistress of the Newcastle Church High School for Girls, when she pressurised her governors into offering her school for use as a military hospital over which she could preside as matron. As this action would have meant the closure of the school, there was a sense of relief when the buildings were deemed unsuitable; the school governors were also able to curb Miss Gurney's excessive enthusiasm for war service by refusing her permission to be absent for half a term to nurse at the Front, though they did allow her pupils to join her nursing division and be active members of Princess Mary's Patriotic Union for Girls.[3] George V and Queen Mary, by contrast, were criticised for not giving up Buckingham Palace and Sandringham for the wounded despite the patriotism of their fellow European monarchs in converting some of their palaces into hospitals and the generosity of most of the British nobility in offering their country houses for that purpose; H.A.L. Fisher, the former First Sea Lord commented that this failure on the part of 'Futile and Fertile', as he dubbed the royal couple, suggested that 'Kings will be cheap soon'.[4]

The reliance on uncoordinated private generosity and voluntary effort was not without its drawbacks. At first the Red Cross, Order of St John and the Soldiers and Sailors Help Society each went their own way without reference to each other and even sent unauthorised medical teams to the Front where they were more of a nuisance than a help. One such team actually found itself left behind enemy lines during the retreat from Mons and its members were suspected by the German Army of being spies because they had no official accreditation as medical volunteers.[5] The growth in private hospitals without regard to military necessity meant that 'nurses are engaged who may never be required in the particular place allotted to them, while, worst of all, stores of surgical material are being hoarded up in scores of homes to such an extent that the market is being seriously depleted'.[6] The advantage of using voluntary organizations, apart from them being well placed to raise additional money, was that it was cheap, and these groups soon set aside their rivalries to cooperate on a more rational basis.Very soon the influx of casualties from Flanders revealed the inadequacies of relying on voluntary effort even if it was the cheapest option.

Poor law infirmaries were requisitioned for military use with scant regard for the needs of their usual patients.There had long been a stigma attached to such hospitals, which had been intended for the treatment of paupers as part of the workhouse. Rather than have a mixture of civilian and military wards in such institutions, as in the voluntary hospitals run as independent charities for the deserving poor, the War Office took over entire workhouse hospitals and systematically removed all traces of their former use so that treatment of war heroes would not be associated with the evils of the Poor Law system.The Brighton Board of Guardians was given no prior warning that its workhouse was required as a hospital for wounded Indian troops or much time to make alternative arrangements for its inmates in November 1914.[7] The Pavilion had already been requisitioned, its oriental architecture considered an appropriate environment for wounded Indians. It was not so easy to accommodate over 1,000 sick paupers dispossessed from the workhouse infirmary and there was an outcry from local residents 'at this profanation of their stately neighbourhood' when some of the former inmates were lodged in 'well appointed hotels'.[8] It was the local cottage hospital at Wimborne that was requisitioned with the result that respectable middle class patients were transferred to the local Poor Law infirmary and suffered the indignities of being classed with the destitute patients and denied access to their own private doctors.[9] The Metropolitan Asylums Board not only gave up four of its infirmaries for use as military hospitals but also had to accommodate Belgian refugees in some of its asylums as well as organising larger war refugee camps at Alexandra Palace and the Earls Court Exhibition Centre despite the call-up of most of its male staff.All was at the expense of the patients for whom their hospitals were originally intended.[10] It was little wonder that more thoughtful commentators thought that 'it is very bad Imperial strategy to neglect the health of the large majority of the nation in order to serve the relatively small Fighting Force'.[11]

Yet the number of available beds for the civilian sick continued to decline. The voluntary hospitals had patriotically offered beds for the treatment of wounded soldiers in special military wards alongside their usual patients, at first free of charge but after the first few months of the war in return for War Office grants which helped to keep many of these hospitals in operation at a time when their income from annual subscriptions was declining due to wartime pressures and prices were rising. However, the beds reserved in the voluntary hospitals for military casualties were often underused and kept vacant during lulls in the fighting. The Board of Management of St Mary's Hospital had placed 100 beds, a third of the total number in the hospital, at the disposal of the War Office on 10 September 1914 'in the event of accommodation in military hospitals proving inadequate' but it was not until 16 November that these beds were occupied when the casualties from the fighting at Ypres and Armentières overwhelmed the military hospitals. Most of these first military admissions were suffering from wounds and frostbite and 'the men as a whole looked rather worn by their hard experiences, but soon settled down.'[12] Smoking, forbidden in the civilian wards, was allowed three times a day and wealthy benefactors took the blue-coated wounded soldiers for drives around the capital, a new experience for many of the men who had never previously visited London. Only after the Somme were the military wards filled to capacity, but throughout 1917 and 1918 there were long periods when large numbers of beds were again left unoccupied until another offensive brought in more casualties. The result was that fewer civilians could be treated than in peacetime. Meanwhile, civilian beds were being closed at the same time that military beds were lying empty because of financial pressures.[13] The pattern was repeated throughout Britain and the other belligerent powers.

It was not only the number of hospital beds that was reduced as a result of the war. The initial rush to answer the call to arms denuded the civilian medical services of doctors and nurses they could ill-afford to lose and such shortages of trained staff became ever more acute as the war went on despite 'the special importance of maintaining the public health at the present time'.[14] By the end of the war over half of the general practitioners in Britain were serving in the armed forces and many trained nurses were tending wounded soldiers both at home and abroad. While doctors called up for military duties were afraid that they would lose their medical practices at home to their rival practitioners still at home, the doctors remaining in Britain complained of having 'had to work even longer hours, endeavouring to cope with the increase of work entailed by the loss of colleagues'.[15] Some patients were unable to find a doctor available to treat them at all.[16] The situation was worst in the industrial towns where most of the doctors before the war had been under forty-one and were liable to be called up, resulting in severer shortages of doctors in such areas than in the country as a whole.[17]

Future generations of doctors were being lost too by the eagerness of medical students to serve their country as ordinary soldiers rather than wait until they had qualified and could use their medical and surgical skills to good wartime use. In this they were following the example of students in other disciplines, whose university careers were massively disrupted by the war. The difference, though, from a classics, history or English student was that a medical qualification could be directly useful in wartime and many people considered that the medical student must put first the competing demands of his 'duty to himself, his family, his Hospital, his profession, his Empire and Humanity'.[18] It was at first left to the individual student to decide what his conscience permitted, although students were needed to fill the places occupied by qualified doctors in peacetime by acting as clinical dressers and even as unqualified house officers on the wards of their teaching hospitals. One compromise was for a medical student to enlist as a surgeon probationer in the Royal Navy, which gave him a period of practical experience aboard a ship or in a naval hospital, considered the equivalent of the clinical clerkships and dresserships of a normal medical school course, though the range of experience was more limited than they would have experienced at home. The problem was exacerbated by the introduction of male conscription in 1915; only medical students in their final years of study and thus close to qualification were exempt from being called up but even so were expected to enrol in an officer training corps as preparation for future military duties.[19]

However, amidst a growing concern about an imminent shortage of qualified doctors, the War Office began to release conscripted medical students to return to their studies.[20] The first to return to their medical schools were men invalided from the army, such as Thomas North who had entered the army as a private in November 1915 after only a month as a medical student, had been seriously wounded on the Somme in July 1916 and returned to his studies in May 1917 still only aged 20.[21] However, many of the returning medical students, now keen to qualify as quickly as possible, feared that they might be accused of shirking. Some students at Guy's Hospital were presented with white feathers after they had discarded their uniforms for civilian suits; in despair, they tried to re-enlist but were not permitted to do so.[22] Opportunities were offered for suitable refugees from Allied but occupied nations to train as doctors. Djurdge Dimitrijevitch was invalided out of the Serbian Army early in the war and, on reaching England as a refugee, was funded by the Serbian Relief Fund to study first English and then physiology at Magdalen College, Oxford before completing his medical studies at a London teaching hospital.[23] Similarly the German Army had released medical candidates to complete their studies, though some of them like Robert Otto Marcus who had studied medicine at Munich preferred to remain in the war because he 'couldn't stand the thought that other people were letting themselves be smashed up for my benefit, while I was enjoying myself going to afternoon concerts and promenading about'.[24] For many of these tough young men who had been seasoned in combat as ordinary soldiers, it was difficult to readjust to life as students on their demobilization to train as doctors in civilian garb. One frustrated, black-browed returning student exploded during a physiology class, 'Damn and blast you. Look, five days ago I was killing Germans. How the hell can you expect me to spend the afternoon tying little bits of cotton and wire to a dead frog?'.[25]

Until the return of the male students, the London medical schools in particular were coming under financial pressure from the loss of income from fees that went with the exodus of students. They needed to find a solution to these problems if they were to survive as medical schools and if enough new doctors were to qualify. In Germany, there was a wartime increase in the number of women studying medicine and Britain followed suit. Of the twelve medical schools of London, only the London School of Medicine for Women attached to the Royal Free Hospital admitted women medical students. Whereas by 1914, most other medical schools in the United Kingdom trained both sexes, the London schools remained resolutely single-sex and the male schools were bastions of a rough and ready masculine culture based on rugby, hard-drinking and hard-living. Now, many of the schools realized that they would have to admit women students if they were to survive.[26] St Mary's Hospital Medical School, Paddington, was one of the first to go down this route but not until other options had been exhausted. In 1915, its governing body preferred to admit an enemy alien, a non-naturalised, middle-aged German citizen, August Appelt, rather than sully its lecture theatres with a female student.[27] Not until a year later, by which time 'the raucous notes of the adolescent male are fast disappearing from within our walls',[28] did it embrace the inevitable and reach an agreement with the London School of Medicine for Women, which had been chafing under the limited clinical teaching capacity of its parent hospital for some time, to admit female students for the clinical part of the medical curriculum. As this was an experiment in co-education, the London School of Medicine for

Women sent many of its best women students to St Mary's in order to create a good impression, but, as 'all the keen young men had escaped to the War and only the lame ducks, the persistent failures at exams and elderly men students were left', the women 'rather showed up everyone's inefficiency'.[29] Certainly, the women outshone their male fellows in the examination hall.[30] Even though the women students were 'no good at rugger, didn't want to indulge in sport, even of the bedroom variety, and were a dead loss all round',[31] most of the other schools followed course and admitted women students but for the whole medical course and on the same terms as male students except for a hard core of medical schools which could afford to remain aloof as citadels of misogyny.[32]

Had it not been for women medical students and house officers, most of the London teaching hospitals would have found it difficult to survive their manpower crises of the war years. The University of London had a long tradition of granting degrees to women and wished to see the wartime expediency of co-education continued in its medical schools once the war was over.[33] The Dean of Charing Cross Medical School admitted that it would be very difficult for a school 'having once opened its doors to women to find any logical reason for closing them again'.[34] It seemed as if the war had widened opportunities for women to become doctors and that the London medical schools had accepted the principle of co-education. It was merely a temporary advance. With the return of male medical students, the backlash began. Ex-servicemen were especially hostile towards women whom they saw as an emasculating force, undercutting them and usurping the career opportunities to which their sacrifice of their careers for the duration of the war had entitled them. At St Mary's, a group of male students got up a petition against women students on the grounds that feminine influence was draining away the athletic virility of the medical school and that 'the recent but, apparently habitual defeat of St Mary's in the Rugger cup-tie, calls for serious consideration', concluding with the strong stance that 'the men do not want the women, they have no wish to be friends, or to co-operate with them in any way'.[35] Within ten years of the end of the war, the position of women medical students in London was back to its state in 1914 with only the London School of Medicine for Women open to them. Only after the Second World War did the London schools again become co-educational.

Yet, women doctors had definitely proved themselves as the equal of their male counterparts in filling the vacancies caused by the war at home and in overseas service, despite entrenched misogynist opposition to them having

any role at all. When Dr Elsie Inglis volunteered her services at the outbreak
of hostilities, she was told to 'go and sit quietly at home, dear lady'.[36] Inglis
was made of sterner metal and instead offered the services of the Scottish
Women's Hospitals, established by the Scottish Federation of the National
Union of Women's Suffrage Societies at her instigation, to her country's
allies. Units fully staffed by women doctors were sent to France, Serbia,
Salonika, Corsica and Russia, but it was at the Abbaye de Royaumont that
the Scottish Women's Hospitals had the greatest success. This hospital, with
its emphasis on scrupulous standards of hygiene, had lower amputation rates
and the lowest mortality rate on the Western Front, in recognition of which
the military authorities began to send the most severe cases there and the
Pasteur Institute in Paris chose it as an experimental unit for an anti-gas
gangrene serum.[37] During the German advance on Aisne in the summer
of 1918 it was the only hospital to remain in full working order with its
operating theatres functioning round the clock to deal with the casualties
flooding in. As the reputation of Royaumont spread among the men in the
trenches, wounded men asked to be sent there and one patient on being
discharged asked if he could be evacuated to 'another Royaumont'.[38] The
Women's Hospital Corps, backed by the Women's Social and Political
Union, organised a hospital at the Hotel Claridge in Paris, which had
an equally impressive reputation and was invited by the War Office to
establish a hospital staffed by women at Wimereux.[39] Marie Curie, the
discoverer of radium, toured the battlefields of France with a mobile
X-ray unit in a converted ambulance, as well as organising 200 fixed
radiological units in military hospitals and twenty mobile cars known as
'les petites Curies'.[40] In Russia women doctors were liable for front line
service from the start of the war. In their service in the war zones, women
doctors proved themselves the equal of men as indeed many of them,
with a background in the suffrage movement, had set out to do.[41] The
Daily Telegraph admitted that 'to the women doctors the war has brought
triumph'.[42] Perhaps even more important than their contribution to
treating the wounded at the Front was the less dramatic but even more vital
role played by women doctors in keeping medical services in existence
on the Home Front, often to the surprise of male observers. When the
jingoist journalists J.L. Garvin and John Bull visited Endell Street Military
Hospital in London, which was staffed entirely by women, they asked 'But
who operates when seriously wounded casualties are brought in?' only to
be told 'the women surgeons, naturally'.[43]

A more traditional role in healthcare for women was as nurses. The sentimentalised image of the nurse treating the wounded soldier became ubiquitous in all countries at war. She was depicted on the battlefield tending the wounded or looking pensive set against a background of war, with wounded soldiers in wheelchairs and as 'the real angel of Mons' and 'L' ange de nos blessés' in the iconography of the war.[44] Queen Elisabeth of the Belgians became known as 'la reine-infirmiére' for her devotion to the care of the wounded during her wartime exile from Belgium and was adopted in this role as a saintly national symbol, the image of the 'Nurse Queen' complementing that of her husband Albert I dubbed the 'Soldier King'.[45] The reality was much less glamorous. Even a seasoned sister in Queen Alexandra's Imperial Military Nursing Service was shocked by the casualties she was faced with at Number 13 Stationary Hospital set up in converted sugar-sheds on the quay at Boulogne, where a soldier 'caked with mud, in torn clothes … and blood stained bandages' was classed as walking wounded 'as long as he could crawl'.[46] As a French military doctor, the writer Georges Duhamel was conscious of the contrast between the peacetime lives of many of these women and their wartime duties: 'beautiful eyes, made for looking out for tennis balls or the nuance of a ribbon, now reflected, with a determined seriousness, the hideousness of the dressing room, of amputated limbs, of wounded heads', yet these nurses offered a reminder of a better world to the men in the wards where 'a scent of woman wafted that had not changed, which was always precious, childlike and heady'.[47]

There was a significant increase in the number of young women taking full nurse training during the war since nursing was seen as vital to the war effort: 'at a time when women are being recruited for munitions, for agriculture, and for many other branches of national work, it is of the highest importance that no time should be wasted in securing those who will be needed for nursing work'.[48] Hospitals were a popular option for those who wished to play their part in winning the war and women now occupied more roles than the traditional womanly role in nursing. The future thriller writer Agatha Christie worked in a wartime hospital pharmacy, which gave her a knowledge of poisons that was to prove invaluable for her successful writing career. In her first best-selling thriller, *The Mysterious Affair at Styles*, in which poisons play a major role, she allows her detective Hercule Poirot to comment on a wartime female pharmaceutical dispenser that 'women are doing great work nowadays'.[49] One woman who actually seized the opportunity offered by the war to realise her ambitions to become a nurse was the King's niece Princess Arthur of Connaught, who willingly submitted to such indignities as being addressed as 'nurse' rather than by her royal title, being chased around the casualty department by drunks, being reprimanded by the matron for revealing too much when she bent over in the ward and catching fleas from her impoverished patients who also tried to offer a tip to a poor, overworked nurse. Despite her insistence on preparing her own trolleys and going about her work incognito in a probationer's uniform, she was conspicuous at her nursing training school, St Mary's Hospital, of which her husband and second cousin Prince Arthur was president, by wearing a military nursing headdress rather than the cap of the other nurses.[50] However, she did qualify as a nurse, becoming the first member of the royal family to qualify as a state registered nurse when state registration was introduced after the war, and took on a more arduous role than the incessant hospital visiting and knitting for wounded soldiers of many other royal ladies from Queen Mary and Queen Alexandra downwards.[51]

Nevertheless, the greatest contribution came not from trained nurses but from the Voluntary Aid Detachments, the VADs, which had been established by the British Red Cross and St John's Ambulance Association in 1910 to assist the professional military nursing service in the event of an emergency. Their employment was not at all greeted with joy by the nursing profession who complained throughout the war about the number of untrained nurses doing the work of trained nurses. As with the employment of unqualified men as housemen in hospitals, the use of untrained nurses was another example of the dilution of labour that was to arouse contemporary controversy among craftsmen in the trades union world.[52] Vera Brittain, working as a volunteer nurse at the First London General Hospital in Camberwell, was well aware that the professional nursing staff were 'still suspicious of the young semi-trained amateurs upon whose assistance they were beginning to realise with dismay they would be obliged to depend for the duration of the war'.[53] She and other VADs worked from 7.30 a.m. to 8 p.m. with a weekly half day off, 'which we gave up willingly whenever a convoy came in or the ward was filled with bad cases'.[54] This they did throughout the sultry summer of 1916 when throughout 'those busy and strenuous days' the wards 'sweltered beneath their roofs of corrugated iron; the prevailing odour of wounds and stinking streets lingered perpetually'.[55] For women from genteel and sheltered backgrounds such experiences were eye opening and shocking.

Many VAD nurses had volunteered their services to serve their country, but if sent overseas might find themselves tending the enemy. For some nurses, especially in the early days of the war, this was difficult since they looked on the enemy soldiers as being 'of the roughest and most objectionable type'; Hilda Speake, a nurse who had fallen into enemy hands when Brussels fell in 1914, was surprised, when called upon to nurse German wounded, that 'the nurses were amply repaid by the smiles on the men's faces when they saw the English nurses'.[56] Vera Brittain's family were more horrified than she was when she found herself nursing in a ward full of German prisoners at Étaples in the summer of 1917.[57] Her attitude was professional and humanitarian in that 'it is hardly possible to feel any antipathy to one's patients in practice however much one may in theory; they are far too ill and utterly dependent on one for that'. Her attitude was shared by the British wounded in other wards that came to visit these severely wounded young men with gifts of cigarettes and fetched them drinks.[58] Edith Cavell recognised that the duty of the nurse overrode nationalistic considerations too with her statement before her execution in 1915 that 'I realise that patriotism is not enough. I must have no hatred or bitterness towards anyone'. Nurse Cavell's execution by the Germans for helping Allied soldiers escape from German occupied territory was greeted with universal outrage simply because she was a nurse, though she had gone well beyond her nursing role in doing so and had used the cover of her school of nursing in Brussels to take on a less than neutral role in helping to return soldiers to combat.[59] Nevertheless she died as a nurse and martyr to German brutality in the popular mind, rather than as simply the patriotic and brave heroine of the resistance that she undoubtedly was.

The men that Nurse Cavell had helped on their way back to fight were the lucky ones. For many wounded soldiers, there was little hope of return to action. Rehabilitation was their only hope if they were to lead productive lives once the war had ended. The novelist John Galsworthy waxed lyrical on the role that a proper rehabilitation scheme could play to 'recreate and fortify' the disabled serviceman 'so that he fits again into the national life, becomes once more a workman with pride in his work, a stake in the country and the consciousness that, handicapped though he be, he runs the race level with his fellows, and is by that so much the better man than they'.[60] The Joint War Committee of the Red Cross and Order of St John had been charged with this duty in 1914. One of its members, the exiled twenty-five-year-old King Manoel II of Portugal, was to make it a personal crusade to alleviate the plight of the disabled after he had first become involved with them when setting up a private officers' hospital in Brighton at the beginning of the war. Not only was he the leading fundraiser for rehabilitation services but he was the motive spirit behind the creation of the Shepherd's Bush Military Hospital in 1916 in premises requisitioned from the Hammersmith Workhouse Infirmary. Manoel had been impressed by the 'curative workshops' set up for the war disabled at the Anglo-Belgian Hospital in Rouen and the Canadian Hospital in Ramsgate and now tried to reproduce them in London. In the occupational therapy workshops at Shepherd's Bush, the patients manufactured all the splints, surgical boots and other appliances used in the hospital and supplied the Ministry of Pensions with orthopaedic appliances.[61] This self-sufficient and economical hospital was staffed by orthopaedic and physiotherapeutic specialists who were able to draw on their pre-war experience of dealing with crippled children when developing forms of physiotherapy for their military patients.

Elsewhere at Chailey Heritage Hospital in Sussex, disabled soldiers were matched with crippled boys to remind them of the value and hope of youth and their own promise as productive members of society.[62] Robert Jones, Military Director of Orthopaedics, set up a further sixteen regional specialist orthopaedic centres and argued that disabled soldiers were 'an essential part of the economic manpower of the nation, independent producers and wage-earners, not helpless dependents'.[63] The aim was to restore the men's self-respect as well as to fit them with new trades, such as tailoring, carpentry, engineering, cigarette-making, French polishing and sign writing, for a role in civilian life, but in the harsh post-war world disabled ex-servicemen found it much harder to make a living at a time of economic hardship.[64]

The plight of the wounded ex-serviceman was not one that would end with the war as many people realised very soon in the conflict, and charity, rather than the state, would bear the brunt of providing aid to them. The return home of blinded soldiers and sailors inspired the newspaper magnate Arthur Pearson, proprietor of the *Daily Express* and *Evening Standard*, to open a hostel where these men could be given the training that would enable them to lead productive, independent lives. Pearson, who had lost his own sight due to glaucoma, was President of the National Institute for the Blind. In 1915, St Dunstan's was opened in Regent's Park, London, as a training centre and workshops for Pearson's 'blind army', many of whom had also lost limbs as well as their sight. By the end of the war over 1,500 men had been trained in the skills necessary for them to work as cobblers, joiners, poultry farmers, telephone switchboard operators and masseurs. This work was to be continued throughout the inter war years and in subsequent conflicts with new generations of ex-servicemen blinded in battle.[65]

Long-term care was also the idea behind the establishment of the Star and Garter Home at Richmond, Surrey, after Queen Mary suggested that the British Red Cross do something to provide a 'permanent haven' for the severely disabled young men returning from the Battle of the Somme in 1916. The Auctioneers and Estate Agents Institute purchased the Star and Garter Hotel on Richmond Hill and presented the deeds to the Queen as a home for ex-serviceman. The average age of the first sixty-five residents admitted in 1916 was twenty-two; some were able to return to their own families, for others the Star and Garter was to be their home for the rest of the lives. After 1924 they enjoyed an impressive new purpose-built home, erected with funding from the British Women's Hospital Committee, which included workshops where residents could make and repair clocks and watches, toys rugs and even socks. Residents were taken on excursions by volunteers from the Lest We Forget and Not Forgotten associations, which also provided entertainments. With continuing royal patronage and a high public profile, the Star and Garter was never short of supporters.[66]

By contrast with the British emphasis on voluntary and charitable provision for the disabled ex-serviceman, Weimar Germany took the attitude that it was the responsibility of the state to provide not only pensions but also occupational therapy, retraining and free medical care for service-related medical problems. There were also quotas for the employment of disabled ex-servicemen in larger businesses and in state employment, which cushioned disabled veterans during the Great Depression. Yet, because the generosity of the public was not engaged as it was by charity in Britain, the disabled ex-servicemen of Germany felt more estranged from the state and society than their British counterparts.[67]

With all this emphasis on the medical needs of the armed forces, the health of the civilian population on the Home Front was neglected but could not be wholly ignored. There were fewer doctors and even fewer hospital beds available for the treatment of such weak and vulnerable social groups as the elderly poor and the mentally and physically handicapped, many of whom had been evicted from the institutions which had sheltered them in order that they could be used as military hospitals or convalescent facilities. Their well-being was not essential to the war effort and little attention was given to their problems. Charities for wounded soldiers, war widows, orphans and refugees caught the popular imagination with the result that less money was given for the aid of other needy social groups.[68] The Royal Edinburgh Infirmary even appealed to the Mid and East Lothian Miners' Association in 1916 to increase its subscription to the charity to mitigate the difficulties arising from the war, an appeal met with sympathy and money since the miners depended on the availability of hospital care if they were injured underground. At the same time the miners of Britain were subscribing towards a Red Cross ambulance convoy for France.[69]

Tuberculosis rates rose during the war, especially among young women. In Germany, 280,000 people died of consumption during the four years of conflict, representing one for every ten military casualties. In Britain mortality rates among young women from tuberculosis reverted to its 1890 rate.[70] The Brompton Hospital for Consumption and Diseases of the Chest, where 700 consumptive servicemen were treated in 1917 alone, saw such a rise in the number of civilian outpatients with tuberculosis that each physician was limited to seeing no more than twelve new outpatients.[71] The reasons for this rise were complex and reflected a number of factors coming together in wartime. Soldiers were crowded together in barracks and army camps, munitions workers lived in cramped, damp hostels and worked in poorly ventilated factories, and refugees spread diseases. A fourteen per cent increase in tuberculosis during the war in Paris was explained by the 'considerable growth in the female workforce, the increased population in Parisian industrial centres and suburbs, from overcrowding', with the munitions workers liable to develop the disease 'through contagion or the reawakening of a youthful bacillus attack'.[72] At the same time that wartime mobility and overcrowding had made the spread of tuberculosis more widespread, there were fewer facilities for its treatment. In France a national committee for the aid of tubercular soldiers was set up to deal with the problem of soldiers discharged with consumption and to prevent its spread among the civil population, but only a quarter of soldiers so discharged ever received treatment. Albert Calmette, with the support of the Rockefeller Foundation, pioneered a scheme in Lille for each soldier to be visited at home for treatment by a specialised health visitor but very few received this service.[73] In Britain priority was given to soldiers in allocating the reduced number of beds available in sanatoria, rather than to industrial workers even though the treatment of the workers would have returned them to work of national importance quicker; one docker in the Port of London complained that he too had risked his health in serving the nation but had to wait for treatment while soldiers took priority.[74]

Food shortages and nutritional deficiencies also affected the health of the people at home, though the health of the people remained remarkably resilient and life expectancy may actually have increased during the war years. Full employment and higher real wages for many sections of the working classes meant that, despite wartime shortages, they were able to enjoy a better diet. Indeed shortages of meat and butter, coupled with a greater consumption of bread and potatoes, mean that the wealthy too were eating a more balanced diet. The reduction in the consumption of sugar meant improved dental hygiene for children. Medical officers of the Local Education Authorities reported that fewer schoolchildren were malnourished in 1918 than in 1913 and that there were fewer 'necessitous children' in receipt of free school meals.[75] Yet the effect of more restricted wartime diets on the health of individuals was mixed rather than universally beneficial. In Germany, gout, that disease of good living, was said to have disappeared among the wealthy middle aged but there was an eightfold increase in rickets and hunger oedema among the poor. More cases of eclampsia were seen among pregnant women in Germany as a result of the starvation diet they faced as a consequence of the Allied blockade.[76] In Russia, obesity, alcoholism, gout, gastritis, appendicitis and constipation were regarded as diseases of the past but there was an increase in enteritis, peptic ulcers and arteriosclerosis.[77]

Paradoxically, despite the reduction in the quantity and quality of medical services available on the Home Front, there is some evidence that average life expectancy rose during the war from forty-six to forty-nine for men and from fifty-three to sixty for women. The poor had had patchy access to medical services before the war so the absence of doctors had little real impact on them. There was a drop in the death rate for women in childbirth in Britain from 181 per million in 1914 to 125 in 1918, but this decline was probably a result of a fall in the birth rate caused mainly by the temporary break-up of families with husbands away at the war. Pregnant women may also have benefited from having their babies delivered by midwives who, unlike doctors, did not use forceps during labour and took fewer risks. At the same time, mortality among girls and young women rose during the war and the care of the elderly was neglected.[78]

Controls on alcohol consumption were seen as essential for the war effort to curb the absenteeism that was imperilling munitions production. David Lloyd George thundered that 'drink is doing more damage in the war than all the German submarines put together'[79] and declared that 'We are fighting

Germany, Austria and drink, and as far as I can see, the greatest of these deadly foes is drink'.[80] Under the provisions of the Defence of the Realm Act, the Central Liquor Control Board took action to deal with the perceived problem. Opening hours of public houses were reduced in industrial areas, sales of alcohol were forbidden to anyone under 18, treating and credit in pubs were banned, and public houses near crucial munitions plants at Enfield Lock, Carlisle and Gretna Green and the naval bases at Inverness and Cromarty were nationalized.[81] In an attempt to give an example to his country, George V took a pledge of abstinence from alcohol for the duration of the war in March 1915 until his medical advisers recommended that he take a 'daily stimulant' for the sake of his health after he was badly injured when falling from his horse during a visit to the Front in October 1915. It was a gesture that was widely ridiculed and rarely emulated.[82]

Alcohol continued to fuel courage at the Front, though as the war had gone on many men had had enough of soldiering. One ditty popular in the trenches expressed the determination not to have 'a bayonet up my arse-hole, I don't want my ballocks shot away' coupled with the desire to remain in England 'and fuck my bloody life away'.[83] Yet had the soldier of the song had his wish, he might have exposed himself to the likelihood of being 'rendered not only ineffective but in some cases killed' through catching syphilis or gonorrhoea.[84] Whereas the French and Germans, with a long tradition of the regulation of prostitution, set up *maisons de tolerances* where their men could have sex with prostitutes who were inspected periodically for disease, albeit with the same unsterilized speculum, the initial British approach was to print in the soldiers' paybooks an exhortation from Lord Kitchener urging his men to stay chaste and shun wine.[85] The American forces too warned their men that 'a man who is thinking below the belt is not efficient'[86] and that 'they had to be 100% efficient to win the war',[87] but also took practical steps to ensure that if their doughboys should be seduced from the path of virtue by 'booze, a pretty face, a shapely ankle' they would 'not take the European disease to America' but would 'go home clean'.[88] Temperance campaigners ensured that the sale of alcohol in, or close to, the military training camps was forbidden, a move that contributed to the climate of opinion that would very soon endorse the Eighteenth Amendment to the United States Constitution enforcing prohibition, though only with the effect of driving minor vice underground where it could become a focus of still greater crime. The Commission on Training Camp Activities headed by the Princeton-educated lawyer Raymond B. Fosdick, bombarded the troops with vivid warnings about the dangers of venereal disease from women less clean than a German bullet.[89] When the French prime minister Georges Clemenceau offered to help establish licensed brothels for his new American allies, Fosdick was warned by the Secretary of War, Newton D. Baker, 'for God's sake, Raymond, don't show this to the President or he'll stop the war'.[90] Despite Woodrow Wilson's high moral tone, American soldiers going on leave were issued, just like the German troops, with prophylactic kits, containing calomel ointment for syphilis, potassium permanganate solution or tablets for gonorrhoea and cotton wool for applying these to the penis as soon after sexual intercourse as possible. The British Army lagged behind in issuing what were known as 'dreadnought packets' for fear that by doing so they might be condoning vice. Soon, like other armies, they had set up ablution chambers, known as 'Blue Lamp Depots' on account of the blue lights they used to advertise their location at night, where a man who had had sex could have his penis irrigated with the chemical protargol and calomel ointment rubbed on his genitals in a procedure that was unpleasant, painful, undignified and not particularly effective. The issue of condoms would have done far more good.[91]

It was not only prostitutes who posed a threat, since any 'bad and diseased woman can do more harm than any German fleet of aircraft that has yet passed over London'.[92] The war had given greater freedom to young women and many of them wanted to enjoy themselves after a hard day's work, mainly as munitions workers though even schoolteachers and flower girls were also out to have a good time with any available man.[93] Such women were considered safer than prostitutes by men on leave – and cheaper since the costs of taking them on a date and buying them a present were much less than those of paying a professional for sex. Dominion troops were especially vulnerable to casual sex with such girls as they were too far from home to have any opportunity to relieve their sexual urges with their wives when on leave. Under pressure from the governments of Canada, Australia and New Zealand, Regulation 40D under the Defence of the Realm Act was introduced and laid down that 'no woman who is suffering from venereal disease in a communicable form shall have sexual intercourse with any member of His Majesty's forces, or solicit or invite any member of His Majesty's forces to have sexual intercourse with her' or would be liable to a fine of £100 or six months' imprisonment.[94] There was an immediate outcry against a measure that was specifically aimed at women, and women's organisations pointed out that 'men expect a certain standard of morality in their wives, and as wives we are entitled to expect the same from men'.[95]

The War Office and Home Office were defensive against such charges and pointed out that catching a venereal disease was considered to be a self-inflicted disease by the armed forces and that soldiers would be punished for contracting diseases under military law. What mattered was the necessity of protecting against something that caused as great 'a wastage of manpower as German poison gas'; rather than making 'vice safe for men', the regulation was intended 'to keep the realm safe by stamping out centres of infection which injure the fighting capacity of the nation'.[96]

Venereal disease had already been a major problem before the war and in 1916 a Royal Commission on Venereal Diseases had recommended a national scheme of free, confidential treatment in a series of local authority provided clinics and diagnostic laboratories.[97] Venereal disease was declared a national emergency, which allowed the Local Government Board to compel the county and borough councils to implement the scheme and by the beginning of 1917 the first treatment centres were opened in London. At first there was a shortage of suitably skilled doctors but the Army Council agreed to release army medical officers to set up the new treatment centres where possible.[98] This indicated the importance of the treatment of sexually transmissible infections in the thinking of the armed forces, but the setting up of this national treatment scheme had been conceived and realized as a civilian scheme and was not specifically a response to the pressures of wartime though the war had raised the stakes considerably and made firm action even more important.

It was not so much venereal disease as the lack of sex that caused problems in prisoner of war camps and in internment camps for male civilians of military age caught behind enemy lines on the outbreak of war. Soldiers in the trenches and the wounded in hospital often had little choice but to satisfy their need for women by playing with their 'wanking warriors' until they could go on leave and enjoy the real thing, but prisoners had no hope of sexual intercourse with a woman until the end of the war whenever that might be. Eric Higgins, incarcerated at Ruhleben Camp set up on a racecourse near Berlin where six men occupied the horsebox space formerly reserved for two horses, was obsessed with the effects of sexual deprivation on the young men with whom he was interned which led to what he called the 'barbed wire disease' or homosexuality. Young men itching to take part in the war and deprived of their usual activities were especially prone to depression and sought any available outlet to raise their spirits and compensate for their night starvation. He despaired that 'against the consequences of unnatural sexual conditions there can, of course, be no ultimate remedy but the restoration of normal conditions' but believed that the 'establishment of such handicrafts as we were able to get into operation was the means of saving many young men from mental and moral destruction'. In fact, Ruhleben contained such a variety of internees that it was able to offer a variety of educational opportunities for its inmates such as lectures on the classics, Renaissance art and science as well as sports and music. Nevertheless, a German sexual specialist, Dr Magnus Hirschfeldt, was brought into Ruhleben to differentiate between the 'cases of inborn psychopathy' and men who were simply seeking any outlet for their frustrations and 'thus prevent particularly among the young men yet imperfectly differentiated, an occasional and circumstantial vice becoming converted into a permanent inversion'.[99] A similar pattern of homosexual relationships serving as a substitute for heterosexual intercourse was later observed in the male-only prisoner of war camps and in the sexually segregated civilian internment camps of the Far East during the Second World War, though in Hong Kong where men and women were interned in the same camp their captors had to insist that 'sexual intercourse is prohibited except between husband and wife or close friends' with the result that lovers found the cemeteries the most congenial place for close relationships to be consummated.[100] Essentially what was needed back in First World War Ruhleben was an antidote to boredom rather than medical intervention, which was for truly medical needs supplied by interned doctors and German hospitals.

There were no such fears of idleness in the munitions factories at home where a greater danger to health came from poor, unsanitary working conditions. One of the most dangerous jobs in the munitions industry was the filling of shells with TNT[101] powder, which could cause toxic jaundice; such workers were nicknamed 'canaries' on account of their faces going bright yellow as a result of the jaundice. At the Ministry of Munitions National Filling Factory at Chittening near Bristol, 1213 women munitions workers filling shells with mustard gas contracted a variety of illnesses including conjunctivitis, inflammation, congestion, nausea and vomiting, a reddening of the skin, blisters and persistent coughs as a result of contact with the toxic substances with which they were working. The Medical Research Committee recommended better ventilation and the wearing of facemasks and protective clothing by the women handling such chemicals but there was little more that could be done to safeguard the health of the workers. At Chittening a small surgery and hospital were opened at the plant for the treatment of the workers.[102] Elsewhere, attempts were made to improve the conditions of the workers by the opening of washing facilities and works canteens offering such basic fare as sausages or mince and mashed potatoes, stewed fruit and milk puddings similar to the food offered by the National Kitchens set up to offer cheap, basic meals for the needy.[103]

The health of the next generation was of greater concern than that of the current generation of soldiers and war workers for the future of Britain. The Bishop of London drew attention to the fact that 'while nine soldiers died every hour in 1915, twelve babies died every hour, so it was more dangerous to be a baby than a soldier'. A tenth of children died before their first birthday and a quarter of those who survived infancy died before they were five. Whooping cough, diphtheria and scarlet fever were childhood killers. Now, according to the Bishop, 'the loss of life in this war has made every baby's life doubly precious'.[104] Great Ormond Street Children's Hospital reminded the public that 'at this critical time with ever lengthening casualty lists and a falling birth-rate, the lives and health of the next generation become of paramount importance as a national asset'[105] although the needs of sick children were often overlooked however essential they may have been for 'the future welfare of the British Empire'.[106] Paddington Green Children's Hospital emphasised that it was treating the children of serving troops and stressed that 'medical and surgical care in infancy and during the early years should be, and must be, efficiently and liberally provided if the coming generation is to replace the terrible losses now being suffered on far-reaching battlefields, both on land and sea'.[107]

Such concerns were addressed with a national 'Baby Week' in July 1917 that aimed 'to save every savable child'.[108] There were calls for more health visitors and infant welfare centres.[109] Comparisons were made with the situation in Germany where the prevention of infant mortality was 'one of the greatest works standing to the credit of a scientific people'[101] though this was disputed by some doctors.[111] Indeed one German doctor, Stephen Westman, declared that the deplorable state of babies and small children, suffering from starvation in the Charité Hospital in Berlin, with 'their big heads and sunken eyes, their faces like those of old people, their chests on which one could count every rib, their protruding bellies and rickety legs', was 'poor testimony to the humanity and culture of which the nations of Europe boasted so much'.[112] Local authorities in Britain were encouraged to provide milk for expectant and nursing mothers and babies and the 1915

Care of Mothers and Young Children Act gave local authorities the power to set up further maternity and infant welfare facilities. The number of health visitors rose from 600 in 1914 to 1355 in 1918. Much of this wartime action, building on pre-war ideas and developments, was consolidated by the Maternity and Child Welfare Act in August 1918. This extension of state welfare provision in the field of child welfare was cemented by the establishment of a Ministry of Health in 1918 to take over some of the powers of the Local Government Board in this field, but the new ministry was of more symbolic than practical purpose since it possessed few new or real powers and was regarded with suspicion by general practitioners fearing it might be the first step to a salaried medical service. A report by Lord Dawson in 1921 anticipated the development of a rationalized, state system of health care under the aegis of the new Ministry of Health, based on district hospitals and primary health centres staffed by general practitioners, but the post-war economic slump ensured that no further action was taken.[113] Nevertheless, the health of children had benefited from a war-inspired confluence of national interest and altruistic concern for the young.

Children's Hospitals were not immune from the fall in charitable income suffered by most hospitals during the war though they fared better in terms of public support due to the public emphasis on child welfare, but shared the same problems of the shortage and escalating price of drugs. The growing internationalism of the pharmaceutical industry in the years leading up to the war had been disrupted by the outbreak of hostilities and had resulted in a shortage of some drugs produced by companies in enemy countries. This led to a search for substitutes for the medicines that could now no longer be imported. With the suspension of German patents and trademarks and the closure of British subsidiaries of German companies, companies such as Boots the Chemist and Howard's of Ilford began to manufacture for themselves aspirin and other synthetic drugs formerly imported.[114] Through its connection with the French company Poulenc Frères, which had been experimenting with arsenical compounds, May and Baker developed an alternative for salvarsan developed by Paul Ehrlich in 1909 for the treatment of syphilis.[115] Meanwhile, with official government support, Burroughs Wellcome developed a generic substitute for the same drug under the brand name Kharsivan.[116] Ehrlich was concerned not at the loss of patent income but by his fears that if other firms were producing the drug under less stringent conditions than he had stipulated for its German manufacture,[117] any substandard batches being distributed might discredit his drug.[118]

The available medicines were of little use towards the end of the war when influenza 'came like a thief in the night', as Sir George Newman, chief medical officer to the Board of Education, described it, and swept through the world, hitting the young and robust the hardest, overshadowing the Armistice to some extent. In San Francisco the end of the war was surreally celebrated by crowds in facemasks. The pandemic struck in three waves, first appearing in March 1918 in the American Expeditionary Force camps in the United States before spreading to Africa and Asia. The second wave swept Africa, North America and Europe, starting off at Brest where the American troops disembarked, in the summer and had become a worldwide pandemic by November. Its third and final wave peaked from February to April 1919. Known as the 'Spanish flu', the disease struck rich and poor equally though young adults were most at risk. It was as lethal at home as at the Front. There was little that the medical authorities could do to prevent the spread of the disease, and the gargles, disinfectants and potions bought by the public had little effect. Timothy Leary of Tufts Medical College near Boston developed a vaccine that was distributed free to physicians in badly affected areas such as San Francisco, but to little practical effect. Schools closed, church congregations dwindled from fear of catching the disease and undertakers did not have enough coffins to bury the victims. A population weakened by four years of war was especially susceptible to the disease but it also affected neutral nations unaffected by the war just as severely.[119] Perhaps the supreme irony was that men who had survived the rigour of combat and overcome severe wounds finally met their doom from influenza. One out of every sixty-seven American soldiers died of influenza or pneumonia in 1918.[120] The surrealist poet Guillaume Apollinaire survived a head wound from a shell-burst and the ruination of his lungs by gas only to die of influenza on 9 November 1918, two days before the Armistice, crying out 'Save me doctor! I want to live! I still have so much to say!'[121] His words may speak for a generation for whom there was to be no business as usual after all they had endured and for whom their promise was to be cut short when medicine failed to save their lives.

4

Spanish Rehearsal

Fascism was hailed as Spain's 'health-giver' at a ceremony to celebrate the 'Day of the Race', the anniversary of Columbus's discovery of America, held on 12 October 1936 in the great hall of the University of Salamanca. Professor Francisco Maldonado likened the role of the Nationalist rebels against the Spanish Republic in 1936 to that of 'cutting into the live healthy flesh like a resolute surgeon free from false sentimentality' in order to eliminate not only left-wing politics but also Catalan and Basque calls for independence which he castigated as 'cancers in the body of the nation'. His remarks were greeted with enthusiasm by his audience, which included General José Millán Astray, the one-armed, one-eyed founder of the Spanish Foreign Legion whose battle cry of '¡Viva la Muerte!' ('Long Live Death!') resounded through the hall. Such sentiments were repellent to the venerable Basque philosopher Miguel de Unamuno, rector of the University of Salamanca, who protested that Millán Astray should not be allowed to dictate 'the pattern of mass psychology' and that 'a cripple who lacks the spiritual greatness of a Cervantes is wont to seek ominous relief in causing mutilation around him'. It was bad enough that 'there are all too many cripples in Spain just now. And soon there will be more of them if God does not come to our aid'.[1] In comparing the disfigured Nationalist hero Millán Astray to his detriment with the great Spanish creator of *Don Quixote*, also a war invalid,[2] Unamuno only narrowly avoided becoming a casualty of the outraged crowds himself through the intervention of Doña Carmen, wife of General Franco, as Millán Astray and his supporters cried '¡Mueran los intelectuales!' ('Death to Intellectuals!'). In Unamuno's more considered view the civil war was 'due to a collective mental illness, an epidemic of madness, with a pathological substratum'.[3] Medicine, used as a metaphor for Civil War Spain, was to be important in the struggle between the opposing Republican and Nationalist forces and to reflect the different nature of the two regimes. Its actual practice in wartime was also to offer many lessons to the participants in the coming Second World War, for whom it was something of a dry run.

At first, though, the calls for radical surgery on the body politic overrode any hopes of healing the nation's divisions as Spain catapulted into civil war. The quality of medical services available to combatants and civilians at the outbreak of the war very much depended upon where they found themselves geographically when the Nationalist military coup was launched in July 1936. Although, not surprisingly, the Spanish Army medical services had declared support for the rising against the Republican government from the beginning, most civilian doctors and nurses continued to practise medicine where ever they found themselves at the outbreak of the civil war and treated their patients impartially whatever political loyalties they may have had.[4] Such professional neutrality was to have its advantages in protecting clinical staff against reprisals when towns fell to the opposing side in the war, though just as significant was the urgent need on all sides for medical expertise which made health personnel too valuable to be squandered for petty political satisfaction. However, Spanish medicine was not immune from politics and many of its practitioners had as passionate partisan sympathies as their neighbours who were fighting either to defend the Republic or against it. The nursing in many hospitals was carried out by Roman Catholic nuns, who now were vulnerable to anti-clerical attacks as a spate of church burnings swept through Republican strongholds. The nuns who worked at the Hospital Marítim d'Infecciosos in Anarchist-dominated Barcelona escaped in the dead of night dressed as secular nurses and accompanied by a doctor who sympathized with the Nationalist cause.[5] Prominent Catholic doctors had their surgeries and homes ransacked and faced lynching or execution at a time when previously dapper men went hatless and tie-less, and once-chic women tried to look shabby in Republican Madrid and Barcelona because to be too well dressed was considered the mark of a bourgeois reactionary.

Survival often depended on arbitrary factors. At the Hospital Marítim d'Infecciosos, the insistence of the medical staff that weapons be left at the hospital door did not prevent one anxious father, the head of a Confederación Nacional del Trabajo committee, and his five henchmen from brandishing pistols at the head of a young doctor and threatening to kill him if he could not cure the man's ten-year-old son of tetanus. The boy was choking on his tongue and his jaw was stiff with the tetanus. The only way that the doctor could stop him choking was to force his way into the boy's mouth, break his teeth and pull out his tongue with a forceps. Had the child died after such radical treatment, the doctor would have been shot; because he lived, the doctor could have enjoyed the power of life or death over any of his personal enemies as his reward had he been so inclined.[6] The story of Dr Udaeta who was killed, together with his twenty-four-year-old physician son, by a militiaman whose wife had died in childbirth while her baby was being delivered by the doctor was widely reported in Nationalist circles as an example of Republican atrocities towards the bourgeois medical profession.[7]

Meanwhile, doctors accused of holding politically liberal views or of being Freemasons were arrested and executed by the Nationalists in a generally much more organised manner compared with the ad hoc purges of the more undisciplined Republicans. Priests and liberal doctors were often old rivals for local influence. At the San Pablo Hospital in anti-clerical Barcelona, a priest, feeling threatened in the midst of the revolutionary attack on the Church, had an argument with a doctor and pulled out a revolver to shoot not the doctor but his patients lying in bed.[8] That particular priest felt threatened in a Republican stronghold and reacted badly. Elsewhere in Nationalist held areas, it was the liberal and socialist doctors who justly feared for their lives. Manuel Montesinos, a socialist physician and brother-in-law of the poet and dramatist Federico Garcia Lorca, was arrested only ten days after his election as mayor of Granada and shot after three week's incarceration in a crowded prison cell.[9] The professor of pharmacy in Granada, José Megías Manzano, one of a number of doctors from the university to be butchered for their political views, was put to work digging graves for his fellow prisoners in the days before his own execution. In nearby Cordoba, the gentlemanly Dr Sadí de Buen, who had directed a campaign for the eradication of malaria in Andalusia, was offered the last rites by a priest before his execution, which he politely refused before handing over enough money from his wallet so that the priest could pay for him his outstanding hotel bill after his death.[10] His fate was shared by many others throughout Spain.

For many doctors with strong political views, there was often no alternative but to escape across the enemy lines to serve the side with which they sympathised in the civil conflict even though this may have meant abandoning career, colleagues and home for the duration of the hostilities.

As the war went on this became essential as the distinctions between military and civilian medicine became increasingly blurred with civilian hospitals tending the wounded and medical staff being called up to treat war casualties. The more politicised society became, the less easy it was to remain neutral. Eduardo Martínez Alonso, a society doctor in Madrid who had enjoyed the favour of Queen Ena before the fall of the monarchy in 1931, narrowly escaped execution and was sent to work with a communist surgical unit near Badajoz for a few months before being imprisoned in Ocaña where he turned his attention to organising a prison hospital. A man whose life he had saved then helped him to escape from imminent execution and, having reached the Nationalist zone, he joined Franco's forces as a doctor.[11] Lluis Trias de Bes, one of the heads of service at the Hospital Marítim d'Infecciosos in Barcelona, had little sympathy with the anarchism that prevailed in the Catalan capital and abandoned his post as soon as the opportunity arose to cross over to the Nationalist zone with which he was more attuned. His former colleagues remained at their posts but after the Republican defeat were dismissed, including the venerable director of the hospital Josep Maria Grau Blanc who had dedicated his life to the hospital since 1914. Grau was replaced as director of the hospital, now given the decidedly right-wing and ardently Roman Catholic name of the Hospital de Nuestra Señora de la Mar,[12] at the end of the war by the more politically astute Trias de Bes who had early thrown in his lot with the victorious Nationalists.[13] Future career prospects indeed depended on backing the right side.

Most Spanish doctors and nurses had no real choice as to whom they treated. It depended upon where they lived and worked, with professional responsibilities and geographical realities overriding personal politics. However, there was a choice for those volunteers from other countries who flocked to defend the Republic against fascism or support the Nationalists in their struggle against communism and anarchism. Although the Civil War was rooted in Spanish political conflicts that went back to the nineteenth century, it was seen by many international volunteers as representative of the international struggle between left and right, communism and fascism, democracy and dictatorship.

Liberal and left wing sympathizers with the Republican cause from the Western democracies rushed to join the Republican army and International Brigades not only as combatants but also as doctors, nurses and stretcher-bearers, and some served with the ambulance units of the Spanish

Medical Aid Committee. Most of the British doctors sent out by the Spanish Medical Aid Committee were young, politically committed and professionally ambitious, although the ambulance driver Wogan Philipps, himself the son of a wealthy businessman, dismissed them as 'terribly bourgeois' which made them 'superior in manner' and 'jealous of each other'.[14] Nevertheless, the thirty-five-year-old, American-born, British-trained doctor Randall Sollenberger died at the Battle of Brunete in July 1937 as a soldier wielding a rifle rather than as a doctor treating wounds so great was his enthusiasm for the military life and the cause he had espoused.[15] Not all of these volunteer doctors, however, retained their initial idealism. Norman King, a member of the Communist Party who had served for three years in the Royal Army Medical Corps, was unhappy when his request to be transferred to an American Unit on the Cordoba Front, where there would be more scope for his experience as an anaesthetist', was turned down by the International Brigade and he felt 'cut off from the British Medical Aid Unit' and that he was 'not getting sympathy from the Lincoln Battalion' to which he had been attached. After only three months in Spain, he took 'French leave' and sought repatriation from the British consul in Valencia.[16]

The nurses sent out with them had much less opportunity to gain experience of new medical and surgical procedures on the battlefield than the doctors, but their professional competence compared with the less skilled and less competent Spanish nurses gave them prestige and authority unavailable to them at home. Penny Phelps in her twenties was put in charge of controlling an outbreak of scarlet fever among the Italian volunteers of the Garibaldi Battalion in the absence of a doctor and briefly held the rank of Lieutenant. Despite an arduous round of inspections of hospital and sanitary arrangements, the fumigation of barracks and clothing, the treatment of minor wounds and a programme of inoculations, she still found time to go for long walks with the 'good-looking' political commissar of the battalion Roberto Vincenzi who talked to her about 'the new world where social justice would prevail'.[17]

Idealism, the thirst for adventure and hope of finding a new fulfilment in Spain motivated these volunteers, for whom 'our moments of tenderness blossom as the ambulance and sandbag'.[18] Many of them had socialist or communist sympathies. Nor were they afraid of actively aiding the cause for which they had enrolled in more than the medical sphere. British nurses were ready to pass on intelligence information and relay information to the press that benefited the Republic such as the group of nurses who reported about German air camps being established along the Pyrenean frontier in 1938.[19] The Soviet Union too sent arms, men and medical aid in the expectation of greater political influence. All of this was gratefully received by the Spanish Republic.

The Nationalists were perhaps more unwilling than their foes to admit foreign medical workers though they had no objection to German and Italian military aid; German and Italian doctors and nurses treated their own wounded and made little significant contribution to the medical needs of their Spanish allies. The Germans indeed were scathing about their Spanish allies in general and were unimpressed by their medical services. With such attitudes, it is not surprising that they preferred to evacuate casualties from their Condor Legion by air back to the Reich for treatment; such air evacuation was on a much smaller scale than that carried out by the Luftwaffe during the Second World War. The Italians, by contrast, preferred to treat their own men closer to the battlefields, although the 1,000-bedded Italian military hospitals at Valladolid and Saragossa were primarily for the use of the Italian forces fighting in Spain not for their Nationalist allies. It did give the Axis powers some experience of medicine in modern warfare as if in preparation for the coming world war.[20]

Individual doctors and nurses also gave support to the Nationalist cause, although perhaps in fewer numbers than joined the International Brigades. Among those who did so was Robert Macintosh, who, shortly after his appointment to the chair of anaesthesiology at Oxford in 1937, inspected Franco's medical arrangements and later recommended another Oxford anaesthetist, Kenneth Boston, for work in the General Mola Military Hospital at San Sebastian with the American surgeon Joseph Sheehan, who had been invited to work there on injuries to the jaw and neck by the Duke of Berwick and Alba. He found that the greatest problem facing the anaesthetist in Spanish field hospitals, apart from occasional lack of any anaesthetics other than cognac, was the problem of supervising partly trained staff while simultaneously attempting to care for large numbers of unconscious patients. His experience of military surgery in Spain led him to recommend the use of barbiturates for relaxing the patient before administering ether, which he considered to be the safest available anaesthetic. His observations in Spain formed the basis of his influential recommendations on anaesthesia in wartime.[21] Many of these foreign Nationalist supporters were motivated by Catholic sympathies and a hatred of Communism, but for others more personal motives were at play. Priscilla Scott-Ellis, daughter of the wealthy Lord Howard de Walden, became a volunteer nurse with Franco's forces as a result of her passion for Prince Ataúlfo de Borbón, who had joined the Condor Legion as a pilot, rather than from any more idealistic motives. Her periods of leave in luxurious hotels with her lover punctuated her bouts of nursing seriously wounded men in the squalor of front-line hospitals.[22]

The Spanish Red Cross was inevitably split according to the political sympathies of its members. There was the additional problem that the Geneva Convention had no legal application to civil conflicts. The International Red Cross Committee sent the thirty-four-year-old Swiss surgeon Marcel Junod as its representative to broker agreements between the Spanish Government and the insurgents that the neutrality of the Red Cross would be guaranteed and that it would be allowed to work in both the Republican and Nationalist zones. Junod had already showed his ability as a diplomat the previous year when he had been sent as a Red Cross delegate to Ethiopia where the Italian Red Cross had declined to co-operate with the International Red Cross Committee and the Ethiopian Red Cross organization had only recently been founded not long before the Italian invasion. The Emperor Hailie Selassie needed to have it explained to him by Junod's diplomatic colleague Sidney Hamilton Brown that the Geneva Convention represented neutral medical care not a pact against aggression. Brown also had to ensure that the Ethiopian brothels and bars removed their traditional signs of a red cross on a white background that would only too easily be confused with the symbol of the Red Cross movement. Meanwhile Junod's task had been to co-ordinate the field units and medical supplies sent to Ethiopia by twenty-eight national Red Cross societies. There he had been shocked by the Italian use of poison gas on the Ethiopians whom they looked on as savages: 'As I came closer, my heart in my mouth, I could see horrible suppurating burns on their feet and on their emaciated limbs. Life was already leaving bodies burned with mustard gas … who was to have pity? Who was to help them in their suffering?'[23]

Junod tried his best. It was expected that his mission to Spain would last for three days but he was to stay for the three years that the war continued. Under his direction, food and medical supplies were distributed to both sides according to strict mathematical formulae based on the populations of the two sides. Attempts were made at tracing missing persons and reuniting families scattered and separated by the random circumstances of civil war since 'for a long time I had realized that this uncertainty was the greatest agony of all' for people who did not know what had happened to their loved ones.[24] His office was thronged with supporters of both sides in the conflict eager to find out what had become of members of their families but not acknowledging that their opponents might have similar concerns and sorrows. One staunch monarchist, Isabella, finally found out that her brother had been executed with ten others by a group of republicans. She showed nothing but contempt and hatred towards Carlota, whose republican fiancé was still missing, as she passed her on the way out. Carlota similarly had no sympathy for her bereaved political adversary and merely commented that 'at least she can visit his grave. But I shall never know, never'.[25] Junod was proud of his achievement in arranging the exchange of prisoners: 'list for list, individually and in small groups, lives were steadily exchanged for lives'.[26] In all his difficult negotiations he had to maintain a show of equality between all warring parties that was to come in useful during the Second World War when his efforts on behalf of prisoners of war in Germany led to his arrest by the Gestapo as a suspected French spy.[27] In Spain, strict neutrality was the key to success.[28]

There was actually very little difference in the medical organisation and practice of the two sides in the Spanish Civil War, which was in itself based on the experience of the First World War. At first the wounded had been left to reach the hospitals themselves for any first aid. This had not mattered in the early days when fighting was confined to the streets, but was not so ideal once regular fighting had started and the wounded had to travel considerable distances to reach a hospital resulting in a high death rate of men from shock. Once they reached the hospital, doctors and nurses often had to search their clothing for hidden ammunition, as 'it is disturbing to have the field hospital incinerator blown up when burning old clothes'.[29] Very soon the hospital was taken to the wounded with the 'exodus of the surgeon from the white tiles and chromium of the hospitals into the whitewash and plaster of farmhouses, or the fading baroque of palaces near the line and just outside the range of the gathering German and Italian artillery' as described by Kenneth Sinclair-Loutit, administrator of the first British Medical Aid Unit who had gone to Spain as a twenty-three-year-old medical student from St Bartholomew's Hospital, London.[30] Large lorries known as 'autochir', were equipped with autoclaves, surgical instruments and portable X-ray machinery to act as travelling front line hospitals.[31] The wounded were evacuated from the battalion first-aid posts to divisional or regimental aid posts and then to mobile front line *hospitales de sangre*, where emergency surgery would be carried out. Finally, the injured were transferred to hospitals in the rearguard. Air ambulances, pioneered by the Spanish Army in Morocco in the 1920s, were used to transfer patients. The Republicans may have possessed the better surgeons but the Nationalist wounded arrived at the hospitals in better condition because of superior transport arrangements from the battlefield to the hospital.[32] The Soviet woman commissar of a medical unit attached to a tank brigade conceded that 'medical transport is a weak spot here' and that the only ambulances available to the International Brigades were either modified trucks or had been 'assembled from odd bits and pieces' with only enough space for four stretchers at most.[33] The Nationalists organised transport for their wounded in a more efficient way.

As in most wars there was a perceived difference in attitude between the situation on the front line and at the staff headquarters in the rear, witnessed no less in medical services than in military attitudes. The left-wing Austrian sociologist and journalist Franz Borkenau visited a front line Red Cross station in Andalusia in September 1936 as fighting raged around the village of Cerro Muriano. Republican militia-men were brought in for treatment for dangerous wounds or shell-shock and 'considered themselves as good as dead, or rather, played dead' because their fighting role was now over. It was left to the doctors, unable to get any answers to their questions from their patients, to find out for themselves what had happened by undressing the injured men and looking for the wounds. Suddenly a bomb exploded a few feet away from the clearly marked first-aid post and everyone, except for Borkenau and two other journalists with him, dived to the floor; despite it being useless to take cover within a building, their training had made it instinctive for them to lie flat on the ground. The wounded remained still, a nurse sobbed and the doctors went on with treating their patients as more bombs fell on the village.[34] It was a great contrast to the attitude of the doctors Borkenau had observed at staff headquarters a few hours earlier. There they were billeted in a hospital 'in a very pleasant sanatorium' though he considered that 'the staff itself was less pleasant'. Despite heavy fighting a few miles away, the staff officers, doctors and nurses were more interested in enjoying a good lunch, telling dirty stories and flirting than they were in their duties or the care of the wounded being brought in. The nurses, 'of more than a dubious quality', neglected their patients 'in the most shameless and repugnant manner'.[35]

George Orwell, fighting with the Republican militiamen in Catalonia, was equally scathing about the competence and honesty of the *practicantes*, hospital assistants, who stole from him every item of value he possessed, including his camera and photographs, when he was admitted to hospital with a poisoned hand. This was nothing compared with the experience of an American volunteer who had been aboard a torpedoed ship and was unable to stop the stretcher-bearers from stealing his wrist-watch as they lifted him into the ambulance taking him to hospital.[36] Orwell later became an object of professional curiosity to the doctors, nurses and his fellow patients when he was shot in the neck by a sniper, the bullet having missed the artery by 'about a millimetre', and was assured by them that 'a man who is hit through the neck and survives it is the luckiest creature alive. I could not help thinking that it would be even luckier not to be hit at all'.[37] Despite him being dopey from the morphia, unable to move and constantly swallowing blood, one medical orderly tried to force a meal of eggs and stew down his throat and seemed surprised when he refused it.[38] The standard of Spanish nursing was indeed generally poor, something Orwell ascribed to the fact that before the war nursing had been the prerogative of nuns. The untrained nurses now tending the sick, he found to be kind but ignorant of anything more than how to take a temperature or tie a bandage. Beds were left unmade, bedridden men with smashed arms were left unwashed for a week and nothing was done to help men with constipation.[39] Martha Gellhorn, an American journalist, dismissed the nurses working in the hospital set up in the Palace Hotel in Madrid as 'peroxide blonds with long, brightly coloured nails'.[40] English nurses too were critical of their Spanish sisters and the conditions they tolerated, such as a ward in which the patients rested on bundles of their clothing instead of pillows, and with half-empty wine glasses and full chamber pots under their beds.[41] More understandable in the heat of battle were conditions in an operating theatre in which the atmosphere was 'stifling and the floor slippery with caked blood'.[42]

The Russian forces fighting in Spain prided themselves that conditions in the Soviet hospitals were far superior to the terrible conditions in makeshift hospitals for Spanish soldiers. By contrast with the filthy and cold Republican hospital established in the grim if imposing surroundings of Philip II's palace-cum-monastery of El Escorial, which was 'overflowing with the wounded', the field hospital for the Soviet tank brigade and members of the International Brigades, set up in a house in a forest nature reserve near Las Rozas, was clean and warm with plenty of double mattresses, clean linen, soap and water. Nevertheless Russian wounded were being treated in hospitals throughout Madrid and it was a matter for propaganda that they should be seen to be receiving attention from their Soviet comrades, so food in short supply to ordinary Spaniards and soldiers, such as tinned milk, cocoa, fruit and chocolate was sent to them from the headquarters of the tank brigade. The commissar of the tank brigade medical unit also visited the wounded tank crews daily and reported back to Moscow on such instances of international socialist solidarity as a dying Frenchman whose last act was to sing the *Internationale*.[43]

In Nationalist Spain, the nuns who had traditionally carried out most of the nursing in hospitals rallied to the cause and served in both military and civilian hospitals, often assisted by untrained volunteers whom they held in low esteem. However, the nuns were unable to cope with the excessive workload the war had brought them and invariably resented the intrusion of lay doctors and nurses into their domains. The result was a shambles and in March 1937 Franco appointed Mercedes Milá Nolla as *Inspectora General de Servicios Femeninos de Hospitales* to take overall charge of all military nursing, whether provided by religious orders, volunteers or the Red Cross. Milá, now aged 42, had studied nurse education at Bedford College in London and was working for the Madrid health service at the outbreak of hostilities. Despite organising hospital services in the capital for the Republic, she had used her Red Cross connections to escape via Switzerland to Salamanca. Her father had been a friend of Franco's and in her new role in charge of military nursing services she was invited to join the Caudillo and his aides for a breakfast meeting every morning. Under her capable if dictatorial superintendence, nursing services were centralised and all local autonomy stamped out. At a local level she gave local command over all nurses to mother superiors who brooked no opposition from secular nurses. Hospital-based courses were organised to train the 5,500 nursing auxiliaries that were recruited to take on the more menial roles, such as preparing dressings and poultices and housekeeping duties, which many of the qualified nurses considered beneath them. Any attempts at interference with nursing arrangements by doctors were repelled. These organisational abilities were to stand Milá in good stead after the war when she was appointed to organise nursing support for the Spanish volunteers sent by Franco to fight alongside the German Army against the Russians in 1942 and in her subsequent appointment as Secretary-General of the Spanish Red Cross.[44] Yet, despite such centralisation and efficient organisation, nursing standards in the Nationalist hospitals were criticised by foreign observers who noted that many of the nurses were expected to learn on the job and if they did receive any instruction it was not from experienced nurses but from the surgeons, many of them as young and inexperienced as the nurses with whom they were working. The result was a sloppiness and a lack of cleanliness in the hospitals that compromised the survival chances of the wounded.[45]

However, it was not only the wounded from the battlefields that were in need of care. Civilians now found themselves the target of major aerial bombardment. Barcelona was bombed almost 200 times in three years of war by planes of the German and Italian air forces based in Nationalist-controlled Majorca; between 2,500 and 3,000 people died as a result of these raids which prefigured the aerial destruction of cities during the Second World War.[46] Fearful observers in other countries heeded the lesson that the bomber would always win through and that war was to be avoided even at the cost of abject appeasement of the dictators. The destruction of the Basque town of Guernica, carpet-bombed by the German Condor Legion for exactly three hours and fifteen minutes on 26 April 1937, became symbolic of death from the air. It was a market day; the cattle and sheep, blazing with white phosphorus, added to the chaos in the burning streets as fleeing men, women and children, including nuns serving as nurses in the hospital, were strafed and grenaded. George Steer, the stylish anti-fascist war correspondent for *The Times* wrote that 'the object of the bombardment was seemingly the demoralization of the civil population and the destruction of the cradle of the Basque race'.[47] Pablo Picasso was inspired to depict the destruction of Guernica in a painting that has come to represent the horror of war and which was only taken to Spain after the death of Franco and once the political wounds of the Civil War were allowed to heal. The British government was influenced by the Spanish experience when it came to planning how to deal with air raid casualties from a world war. In March 1938 British officials estimated that one ton of bombs would cause seventy-two casualties based on the effects of the bombardment of Barcelona. Later it was realised that the true casualty ratio in Barcelona was actually 3.5 people per bomb, but the British plans continued to be based on the earlier, more drastic and more frightening figures.[48]

Whilst there may have been little difference in medical practice between the opposing sides, the main medical advances that came from the war were from the Republicans, chiefly because the long established and flourishing centres of medical research in Barcelona and Madrid remained under government control until the end of the war. There the challenge of dealing with the effects of battlefield casualties and air-raid victims combined with the idealism of a number of young doctors to produce innovative medicine. By no means did the least of the achievements of Republican Spain lie in the field of social medicine. Barcelona led the way towards a socialized system of medicine which saw unprecedented collaboration in the provision of universal and free medical services between the 1,000 doctors, 3,200 nurses, 330 midwives and 600 dentists of the city.[49] Despite competing demands for doctors and medical services at the Front, there were over a thousand more beds for sufferers from tuberculosis in Republican Spain in 1937 than there had been before the war. By that time there were as many child-welfare centres in the areas held by the Republic as there had been in the whole of Spain previously. Inoculation against smallpox, diphtheria and typhoid was made compulsory in 1937. Abortions in the first three months of pregnancy were legalized in January 1937, provided they were carried out with full medical care, something that was anathema to the devout Roman Catholicism of the Nationalists.[50] Even as the war raged close to the capital, a modern maternity hospital with the latest in facilities was opened in Madrid. Meanwhile a scheme was organized for the evacuation of expectant mothers away from the war zones where they could find comparative peace and quiet and also have first call on the scarce quantities of milk as yet still available in rural areas far from the fighting.[51] Workers were now entitled to full pay if they were off work as a result of sickness and permanent invalids were entitled to seventy-five per cent of their former salary. Such a generous provision had to be paid for and in anarchist Barcelona profits from collectivized industries and businesses were used for this purpose. Surplus profits from the collectivized cinemas and theatres were also used to build a school and a clinic.[52]

As well as improvements in the provision of medical services, there were also major advances in medical and surgical treatments among the Republicans in response to the challenges of dealing with battlefield and air-raid casualties. Foremost among these was the work on war wounds and fractures of Josep Trueta Raspall, professor of surgery at the Hospital de la Sant Creu i Sant Pau in Barcelona. Faced with large numbers of casualties, such as the 2,200 wounded brought into his hospital over two days of bombing in March 1938, Trueta devised a new method for the management of serious injuries. He revolutionized the treatment of fractures with what was known as the 'closed method of treatment'. The wound would be operated on as soon as possible within eight hours. All dead, dying, contaminated or damaged tissue was removed, though skin and bone were conserved wherever this was possible, and the wound was left exposed and unsutured. It was cleansed with soap and water using a nailbrush. After this débridement had taken place, the bone was set and the wound packed with dry, sterile gauze and drained. Then the limb was encased completely in a plaster cast so that it would be immobile until the bone had knit. Whereas older methods of treating fractures had relied upon frequent dressings and examination of the wound, Trueta insisted on leaving it to heal on its own without the use of any antiseptics. The cast was only changed if it became wet and soft or too smelly. Generally, the patients were nursed on open balconies because of the smell that emanated from their wounds. They themselves preferred the smell to the dreaded pain that had previously accompanied the daily changing of dressings and use of antiseptics.[53] Trueta's results were remarkable. Whereas septicaemia and gas gangrene had once been common in Catalonia, they were now so rare that surgeons visiting Barcelona in 1938 believed that Spain was free of the anaerobic bacteria that carried gas gangrene. Trueta recorded only one case of gangrene in 1073 patients treated,[54] while another surgeon using the same technique recorded only twenty cases among 5,000 patients.[55] Even so Trueta had to battle to get his ideas accepted by conventionally minded army surgeons resistant to change. Trueta's ideas were to gain greater acceptance in Britain after 1939, when he published a book on the treatment of war wounds and the closed method of treatment of fractures was to come into its own in the Western Desert during the Second World War where the Tobruk Splint, a conventional Thomas splint of the type used in the First World War but reinforced with plaster of Paris, was used to immobilize limbs without obstructing circulation. Trueta was also aware that his methods developed in wartime were also applicable in peacetime orthopaedic surgery since 'open fractures produced in road accidents or in industry do not differ essentially from those produced by aerial bombs or falling masonry'.[56]

Other procedures might be necessary before Trueta's methods could be followed if the injured had more problems than just fractured limbs. On the battlefield the Catalan surgeon Moises Broggi, serving with the International Brigades, noticed during the Battle of Belchite that casualties with severe facial injuries and fractures were dying while waiting on a stretcher for treatment. These deaths were usually as a result of choking on blood in the airways. In order to avoid this happening, Broggi began to perform emergency tracheotomies so that the airways could be suctioned and respiration restored. Once the patient had been stabilized, it was possible to begin débridement of the wound. It was a simple medical management technique that was to save many lives during the Civil War and be adopted in the Second World War.[57]

The battlefields of the Civil War also saw the introduction into military medicine of the sulphonamide drugs that were to prove themselves in the campaigns of the Second World War. Trueta only ever used sulphanilamide on rare occasions because he believed that chemical agents could never be a substitute for effective and competent surgery. Other military surgeons welcomed them as a means of controlling infection. Colonel Joaquin d'Harcourt Got, head of the Republican surgical services, who had opposed Trueta's recommendations about not changing dressings daily, had some success in treating cases of septicaemia with sulphanilamide in cases of wounds where further surgical treatment would have been useless.[58] The sulphanilamide drugs had been discovered by Gerhard Domagk, research director of the chemical combine I.G. Farbenindustrie research institute for pathological anatomy and bacteriology at Wuppertal. As a result of his experiences as a medical orderly during the First World War, Domagk 'swore, in case I would return to my home alive, to work and work as hard as I could in order to make a small contribution' in the fight against 'bacteria, those horrible enemies of the human race that kill so insidiously'.[59] The main products of his firm were azo dyes used for colouring textiles so it was inevitable that he should investigate their potential to kill bacteria. In 1932 he found that when he administered the red dye prontosil rubrum to mice infected with haemolytic streptococci he was able to cure them. Results were good when prontosil was used on human beings, including Domagk's own six-year-old daughter when she fell seriously ill with a streptococcal infection and her life was at risk. Researchers at the Pasteur Institute established that the sulphonamide molecule within the compound, rather than the dye itself, was bacteriostatic, which meant that it did not kill the bacteria but rather prevented them from growing which gave the body's own immune system the opportunity to destroy them.[60]

Since prontosil could not be patented because its active constituent sulphonamide had been synthesised as long ago as 1907, it could be developed as a drug effective against more than just streptococcal infections by other chemical and pharmaceutical companies. The British firm of May and Baker developed M and B 693, which was effective against a range of bacteria, in 1938. However, it did not work so well on localised areas where pus had formed and it was often found to be more efficacious to give it five days after the infection had started rather than immediately. There were also nasty side effects such as rashes and vomiting which made it a far from pleasant treatment for the patient. However, its value in the treatment of infection on the battlefield was first shown during the Spanish Civil War and it came into its own during the Second World War when it was used by both sides to treat infected wounds. American troops even carried packets of sterile crystalline sulphanilamide with them to be sprinkled on to a wound before a field dressing was applied. Other armies preferred to apply sulphanilamide dressings in casualty stations.[61] Domagk did not go without a reward for his discovery, despite there being no royalties from it for his firm, although it was to be many years before he was able to collect his honour. Awarded the 1939 Nobel Prize for Medicine, he was forbidden by the Nazi government from accepting it and was even detained by the Gestapo to prevent him from going to Stockholm to collect it.[62]

Great advances were also made in the use of blood transfusion to treat casualties suffering from a severe loss of blood and from shock compared with the primitive procedures of the First World War. Now, for the first time, it was possible to give the wounded in forward medical posts blood that had been donated by civilians and then stored until it was needed. The Nationalist forces followed the practice of their allies in the German Army in carrying out transfusions only in fully equipped hospitals behind the lines but the Republicans actually made blood supplies readily available for urgent use in the front line. Dr Carlos Elosegui started up a blood transfusion service for the Nationalists in San Sebastian and Burgos in September 1936 but it was not until 31 March 1937 that it received official sanction from Franco's government.

The Republican success with front line blood supplies was the achievement of the Catalan doctor Frederic Duran i Jordà, who had realized the importance of large-scale blood supplies for both the wounded and for air raid casualties from the outset of the civil war and set up the Barcelona Blood Transfusion Service, which, with its counterpart in Madrid, was praised by *The Lancet* as being one of the 'magnificent blood transfusion centres in Republican Spain' that were 'clearly a great advance on any system that has been advocated in this country'.[63] Between August

1936 and January 1939, over 9, 000 litres of blood had been collected in some 20,000 bleedings from a list of 28,900 donors, and over 27,000 tubes of blood had been prepared for forward use by the Barcelona Blood Transfusion Service.[64] It was an impressive feat that owed much to the pioneering spirit of Duran himself.

While tending the wounded at Hospital 18 on the slopes of Monjuïc on the outskirts of Barcelona, thirty-one-year-old Duran had become aware that the amount of blood that could be administered by a direct arm-to-arm transfusion from donor to recipient, which was the most common technique then used, was often less than the amount needed by the patient. The solution to the problem lay in recent developments in the storage of blood products. In Moscow in 1930 the surgeon Serge Yudin had used sodium citrate to store blood collected from corpses, which he had then used for transfusions. It was a method that most people found distasteful, but it did show the potential for building up supplies of blood ready for when they were needed. John S. Lundy of the Mayo Clinic began to store citrated blood from live donors in 1935 and in 1937 a blood bank was opened by Bernard Fantus in the Blood Preservation Laboratory at Cook County Hospital, Chicago.[65] Using these new storage techniques for his innovative blood transfusion service, considered to be 'work of great scientific and military importance',[66] Duran was able not only to supply blood to casualties near Barcelona but by September 1936 was able to send seven litres of blood in a refitted refrigerated fish truck for use on the distant Aragon Front.[67] Duran took great care to ensure the purity of his blood supplies. Donated blood was tested for syphilis and malaria. In order to screen out tuberculosis sufferers, he acquired X-ray apparatus equipment. Duran designed a special ampoule to avoid any contamination of the blood during collection, storage, transit or transfusion. Sterile pressurised air was used to force the blood into the patient being transfused. This method was based on a system called *Autoinyectable Rapide* (fast autoinjectable) originally developed for the storage and infusion of saline and glucose, but which now proved ideal for safe blood transfusion. A sterile needle protected by a glass cover was attached to a two-way valve on the ampoule for quick and rapid transfusion. More attention was paid to the compatibility of blood groups and universal-donor group O was recognized as being safe to use on all patients if their blood group was unknown in the heat of a battlefield when there was never time for cross-matching. Each flask of blood consisted of six different specimens of blood from the same group in order to reduce the chances of allergic reactions to something in one particular donation and also to make allowances for errors in blood typing. The chilled blood carried by the mobile medical units could be stored safely at temperatures of one degree centigrade for eighteen days and was heated to forty degrees centigrade before injection. Reactions to the transfusions were rare. Dr Josep Vives Mañé was so impressed by the results of over 130 transfusions using the Duran i Jordà method that 'we think that at the front it is irreplaceable'.[68]

Yet Duran was not alone in organising blood transfusion services for the Republican forces, although his organization in Barcelona continued throughout the war to supply blood by delivery van to all the fronts. Other doctors observed what he had created and copied it. Services were established on other fronts. The Canadian Surgeon Norman Bethune set up a unified blood transfusion service serving 100 hospitals and casualty clearing stations for the Madrid Front. However, his heavy drinking, womanizing and erratic behaviour resulted in his transfusion units being taken over by the Republican government and Bethune's return to Canada. He was to utilise his Spanish experiences in fighting against the Japanese for the Communists in China where he died in 1939 from septicaemia from a cut when he was operating.[69] Reginald Saxton, who had been a young general practitioner in Reading before he had joined the British Ambulance Unit in Spain, helped to organise the Madrid Blood Transfusion Institute under the aegis of the *Sanidad Militar* of the Spanish Republic. By September 1937 it was supplying in the region of 400 litres of preserved blood each month for use with the casualties from the fierce fighting raging around the Spanish capital and was under pressure to increase its output as the preserved blood only lasted for three weeks. Blood donors, aged between eighteen and fifty, were issued with special ration cards that allowed them to buy extra food as an incentive to give blood and, when these were available, were also given rice or condensed milk as a treat when they made their donation.[70] Nevertheless, despite such incentives to give blood, most donors were motivated by humanitarian reasons, and, as in Duran's service in Barcelona, 'there are many among their number with whom it has become a veritable obsession to give blood, and these present themselves long before the expiration of the period' of three weeks normal between donations.[71]

While great attention was paid to repairing the ravages of war on the body, some observers seemed to think that psychological damage was not so great a problem. Franz Borkenau commented that 'to a surprisingly small degree is the Spanish Civil War a psychological crisis', a situation he explained by the fact that 'the Spaniards, amid their terrible ordeal, keep quiet and poised as individuals, because they are basically healthy'.[72] It was not a view shared by some of the combatants in the war. A commander in the Spanish Republican Army told the psychiatrist Emili Mira i López that 'I think that during war everybody is upset, nervous, jittery and perhaps slightly crazy. It is no wonder, then, that you do not find an increasing number of insane. You simply lack a normal background for comparison'.[73] Mira, professor of psychology at the Autonomous University of Barcelona, had the experience to be aware of the psychiatric problems of both combatants and civilians in wartime. Early in the Civil War he was appointed director of the Institute of Professional Adaptation for Women, an organization instituted by the Catalan government to prepare women to take over the jobs of men fighting at the Front, and in 1938 was appointed as Chief of Psychiatric Services of the Republican Army. With such a background of wartime service, it is little wonder that he believed that one of the major roles of psychiatry in wartime was to ensure that the population was able to contribute to the war effort to the utmost of their ability and mental energy. Morale was to be maintained, mental breakdowns and exhaustion avoided and soldiers and civilians kept fit for their wartime roles. Despite resistance to the idea of any psychological examination of recruits, Mira was concerned about screening out men with nervous or mental temperaments and disorders that might make them inefficient in the field. He got new recruits to fill out questionnaires that would offer clues to their level of intelligence and political awareness, their psychological strengths and weaknesses, and their susceptibility to war neuroses. Men who did break down were to be isolated from their comrades in arms so as to prevent a breakdown in morale. Drunkenness as a psychopathic reaction was treated harshly and Mira recommended that anyone found to be habitually intoxicated was to be marked out and closely watched by the regimental physician. Men addicted to alcohol were to be separated from their drinking companions and given a solution of the liquor ammoniae anisatus to try to condition an aversion to the taste of alcohol. In a hard-drinking environment, attempts to control alcoholism could have little hope of success. For men recovering from shell-shock and battle fatigue, recovery and retraining centres were established to prevent them from relapsing once they returned to action. Emphasis was placed on games and activity involving teamwork. However little sympathy was given to people he perceived as being shirkers or as having 'hysterical fits with a selfish purpose'.[74] Generally, though, psychiatric casualties were low in the Republican armies compared with the incidence of psychiatric disturbance among a fearful civilian population with less physical stimulation and less control over their destinies.[75]

With regard to civilians, Mira was only too aware that a long-drawn-out war with no end in sight could sap morale, especially when there no longer seemed to be any hope of external aid to sustain them in the face of lack of sleep, food, clothing and armaments and the loss of their homes. This was especially noticeable in the last winter of the war when 'the agony of the Spanish people is to enter a new period of intensity'.[76] The influx of three million refugees into Government territory, mainly women and children fleeing from the effects of aerial bombardment and a food blockade, put increased pressure on already scarce resources. The ever-expanding Nationalist zone had from the outset covered the major food producing areas of Spain, whereas the Republican Government zone was more susceptible to starvation and malnutrition. Yet it was remarkable that until late in the war, when smallpox and typhus epidemics broke out, there were few major outbreaks of disease.[77] At the beginning of the Civil War there had been fears of epidemic disease; refugees from Spain arriving in Britain were medically inspected 'for fear that they may bring infection due to the unsanitary conditions in parts of Spain following the Civil War'.[78] However, when 4,000 Basque refugee children landed at Southampton in 1937, they were found to have body lice but otherwise to be free from the expected malnutrition or other deficiency diseases.[79] Now, as the Nationalists advanced, starvation went ahead of them in Catalonia and Madrid. By the end of the war, there were between 300 and 400 deaths from starvation each day in Madrid. Daily rations were reduced to two ounces of lentils, beans or rice, occasionally supplemented by sugar or salt cod when available. Lentils were renamed 'Dr Negrín's little victory pills' in honour of the prime minister.[80] Even after the fighting had ended 'food, particularly bread, is still the main preoccupation of Barcelona'.[81] During the fierce fighting around the capital, Franco's Moroccan troops were just as hungry as the beleaguered *Madrileños* and ate the inoculated animals kept for experimental purposes in the laboratories of the Clinical Hospital in the University City quarter as they fought their way through the building; it was as fatal for them as the bombs placed by the Republican Thaelmann

Batallion in the lifts of the hospital so as to blow up the Moroccans on the next floor.[82] Previously, Dr Grande Covián had studied the effects of nutritional deficiencies on over 3,000 cases, suffering from such diseases as pellagra and thiamine deficiency. Malaria had always been rampant. Scurvy alone was never very common if only because oranges were one of the few things never in short supply.[83] Foreign aid became ever more important to the Republicans as defeat loomed ever closer. British diplomats in Barcelona reported in December 1938 that 'the lack of all kinds of medical supplies horrified me during my visit to the southern zone'.[84] A British aid worker Dr Audrey Russell met a four-year-old girl carrying home a tin of milk and asked her whether it was for her only to be told 'No ... I am too old for milk. I am taking it for the babies'. Republican supporters urged that 'it is a moral obligation for us to see that food reaches these innocent victims of the new reign of madness and terror that has descended upon the world'.[85]

Foreign aid could not stave off the final agonies of the Republic and by the end of March 1939 Spain was in Nationalist hands. Many of the leading pioneers in medicine from the Republic fled their homeland taking with them that expertise in war medicine that was to become so useful to the Allied cause in the Second World War that was to break out within six months. The unlucky were interned with their erstwhile comrades in unhygienic camps in France where there were only two small wash troughs for 1,400 men and most men only managed to get a shower for the first time after several months of imprisonment; here interned Spanish and International Brigade volunteer doctors tended the sick and wounded in hospitals that only differed from the barracks, where the internees slept on straw sacks, in so far as they had windows.[86] More prominent figures were offered refuge in the Western democracies. Trueta crossed the Pyrenees to take refuge in Perpignan before being invited to London to advise on air raid precautions. He remained in Britain and subsequently became professor of orthopaedic surgery and traumatology at the University of Oxford. His views on the treatment of war wounds became the orthodoxy in the Second World War.[87] Duran was invited to Britain by the British Red Cross and sponsored by the physiologist Janet Vaughan of the Royal Postgraduate Medical School at the Hammersmith Hospital. Vaughan had known Duran in Barcelona and realised that he could give advice on the storage of blood that would be invaluable for Britain in the imminent war.[88] Mira too went to London, after two months of exile in France, and was given a fellowship from the Maudsley Hospital. He then left for the United States at the beginning of the Second World War and ended up in Argentina because his wife could not stand the thought of being involved in another war.[89]

It was not only Spanish exiles whose medical experiences were to prove useful lessons for the Allies during the Second World War. Volunteers who had rallied to the defence of the Republic also brought useful experience back to their own countries. Frank Copeman, the former commander of the British Battalion, found himself in the unlikely situation of lecturing to the Royal Family at Windsor on air-raid precautions.[90] The Home Guard medical service was set up once the war had started by men who had served in the International Brigades and knew how to rely on improvised medical services.[91] The medical press in Britain was also full of papers and editorials on the medical aspects of the Civil War, although predominantly from the Republican rather than the Nationalist viewpoint, a bias arising not just from political prejudice but from the impact that Republican improvisations had made on medical thought and practice. These offered lessons as a world rather than just one nation hurtled towards war.

Healing for Victory

Had a surgeon from a casualty clearing station on the Somme of 1916 been transplanted to a field surgical unit in Normandy in 1944 he would have found much that was all too familiar and he may well have wondered just what had changed in the years that had passed. Surgery on the battlefield was still primitive and instruments continued to be sterilised over a primus stove against a background of the constant explosion of mortar shells. Mud was everywhere.[1] The doctors concerned, such as surgeon J.C. Watts, 'were learning medicine the hard way, under terrific pressure … I was astonished to see the rapidity with which the green team could settle down and almost become veterans in an afternoon'.[2] Bill Helm, a recently qualified doctor, was working in an Advanced Dressing Station near Caen, which was receiving about fifty wounded to be assessed every ten minutes. Some of this 'group of terrified disorientated lads, jittering and yelling in a corner' were dying and some needed urgent blood transfusions. A 'tough and dirty bunch' of SS prisoners was brought in to join the chaos, among them a young Nazi with a broken jaw and already close to death who murmured 'Heil Hitler' before fainting. Helm remembered his father's advice from the First World War that it was better to leave a casualty with severe fractures where he lay until he could be given medical treatment rather than move him without a splint when an officer who had lost a foot and broke both his legs was brought in but by then a transfusion was too late to save his life.[3] The chaos and confusion above all remained the same.

However, to think that nothing had changed would have been illusory. The lessons of the First World War had been learned well. Surgical units were located as close to the battlefront as possible and patients were evacuated to base hospitals at the earliest possible opportunity. Wounds were now routinely excised, primary suture was delayed, injured limbs were immobilised using the Thomas Splint, surgery performed on abdominal and chest wounds as soon as possible and meticulous attention paid to the care of head injuries. However, whereas in surgery the Second World War was marked by consolidation of the innovations of the 'last lot', great advances had been made in the latest war in the fields of blood transfusion, aviation medicine, the treatment of burns, plastic surgery, military psychiatry and the development of antibiotics which would have amazed the veteran of 1916.

The British Army Medical Services were much more responsive to changing patterns of warfare than they had been in previous wars. The increased mechanization of warfare and the faster pace of fighting demanded more mobile and flexible medical units than those of the First World War. General hospitals and casualty clearing stations were too unwieldy and were replaced by smaller, more mobile, motorised field ambulances, which could follow armoured divisions quickly. Forward treatment, which had been pioneered by Arthur Bowlby in the last war, continued to be the basis of medical provision but was carried out in the field hospitals rather than at casualty clearing stations that were more suited to the static conditions of trench warfare. The confusion surrounding the fall of France and the evacuation of British forces from Dunkirk revealed the inflexibility of the casualty clearing stations which could not keep pace with the new situation created by the rapid, unexpected German advance. Casualty clearing stations were attacked by the Luftwaffe, overrun by the enemy or abandoned with all their equipment.[4] Wounded men were evacuated back to Britain before their injuries could be adequately treated and by the time that they were eventually seen the 'infection of their wounds was already of many hours standing'.[5]

The lesson was learned in good time for the campaigns in the Western Desert, where long communication lines made static hospitals almost redundant and field ambulances needed to be ever more mobile. Medical officers were issued with armoured scout cars so that they would always be able to keep up with rapidly moving tanks and be in a position to reach the wounded. Specialist surgeons were now able to offer earlier and more effective treatment.[6] One soldier is said to have reassured a comrade going up the line into battle that 'Half Harley Street is just in front of us'.[7] During the Burma Campaign, Corps Medical Centres, consisting of smaller specialist treatment units, were created. When the army advanced, the separate medical units moved forward and reconfigured themselves to form new centres. The lightly wounded were treated by these units and anyone requiring more complex operations would be flown immediately to base hospitals by air transport. This soon became the pattern in all theatres of war.[8] Once evacuated for treatment, the wounded could benefit from modern medical advances.

Much continued to depend on the calibre of the medical officers in charge of the field ambulances. In the heavy fighting against the Japanese during the Bishenpur and Imphal operations of 1944, Captain Henry Cockburn of the Royal Army Medical Corps soon found himself dealing with the casualties from three battalions only to learn that the field ambulance of yet another battalion had been put out of action by the enemy advance. Although the battle was still raging, Cocky, as he was universally known, organised search parties to bring in the wounded. By now the road to Imphal was blocked and the field ambulance was under continuous fire. Undaunted, Cockburn inspired the orderlies to form digging parties and was able to get all of the 200 casualties in his care under cover. He also ran the bullets of Japanese snipers to visit unit medical officers to ensure that the sick and wounded were receiving prompt attention and were being evacuated in good time for further treatment. All of his duties were performed 'with a selfless cheerful devotion and efficiency, often under fire, which inspired confidence in the troops and was a material factor in maintaining their high morale'.[9] His self-deprecating comment on being awarded the Military Cross was that as they were giving them out he thought he might as well accept one.[10]

The German medical services lagged far behind the British services. Axis standards of military surgery were inferior to those enjoyed by the Allies. German base hospitals were often dirty, short of supplies and full of amputees. Sometimes scissors had to be used as scalpels. Field hospitals were less mobile than those of the Allies and short of equipment and drugs. This lack of concern for military medicine had been apparent as early as the Poland campaign of September 1939.[11] It was especially pronounced on the Eastern Front after the German attack on Russia in 1941 when communications lines became overstretched. One soldier Leo Mattowitz found conditions in the field dressing station, full of men like him with spotted fever and the wounded 'falling over with their feet frozen, toes, socks hanging on them', as appalling as in the lice-infested trench where he had lain among corpses who had first appeared to him to be 'lengths of wood'. Evacuation back to Germany in a freezing hospital train was no pleasanter with men expected to die being offloaded at various stations en route to join the layers of bodies 'all of them frozen solid'.[12] It was widely believed that the Nazis had given little priority to the medical care of their troops:

'evidently the Nazis gambled their all on the science of killing, ignoring or under-estimating the value of preserving their own Army in the field'.[13]

The Russians were little better. The Red Army had a Military Sanitary Department with mobile medical teams but standards of care were primitive and brutal. The suddenness of the German attack in 1941 left Soviet medical arrangements in disarray; hospitals, equipment, drugs and transport were destroyed by bombing and doctors and nurses killed.[14] As the war went on, the hospitals continued to reek of blood and gangrene. Mutilated bodies were dumped in piles outside the hospitals and had cold water poured over them to separate the living from the dead. During the Battle of Stalingrad, casualties were ferried across the river for safety only to be left to die on the river bank for lack of attention. Severed arms and legs were thrown into bins outside operating tents in the field hospitals after being guillotined from a soldier dosed with too little morphine to deaden the pain. It was little wonder that Red Army soldiers made pacts with each other to assist their comrade if he were to be wounded in battle.[15] It was a far cry from Anglo-American medical arrangements with their forward surgical teams and swift airborne evacuation of casualties.

Aircraft were not only evacuating casualties but were also increasingly being used to airlift in medical teams for the rapid treatment of casualties. Parachute landings needed a different approach to the provision of advanced medical support from an army landing by sea or advancing by land. The Airborne Medical Division was formed in 1941 to meet the new needs of the 'cavalry of the air' with special techniques and equipment geared towards airborne attack. The first parachute field ambulance was formed in 1942 and by the end of the war there were five such parachute field ambulances and five air landing field ambulances. High standards of physical fitness were demanded from the nursing orderlies staffing these units and some were recruited from non-medical units and had to be retrained in medical duties. All were volunteers and about a third of them were conscientious objectors.[16] Surgeons, anaesthetists and orderlies jumped with the parachutists. Their equipment, including specially designed folding stretchers, trestle operating table, instruments, dressings, plaster of Paris, sterilisers, reinforced plasma containers, drugs and anaesthetics, was all dropped with them, so that they would be ready to treat the parachutists almost from first landing, though casualties among the medical teams themselves could be high. Much of the equipment had been designed by Major R. West of the Airborne Force Development Centre, which had been established in 1943. Specially modified jeeps capable of carrying stretchers and heavy medical supplies were landed in Sicily in 1943 by gliders.[17]

Aviation medicine as a discipline advanced enormously during the Second World War. It had been during the First World War that aerial combat had become a significant feature of modern warfare, and with it recognition of the special medical needs of airmen. At first there had been little acknowledgment that there needed to be minimum physical standards laid down for the aspirant airman if he were to be up to the demands of flying a fighter aircraft. Casualty rates and the loss of planes had been high in the fledgling Royal Flying Corps. One airman with poor eyesight, Second Lieutenant Bailey, did not normally wear spectacles but for flying had 'specially made goggles with magnifying glasses in them'; however, he was unable to see properly for landing his aircraft, the cause of a fatal crash. Eventually, by 1917, the medical evidence pointed to the need for much higher standards of vision than those initially laid down for pilots and observers despite 'the many complicated processes and the elaborate physiological and material mechanisms involved in modern Air Flying in War'. Alongside the recognition of the importance of good vision came the realization that 'co-ordination of hand and eye and other neuro-muscular adaptations are necessary' for success in the air. At the same time, it was decided to disqualify any candidates for the air force suffering from heart disease or syphilis.[18] It was not only the weeding out of unsuitable recruits that attracted the attention of medical researchers but also the physiological effects of flying at high altitudes where a lack of oxygen could result in unconsciousness. The physiologists J.S. Priestley and J.G. Haldane carried out exhaustive tests on acclimatisation to a lack of oxygen, Haldane spending fifty-two hours shut up in a respiration chamber to assess the effects of lack of oxygen on himself, but found that the only effective way of preventing altitude sickness was 'an artificial supply of oxygen' and the use of oxygen masks.[19] Haldane put the onus on the aviator to keep himself fit to cope with such problems: 'by keeping in good training, and in particular by practising walking, running or rowing, airmen can render themselves less liable to be affected by diminished air pressure'.[20] Martin Flack devised a test, the 'Flack Test', to identify men with a large lung volume and slow respiration rate who were less sensitive to the effects of altitude, which was used in the selection of flying crew up to the Second World War.

Aircraft flew at even greater altitudes during the Second World War than they had done in the First, yet oxygen equipment had hardly advanced in the intervening two decades. It was not until the establishment of the Flying Personnel Research Committee in August 1939 that aviation medicine assumed any importance in British military planning. Over the next six years much was to be achieved and the War Cabinet Scientific Advisory Committee was in 1944 to endorse the creation of an Institute of Aviation Medicine at Farnborough as 'of first rate importance, not only for the continuation of research in the physiology and medicine of aviation for the Royal Air Force, but also for the Fleet Air Arm, for paratroops, and for civilian aviation'.[21] One of the major tasks faced by the Royal Air Force physiological laboratories at Farnborough was to find a more effective answer to the problems of high altitude flying.[22] Oxygen bottles were heavy and delivered a continuous flow of oxygen even when it was not needed with the result that some aircraft could not carry sufficient oxygen supplies for a long sortie. Within a few months a research team led by Bryan Matthews, head of the laboratory, had devised a new oxygen supply system for the RAF, the 'Oxygen Economizer' or 'Puffing Billy', which used a rubberised bag and valves to control the flow of oxygen. By the end of 1941 the system was fitted in all new Spitfires and long-range bombers.[23] New, better fitting oxygen masks were also designed. A special one was made for the Prime Minister Winston Churchill's flight to Moscow in August 1942 to allow him to smoke his trademark cigars while the oxygen was delivered to his nose through what he called 'this damnable muzzle'.[24] The services of a Savile Row tailor's cutter were sought to help develop a pressure suit in 1941 as a possible solution to the problem of decompression sickness or 'the bends', though experiments in a decompression chamber showed that lightly built, fit young men were less likely to get 'the bends' than older, heavily built men.[25] Attempts were made to improve the night vision of pilots using glucose, alcohol, caffeine, quinine, strychnine, nicotine and massive doses of vitamin A but without much success, although popular myths about aircrew being able to see in the dark through eating lots of carrots was to be a good cover for the development of radar.[26] Once again the onus was on the men of the RAF to keep themselves at a level of fitness equal to their glamorous reputation as the 'Brylcream boys'.

The down side to the daredevil image of the airman was a high casualty rate that went with their dangerous role. In the summer of 1940 hospitals throughout the south-east of England were filled with aircrew from the Battle of Britain, raging in the skies above, 'with hands and faces coagulated, many under bad conditions, and usually already septic'. In many cases over a third of the skin covering the pilot's body had been burnt right away.[27] The pilot Richard Hillary remembered a 'terrific explosion which knocked the control stick from my hand, and the whole machine quivered like a stricken animal' just before he passed out when he was shot down. He regained consciousness and looked for his wristwatch only to see that his hands were badly burnt, 'down to the wrist the skin was dead, white and hung in shreds', and then he 'felt faintly sick from the smell of burnt flesh'.[28]

Such severe injuries were open to infection. The bacteriologist Leonard Colebrook doubted that 'we shall ever be able to prevent streptococcus infections of burns altogether as this organism is so ubiquitous and grows so readily in serous fluids'.[29] In the Burns Unit that he set up in Glasgow, he first used the sulphonamide drugs and later penicillin to control the bacterial infection as far as possible, although where the burns had become infected skin grafts often failed to 'take' successfully.[30] Moreover, the surgeon Archibald McIndoe was adamant that while 'in peacetime, early operation and treatment undoubtedly reduced its incidence', this experience in treating sepsis showed that 'this has not proved to be so in wartime', possibly because of 'reduced personal hygiene under wartime conditions, delay in transport to proper facilities, or, what is more likely, to differences in the mode of burning'.[31] Flame and blast burns were more common in the RAF and among the crews of tanks than steam burns. In the stifling confinement of the tanks, the crews wore as little clothing as possible, which made the burns even more extensive and horrific when the tank was hit.[32] Each tank crew was provided with tannic jelly preparations in its first aid kits and it was observed that men who had used these jellies usually did better than those who had ignored them since the burnt area had usually coagulated under the caked-on black 'cement' caused by the tannin within three to five days and the loss of blood serum had been stopped. Morphia would be injected to deaden the pain.[33] McIndoe, however, was concerned that the use of tannic acid on the hands, especially the fingers, could result in 'severe crippling in the case of second and third degree burns' and was in favour of treating such injuries with saline packs or hand baths.[34] It had been noticed that burns casualties evacuated from Dunkirk who had 'been immersed in sea water suffered less from infection than had been expected'.[35]

The Medical Research Council also advised against applying tannic acid to facial burns because deep black stains could be left on the skin. Instead it recommended the use of gauze impregnated with sterilised Vaseline for the face. Once the patient reached hospital, the burnt area would be dusted with an antibacterial sulphonamide powder and a coagulant, made up of silver nitrate and tannic acid or gentian violet, would be applied to all areas other than the face, hands and feet which were not to be tanned and were instead dusted with sulphonamide powder and covered with gauze soaked in paraffin.[36] Later penicillin was to make a difference, but in the meantime alternative treatments were sought.[37] A prescription for a paste for burns was unearthed from an old pharmacopoeia from St George's Hospital, London, but was rejected because one of its ingredients, 'oleo-resin', was no longer available and in those heavily food-rationed days another, suet, 'would be prohibited under present conditions'.[38]

Infection, however, was not the main problem for 'in the RAF pure shock, as a result of extensive burns, continues to be the most common cause of death'. It was widely believed that 'early operation with the use of an anaesthetic and cleansing of the burned areas' would limit the occurrence of secondary wound shock, but McIndoe's experience with Battle of Britain casualties led him to consider that 'since coagulation is rarely applicable to RAF casualties and sepsis can be controlled by other methods, it has now become a rare occurrence for burnt airmen to go to the operating theatre, and anaesthetics are rarely used'.[39] What was best for treating secondary wound shock was a transfusion of saline and blood plasma to replace loss of fluids and proteins by the burns victim. This method had been developed in the 1930s but came into its own during the war. Its success depended on the availability of blood banks and blood transfusion facilities, one of the main lifesaving developments of the war.[40]

Towards the end of the First World War citrated blood had been stored before major battles ready for use when needed. In 1938, the Army Blood Transfusion Service was set up, the first such organisation in any military medical service. It was set up by doctors confident in the knowledge that refrigerated citrated blood could be kept for several weeks. Under the leadership of Brigadier Lionel Whitby, the Royal Army Medical Corps set up blood banks, containing stores of blood and dried plasma, which were released and made available when needed. Whitby had himself been seriously injured in 1918 and had received a lifesaving blood transfusion before having his leg amputated through the thigh by the surgeon Gordon Taylor, normally a specialist in abdominal surgery, who had then encouraged him to study medicine after the war. Whitby's personal experience of the value of blood transfusion in one war was to inspire him to ensure that it was to be a lifesaver in the next.[41] However things did not go as smoothly as they might during the Norway campaign of 1940, the first major engagement of the war that British forces were involved in. There the only facilities for blood transfusion were available at the general hospital at Harstad and at only one of the British casualty clearing stations. This meant that wounded men were often left waiting for a considerable time before they received their necessary transfusion to alleviate their wound shock, a catastrophe that convinced the military doctors that prompt transfusion and resuscitation were essential if lives were to be saved.[42] An even greater test came in France when, in the nine days following the German invasion, the Blood Supply Depot at Bristol supplied no less than 990 bottles of whole blood and 116 of plasma. In the chaotic conditions surrounding the fall of France, many of the wounded who could have benefited from transfusion did not receive it in time because of the breakdown in the military chain of evacuation and the rapidity of the German advance.[43] By 1941, in North Africa bottled blood was being stored in refrigerators at base transfusion units and distributed by air to mobile blood transfusion teams under the command of Colonel G.E. Buttle. The surgeon J.C. Watts, serving with the Eighth Army, observed that whereas 'in 1940 transfusion had involved finding a donor, cross matching his blood to ensure against incompatibility, then withdrawing the blood into a complicated transfusion apparatus', time-consuming tasks performed by the field surgeon himself, now 'thanks to the masterly organization of Colonel Buttle, each group of surgical teams had a field transfusion unit attached, with highly trained personnel and supplied with bottles of blood by air'.[44]

Other armed forces took longer to establish front line transfusion services. As late as 1942 in North Africa, the United States medical services had to rely on plasma, which was of little value when dealing with severe blood loss, but from 1943 began to set up blood banks on the British model.[45] German techniques of blood transfusion were not as advanced as the British ones and it was only after the capture of dried blood serum from a British Army hospital at Tobruk in 1942 that these methods were refined and improved. However, very little attention was given to ensuring that blood reserves would be adequately collected and stored in advanced areas and the German blood transfusion organisation was to be disrupted by the heavy Allied bombing of Germany in the later stages of the war.[46] The superiority of British blood transfusion services was a source of pride to the British Army Medical Services which could claim that 'the German doctors themselves envy us our blood transfusion' and that 'what you the donors have done and what the doctors and scientists have done with your gift has been one of the greatest life-saving measures ever provided for any Army'.[47]

Had it not been for blood transfusion fewer men would have survived their wounds to receive further treatment for their injuries. In the RAF, 'the death rate will always be high, owing to the severity of the burns and their association with other injuries. The majority of fatal cases never reach hospital'.[48] Yet soldiers, sailors and airmen suffering from horrific burns and injuries were indeed filling the hospitals. Reconstructive surgery had been pioneered by Harold Gillies during the First World War and was to come of age during the Second World War. Then the surgeons had never operated in forward areas, but by 1940, it was realised that it was 'only by the early treatment of these cases that serious deformity and loss of function can be obviated or mitigated'.[49] Minor maxillo-facial surgery was now being carried out on badly injured soldiers in forward areas by surgeons and dentists before they could be transferred to specialist hospitals for more advanced dental treatment, skin and bone grafts. The *Vogue* photojournalist Lee Miller was shaken when one badly burned man awaiting surgery in an evacuation hospital in Normandy in August 1944 asked her to 'take his picture as he wanted to see how funny he looked. It was pretty grim and I didn't focus good'.[50]

Foremost among the hospitals where plastic surgery was being developed was the Queen Victoria Hospital at East Grinstead where Archibald McIndoe was to build on and, in popular repute, overtake the pioneering work of his cousin Harold Gillies, who continued with his reconstructive surgery at Park Prewitt Hospital near Basingstoke during the Second World War. McIndoe, a thickset, short-sighted, aggressive New Zealander, believed that 'with efficient and adequate treatment it is possible to push the frontier between the fatal burn and that from which recovery may be expected further and further into the territory of presumptive death' and that 'successful treatment is dependent on close organisation, intelligent medical and nursing co-operation, and adequate equipment'.[51] These principles he put into practice at East Grinstead.[52] The first stage of treatment for a burned airman under his care was for the wound to be cleansed and dressed with Vaseline or saline packs to keep it moist. The patient was regularly bathed in warm saline solutions kept circulating at just above normal blood temperature, which kept the wound flexible and promoted granulation or the creation of a surface suitable for skin grafting. McIndoe claimed to have pioneered the use of brine, but saline baths had been used earlier for the treatment of mustard gas casualties in the First World War. The baths were specially made of ebonite, an artificial form of ebony with an enamelled finish, so that they would not be corroded by the saline and had wheels fitted so that they could be moved around. The beds too were specially adapted with removable headrests that would allow dressings to be changed from all angles. Woollen blankets harboured infection and were not used. Special anaesthetic masks were designed to cover the whole face and so avoid putting too much pressure on open burn wounds. All of this demanded intensive nursing care, though McIndoe, a man driven by his devotion to his work and his patients, was not the easiest of people to work for and often bullied his staff in pursuit of excellence.[53] Yet his reputation and brilliance spread beyond East Grinstead. As a prisoner of war at Kloster Haina, David Charters performed plastic surgery with primitive tools and worked using diagrams and notes from McIndoe on the replacement of eyelids.[54] Back at home, McIndoe had created the environment, 'with a very strong staff, highly organised, well equipped and practically self-contained', in which he could reconstruct faces.[55]

Richard Hillary had been proud of his golden good looks before his Spitfire was brought down in September 1940. His eyelids and lips were burned away. When he arrived for his first operation at 'the beauty shop' at East Grinstead, he had drunk so much whisky to prepare himself for what was ahead that McIndoe suggested that a stomach pump might be needed before Hillary could be prepared for an operation to give him new upper eyelids from skin taken from the inside of his left arm. When his dressings were removed, his new eyelids were 'a couple of real horse blinkers' and the only way that Hilary could see ahead of him was to turn his face towards the ceiling. Soon, the skin had shrunk and he could move the new eyelids up and down. McIndoe next fashioned him a pair of lower eyelids but when the dressings were taken off he looked like an orang-utan. He was, though, for the first time since his crash able to close his eyes and no longer had 'to sleep with them rolled up and the whites showing like a frightened Negro'.[56] His next operation was to give him a new upper lip, using skin from the inner arm rather than from the leg on the assumption that he wouldn't have to shave if the lip came from smoother skin. He was disappointed by his new lip, which was completely white and had no central ridge. He also caught a streptococcal infection and had to be treated with Prontosil. Feverish and resentful of his facial disfigurement, he vented his rage on one of McIndoe's assistants. The ward sister calmed him down and McIndoe arrived in his theatre gown to encourage him to continue with the treatment despite the setbacks.[57] The fact that there were other men in the ward with worse injuries than his own shamed him, but his appearance continued to displease him as the scars were only too visible on his face. His burned hands were like a bird's claws and he was unable to use the cutlery in the officer's mess, yet he returned to flying only to die in another crash.[58]

There were limits to what the surgeon could achieve without the determination of these young men to live as normal a life as possible despite their disfigurements. McIndoe told the press that 'this is the happiest hospital I've ever had ... the patients are so cheerful that they do as much to heal themselves as I do for them'.[59] Most of the patients wore civilian clothes when they were able to get out of bed and dress themselves. Officers and other ranks shared the same ward and mixed socially without regard to rank. Crates of beer were secreted under the beds and the anaesthetist John Hunter made wagers with the men that he would buy them a drink if they were sick after he administered the anaesthetic. Popular entertainers such as Flanagan and Allen, Tommy Trinder, Joyce Grenfell, Douglas Byng and Frances Day regularly performed for the men and even the Hollywood film star Clark Gable visited them. The men were encouraged to visit the pubs, restaurants and cinema in the nearby town of East Grinstead and their acceptance by the local people despite their disfigurements helped to reintegrate them into the wider world. The men themselves formed the Guinea Pig Club in 1941 with membership confined to airmen treated at East Grinstead and the staff who operated on them, an association that still continues to give the dwindling number of survivors mutual support. It received its name from the comment of a pilot about to be taken to the operating theatre: 'What a life! We're nothing but a plastic surgeon's guinea pigs'.[60]

It was important that people with horrible disfigurements only partly made good by reconstructive surgery should be accepted by the public. In 1941, a film was made about plastic surgery in wartime to highlight what was being done for the victims of air raids as well as military casualties. The tone was upbeat as the surgeon reassured the audience that one young seaman who had been burned badly during an air raid while on leave would recover: 'he has taken a good long time to heal and we expect now to make him a very satisfactory repair of the upper lip and the cheek from his forehead'. Such techniques as skin grafting, the making of a new thumb by joining up the second fingers and the forging of a new nose from a flap of skin from the forehead were patiently explained in the hope that anyone seeing the results would be more understanding and sympathetic. One man, badly injured in a raid on Coventry in November 1940, casually told the camera that 'you'll notice my ear's gone – well my left hand pretty nearly went too'.[61]

Such insouciance and wartime cheerfulness was a front for public consumption. Privately, it was recognized that the wounded might have psychological problems in adjusting to disfigurement and to everything that had happened to them. The extent to which soldiers might be affected by the trauma of combat was believed to depend on the individual's predisposition to nervous disorders, conditioned by hereditary and upbringing, with men of a depressive, anxious or timid character being unable to stand up to stress although mild psychotics and higher grade mental defectives were believed to be open to training that could make them into good soldiers.[62] The psychiatric health of recruits came to be seen as just as important as assessing their physical health in determining who was fit for armed service. The Medical Director General declared that 'the first and main duty of the Medical Service is the maintenance of health and fighting fitness. The most important work in this connection is the maintenance of mental health, i.e. happiness, contentment and morale'.[63] In 1942, intelligence aptitude and psychological tests were introduced to identify which individuals were best suited to particular branches of the services and who might break down in battle. Both the German and American armies already subjected their recruits to such a battery of tests, which by the 1930s had become linked with modernist efficiency in many branches of industry. Psychology was seen as important in showing 'the aptitudes and abilities of soldiers for the many jobs to which the Army may assign them' and maintaining 'efficiency, both physical and psychological'.[64] However, there was great scepticism about the psychological tests designed to reveal the personalities of prospective officers; they were seen as too subjective and could lead to the loss of good officer material that did not fit into a preconceived pattern. Churchill was dismissive of psychiatrists and the Brigade of Guards, preferring to rely on such traditional values as character and upbringing, refused to join in the General Service Selection Scheme.[65] Some doctors continued to judge the calibre of the recruits they were examining by outward physical signs, one doctor commenting on the 'immense improvement in the health and muscular development in the young men' and their 'real beauty in features and appearances' compared with the recruits of 1914 but ignoring the need for mental strength in battle.[66] The Navy prided itself on the good psychiatric health of its men, which 'may be attributed to the good material which was until recently self-selected by expressing a Naval preference at recruitment.'[67]

The American armed forces put their recruits and draftees through rigorous physical and psychological examinations designed to weed out the unsuitable. Nearly 18 million young men and women were examined throughout the course of the war. Most of them were found fit for service, although sometimes remedial work might be necessary to render them so. In total, 2 million men were rejected for neuropsychiatric reasons that included homosexuality, while 4 million were unfit because of rotten teeth, poor eyesight and illiteracy. For those whose deficiencies could be made good, 25,000 army dentists extracted 15 million teeth and fitted 2.5 million sets of dentures, army optometrists supplied 2.25 million pairs of spectacles and special literacy classes were arranged for almost 1 million recruits. A quarter of all draftees of African American extraction were found to have syphilis, which would have disqualified them from service had they not been treated with neo-salvarsan. For many of the recruits it was the first time that they had received proper medical treatment.[68] Their diet was also greatly improved, with garrison rations giving them 4,300 calories daily; even field rations contained food supplying 3,400 calories together with a stick of chewing gum and four cigarettes. This made GIs stationed in Britain the envy of their heavily rationed allies. They were even allocated 22.5 sheets of toilet paper a day compared with the British Army ration of three sheets.[69] It was little wonder that American servicemen in Britain were warned about the privations suffered by British soldiers and civilians: 'one of the things the English always had enough of in the past was soap. Now it is so scarce that girls working in the factories often cannot get the grease off their hands or out of their hair. And food is more strictly rationed than elsewhere'.[70] Physically and psychologically, the Americans prided themselves on the superior fitness of their forces.

Many officers were unsympathetic towards any sign of mental breakdown. One battalion commanding officer asked the psychiatrist P.J.R. Davies, 'Why should I send these men to you so that they will survive the war and go home and breed like rabbits, whilst all my finest men are going to risk being killed?' Of more than 350 men seen over a seven-week period by Davies, serving in India and Burma, more than half were 'definitely unsuitable for battle'. The 'dullards, many of them with superimposed anxiety or hysterical symptoms' were transferred to the Pioneer Corps, whereas some of the more severely traumatised 'dullards and a handful of psychopaths' were admitted to hospital.[71] In peacetime, all soldiers who became psychologically disturbed would be discharged to a civil mental hospital, but from 1940 they were kept in the forces wherever possible 'to enable proper diagnosis to be made, active treatment to be given, short psychotic episodes recover and the question of attributability to be explored very carefully in each individual case'.[72] Nevertheless between September 1939 and June 1944, 118,000 psychiatric cases were discharged from the British armed services.[73]

Psychiatrists were now appointed in forward areas to deal as swiftly as possible with combat neuroses, manifesting themselves by such symptoms as screaming, tremors, hysterical laughter or tears and even staring cataleptic states. Army Rest Centres were set up close to the battlegrounds. The most common treatments were rest, reassurance and mild purgatives or strong sedatives. The role of the psychiatrist was to return as many exhausted men as possible to active service by 'debunking battle noise, the tank and the morale-destroying aspects of the dive bomber'.[74] There was a danger of labelling the survivors of armed combat, most of them 'unshaven and unwashed, red-eyed, covered in dust or mud from head to foot, scarcely able to keep their eyes open', as simply suffering from 'physical exhaustion' when there was little time available to give them a full assessment, though not labelling a man with a psychiatric diagnosis paradoxically often enabled those suffering from battle stress to recover more quickly.[75] Of course there was always the danger of a man being caught up in what Joseph Heller was later to call 'Catch-22'. An American airman could be grounded for showing signs of nervous exhaustion yet if he asked to be released from flying any further missions because of his mental state he would be regarded as fit to fly on the grounds that 'anyone who wants to get out of combat duty isn't really crazy'.[76] The other side of the paradox was that if a man was labelled as neurotic or hysteric, he would consider himself to be mentally ill but if his condition was just left without professional categorisation he would be more likely to overcome the effects of stress.

Even more important than psychology in maintaining good morale and mental fitness among the troops was the leadership of the good officer. Alongside good leadership often went an efficiency allied to an appreciation of hygiene and sanitation that maintained good physical health. The greater attention paid by Field Marshall Bernard Montgomery to matters of military hygiene than by his great opponent Erwin Rommel was reflected in the higher sickness rates among the Axis forces in the Western Desert than among the British. In the months leading up to the Battle of El Alamein, a fifth of Rommel's Afrika Korps were struck down with dysentery and their Italian allies were in no better condition, their positions being 'obvious from the amount of faeces lying on the surface of the ground'. British doctors observed that 'the enemy appears to have no conception of the most elementary sanitary measures and has a dysentery rate so very much higher than ours that [it] is believed that the poor physical condition of these troops played a great part in the recent victory at El Alamein'.[77] At Guadalcanal in late 1942, the Japanese were so malnourished and ravaged by dysentery that their defeat by the Americans was inevitable once military hygiene broke down. The hair and nails of many soldiers stopped growing and the buttocks of some of the men had wasted away to such an extent that their anuses were completely exposed.[78] An indifference to hygiene also accounted for the high mortality rate from diseases, including malaria, among Orde Wingate's Chindits in the jungles of Burma.[79]

There was now a strong insecticide available that was effective against mosquitoes, flies and body lice, all of which spread disease. DDT (dichlorodiphenyl-trichloroethane) had first been synthesized in 1874 but it was not until 1939 that its use as a powerful insecticide had been discovered by Paul Müller, managing chemist of the Swiss Geigy Corporation. Its first large-scale deployment came in early 1944 when a typhus epidemic broke out in Naples. The city was declared out of bounds to Allied troops, who were inoculated against the infection and had their kit regularly disinfected. Medical teams were sent into Naples with supplies of DDT to disinfect the civil population. Crowded air-raid shelters were suspected of being breeding grounds for the epidemic and mass delousing of their inhabitants, many of them refugees or people made homeless by the bombings, was made compulsory.[80] The insecticide was also used to control malaria in Italy and other theatres of war. In Italy many soldiers wearing shorts were bitten by mosquitoes and failed to take the drugs Mepacrine or quinine or use anti-malarial creams. Indeed 'men who had been in Sicily swore that anti-mosquito cream actually attracted mosquitoes'.[81] With the introduction of DDT, it was possible to disinfect kit and buildings with it and to spray malarial areas with from aircraft; such aerial dusting had to be carried out weekly 'or it will be impossible to control dangerous mosquito breeding'.[82] It was boasted that 'power sprays, DDT, aerosol bombs, an effective repellent – these, and the jeep, have made it possible for an Army to protect itself from malaria under the most difficult conditions'.[83]

Quinine, extracted from cinchona bark, had been used as a prophylactic for the prevention of malaria since the nineteenth century, but the Japanese occupation of Java had cut off the main source of supplies. Luckily, an alternative was available in the form of the synthetic drug Mepacrine, also known as Hydrochloride Atrebrin. This had been synthesised by German chemists in the early 1930s but the formula had been sold to America. Mass production was got under way soon after America's entry into the war and by 1942 Mepacrine was being made available to front line units in malarial areas. However, few soldiers, unless they went down with malaria, could be bothered to take it regularly and it was believed that it and quinine reduced sexual potency. It was only when decisive commanders insisted on the use of the available preventatives that malaria could be controlled. After the retreat from Burma in 1942, British forces were riddled with malaria and during the Arakan campaigning in Burma in 1943 very few troops escaped infection. Field Marshall William Slim, commanding the Fourteenth Army, made it a military offence to refuse to take Mepacrine and established treatment centres near the front line, thus both controlling the disease and gaining a military advantage over the Japanese as their drug supplies and discipline collapsed later in the war.[84] In Italy, General Alexander and his staff refused to take Mepacrine themselves even though it was a court-martial offence for the troops under his command not to take the drug. It was his advice and that of George VI that Winston Churchill was inclined to follow rather than that of his doctors in August 1944 when he refused to take the yellow pills that would save him from malaria, since 'even though he has only to press a bell to bring into the room the greatest malarial experts in the world … he turns his back on science and asks the King whether he ought to take Mepacrine when he visits Italy'. His physician Lord Moran only managed to persuade him to follow the instructions of the doctors by wondering aloud 'if General Alexander's views on medical matters have the same value as mine on military affairs'.[85]

In the Italian campaign, venereal disease rather than typhus or malaria was the major problem, as indeed it had been throughout the war. During the tedious long-drawn-out months of the Phoney War, British troops stationed in France had sought whatever amusement they could find whether it be with Polish immigrant workers, French shop girls or in the licensed brothels set up by the French Army.[86] On their enforced return from Dunkirk, they may have left most of their equipment behind them but they brought an upsurge in the incidence of venereal disease in Britain that was not so welcome and put a considerable strain on the local health authorities in the areas in which they were now billeted. The French Army and the German Wermacht, believing that sexual intercourse was essential for morale and for stopping frustrated soldiers turning to what were seen as such unnatural vices as homosexuality, might both have considered licensed brothels and the regular medical inspection of prostitutes to be the best means of controlling venereal diseases, but to the Allies this was unacceptable.[87] Anglo-American propaganda seized on the opportunity to contrast the wanton promiscuity of the Axis Powers with the greater purity and self-discipline of their own ideal of the good citizen and soldier, safely ignoring the practices of their own continental allies. Allied servicemen were told that in Germany 'venereal diseases strike at every fourth person between the ages of 15 and 41'.[88] Soldiers were reminded that 'you were transported thousands of miles to fight the Germans or help your comrades to do so' but if they were incapacitated by venereal disease 'they were not only useless … but are doing about as much as you can to prolong the war'. They were even told that 'a man can endure the hardships of war better if he does not go with a woman'.[89] It was not altogether convincing and what really made a difference to whether the real serviceman lived up to the chaste, ideal warrior was whether there was an opportunity for sexual intercourse or not. Men serving in populous areas such as India or Italy, which had the highest VD rates with 70–80 men per 1000 infected, were more likely to pick up a sexually transmitted infection than their comrades in the jungles of Burma.[90]

The arrival of American servicemen in Britain in 1942 had brought to a head concerns about the menace of venereal disease in wartime Britain. The United States Army and Air Force were alarmed that their 'young inexperienced men who had probably never spent much time in a large city' were at the mercy of sexually voracious British women while on leave in London and that 'it was natural that they would form an easy prey to the less desirable characters' of the capital. Only reluctantly was it conceded that 'many of the United States soldiers over here tended to show a lack of self-control and restraint'.[91] The Foreign Office was sympathetic to calls for the removal of the so-called 'Piccadilly Warriors' from the centre of London since open prostitution was having 'a really damaging effect on American opinion about this country'.[92] In November 1943 a new regulation was added to the 1939 Defence of the Realm Act to allow for the compulsory tracing of contacts and treatment of anyone found to be infected with syphilis or gonorrhoea. It was intended 'to bring under medical care those infected persons who … remain a constant source of danger to the health of the community and a drain on the man-power and woman-power of the nation in its war effort'.[93]

It was during the North African and Italian Campaigns of 1943–4, that the problem of venereal disease among the armed forces finally seemed to be getting out of control. Soldiers were not only catching infections in the many brothels of Naples but were also seduced by casual encounters on 'the doorstep' where they had 'bottles of wine thrust into their hands by these harpies or their agents'.[94] Attempts to put the brothels off-limits and suppress clandestine prostitution by the United States and British military authorities proved fruitless as did threats to punish diseased men with loss of pay. The Green Cross Chambers, disinfection chambers where a man could be treated with douches of potassium permanganate and perchloride of mercury and have his genitals rubbed with a calomel cream after intercourse, were so uninviting as to be hardly ever used.[95] There was a danger that men could get jaundice if the syringes used to inject them with salvarsan were inadequately sterilised between injections, a problem exacerbated by the rising number of VD patients at a time when new syringes were in short supply and there was too little time to disinfect them between patients.[96] It was claimed that ENSA performances in Ghent were of an unusually and exceptionally high standard so as to be a more attractive alternative to the delights of the Belgian brothels, but in Naples even the singing of a hugely popular entertainer such as Gracie Fields, said to have been the highest paid pre-war film star in the world, was no distraction from the allure of the prostitute.[97]

Within two months of the Allied invasion of North Africa, thirty out of every 1000 troops were contracting venereal diseases. In some units a tenth of the men were incapacitated at any one time by syphilis and gonorrhoea. More men were out of action as a result of such infections than because of wounds.[98] Something had to be done urgently. Fortunately there was a new wonder drug, penicillin, being tested on some of the wounded in North Africa at just that time by Howard Florey of the University of Oxford and Hugh Cairns, consulting neurosurgeon to the army. In August 1943, they tried this new drug out on ten cases of gonorrhoea with amazing results. The infection cleared up within twelve hours. Syphilis took a little longer but still only a week. Men could quickly return to duty, whereas even once a wound infection had cleared up there would still be a lengthy period of healing and rehabilitation before the casualty could return to his unit. It was obvious to the War Office that the new drug should be used to treat the biggest drain on military manpower but there were concerns about what would happen if it got out that penicillin was being denied to war heroes so that it could be given to treat sexually acquired infections that were considered to be self-inflicted wounds. The matter was referred to the Prime Minister Winston Churchill, who scrawled across the memorandum presented to him 'this valuable drug must on no account be wasted. It must be used to the best military advantage.'[99] They were fine words, but just what did this enigmatic pronouncement mean? After much consideration, it was decided that the treatment of venereal cases was the best strategic use of the drug. Such soldiers could be got back into action, in more ways than one, much more quickly than the wounded could be healed and this would make a big difference to military manpower.[100]

By June 1944, penicillin was the drug of choice for the treatment of early syphilis for both the American and British armed forces.[101] In offering a quick fix to the problem of wastage of manpower due to venereal infections, penicillin in the longer term was to encourage a loosening of the moral code and greater promiscuity. The Spanish physician Martinez Alonso put it succinctly when he wrote that 'the wages of sin are now negligible. A few shots of penicillin put you on your feet in no time (or whatever position you may want) and you can start all over again'.[102] With the loosening of military discipline during demobilization at the end of the war, the American forces feared a major epidemic of venereal diseases as a new generation of more self-confident teenage girls dubbed the 'bobby soxers' made a play for the men coming out of uniform, but this was averted only thanks to the greater availability of penicillin.[103] Similarly it was only the prevalence of venereal disease in the Germany of Year Zero that persuaded the Allied occupying powers to allow penicillin to be released for the treatment of German civilians. Although fraternization with the former enemy was forbidden, servicemen were seeking out the services both of professional prostitutes in the ports and cities and of the desperate and displaced young women who had turned to 'hunger prostitution' as a means of survival. Fears that the troops stationed in Germany would take syphilis and gonorrhoea home with them, together with newly emerging virulent strains of the streptococcus bacterium, and thus cause epidemics in austerity-weary Britain, forced a reversal of the policy that the Germans did not deserve the benefits of antibiotics in punishment for their war guilt.[104] Disease respects neither political nor national boundaries.

The drug that had seemingly saved the world from the scourge of venereal disease, penicillin, was undoubtedly the major medical breakthrough to come out of the Second World War. This 'miracle cure' had been discovered by the Scottish bacteriologist Alexander Fleming at St Mary's Hospital, London, in 1928, but it was not until 1941 that it was brought into therapeutic use. Fleming, an observant and meticulous scientist with an eye for the unusual, had noticed a fungus growing on a culture plate of *Staphylococcus aureus* which seemed to be preventing the growth of the bacteria. His further investigations of this phenomenon showed him that the mould, *Penicillium notatum*, was producing a substance he named penicillin, which might have a therapeutic potential one day.[105] Fleming, whose ingenuity had been so invaluable for the study of wound infections in the First World War, enjoyed the intellectual freedom to pursue his observation, but lacked the greater range of expertise, knowledge and experience and the backup of colleagues in other fields needed to develop his discovery into a practical tool of healing. Working with two research assistants, whose knowledge of chemistry was not much greater than his own, he was unable to stabilise the penicillin, which meant that it soon lost any power to do any good, or purify it so that it would be safe to use. It was only when a research team at the Sir William Dunn School of Pathology at Oxford began work on penicillin in 1939 that conditions were in place for these problems to be overcome. That work was to be rewarded, jointly with Fleming, by a share of the 1945 Nobel Prize for Medicine for the leader of that team, the brash Australian pathologist Howard Florey and the volatile German-Jewish refugee biochemist Ernst Chain. However, the key to the Oxford success had been multi-disciplinary teamwork, the bringing together of expertise from different fields to solve a common problem.[106]

The Oxford team had begun work on penicillin in the early days of the Phoney War, with a small grant of £25 from the Medical Research Council and a larger sum of $5000 from the Rockefeller Foundation for one year. Normally, Florey could have expected to receive funding for three years but to even receive a grant for one year was considered by the Foundation Trustees to be very much 'an act of faith, particularly so in the winter of 1939–1940, as England was moving deeper into the orbit of war'.[107] Initially, they were simply interested in it as an academic study of the antibacterial properties of a fungus. Chain was always adamant that 'the possibility that penicillin could have practical use in clinical medicine did not enter our minds when we started our work'.[108] However, as their research progressed and the threat of invasion loomed during the dark days of Dunkirk and the Battle of Britain summer, the practical potential of penicillin became more apparent. The turning point came on Saturday 25 May 1940 when tests on mice showed Chain and his colleagues that 'we had stumbled upon one of those very rare drugs which would not only kill bacteria in a test tube, but also in the living animal without harming it. We realised at once that penicillin could play a vital role in war medicine'.[109] So important had this work become that Florey, Chain, the biochemist Norman Heatley and the pathologist Gordon Sanders smeared spores of *Penicillium notatum* into the linings of their suits so that in the event of an invasion they could attempt to escape with the mould and continue their work overseas out of Nazi hands.[110]

Already wartime conditions had made the task of the researchers at the Sir William Dunn School of Pathology more difficult than it would normally have been. Norman Heatley, like Fleming before him, was a brilliant improviser and rose magnificently to the challenge of devising methods of stabilising, purifying and assessing the activity of penicillin using whatever came to hand at a time of shortages of material due to the war. Flasks, flat-sided bottles, biscuit tins obtained from the Huntley and Palmer factory at Reading, petrol cans and hospital bedpans were pressed into service for growing the mould, until special ceramic culture vessels based on the design of a bedpan, which had proved the most productive of the makeshift culture containers, could be made.[111] Rough and ready production equipment worthy of Heath Robinson was cobbled together from oil cans, food tins, bathtubs, dustbins, milk churns, refrigerator coolants, library book racks and centrifuges, prompting Chain to comment rather unfairly that 'a little less improvisation and more professionalism would have profited our work'.[112] In fact sound ideas lay behind the process by which penicillin was extracted in to amyl acetate and then back extracted into water by use of a counter current system. Impurities were then removed with the newly developed technique of alumina column chromatography. The penicillin was concentrated, at first by vacuum distillation and later by the relatively new technique of freeze-drying.[113] Six 'penicillin girls' were employed to maintain production in cold, damp, smelly unpleasant conditions for a lower wage than they could have earned by simply serving in a canteen let alone doing factory work in nearby Cowley.[114]

In wartime Britain, munitions took priority over pharmaceuticals and it proved difficult to get mass production underway with the result that the facilities at Oxford were to remain the largest penicillin extraction plant in the United Kingdom until 1943. Florey had approached the Wellcome Laboratories in Beckenham for help with production in 1940 but that pharmaceutical plant was already overextended in producing vaccines, antitoxins and blood plasma for the war effort[115] without taking on cultivation of a mould 'as temperamental as an opera singer'.[116] By 1942, ICI had set up a pilot plant at Trafford Park, Manchester, and Kemball Bishop, based at Bromley-by-Bow in the East End of London, began to cultivate batches of the crude mould to send to Florey at Oxford, after sending a biologist V.J. Ward and organic chemist John Gray Barnes, an Oxford athletics blue calculated to represent the acceptable face of commerce to the university, to Oxford to learn about production techniques.[117] Despite the regular night raids on the heavily bombed East End, the factory never suffered a direct hit, though the resulting contaminants ruined many batches and the staff working on penicillin production or firewatching sometimes saw their own homes burning from the roof of the works they were protecting.[118]

Frustrated by the lack of resources for penicillin production in wartime Britain, Florey and Heatley set off to North America in July 1942 to try to interest pharmaceutical and chemical companies there in the new discovery. At that time the United States was still at peace and, more crucially, had an immense industrial capacity. However, it was only after Pearl Harbor and the entry of the United States into the war that American industry showed any real sense of urgency. At first, the hard-headed industrialists heading these companies had not become involved for fear that if penicillin could be easily synthesised their investment in production from the mould would be obsolete overnight. Luckily, the Federal Government was more interested and the newly formed Office of Scientific Research and Development, set up specifically to prepare scientifically for what was now seen as inevitable involvement in the world war, had attempted to mobilise industrial support for ' a concerted programme of research on penicillin involving the pooling of information and results' and had directed Heatley to work on improving production methods at the US Department of Agriculture Regional Research Laboratories at Peoria, Illinois, which had been a centre of whisky production before Prohibition and thus had a knowledge of fermentation techniques.[119]

At Peoria a programme to increase penicillin yields that now began under the direction of Robert Coghill, Chief of the Fermentation Division was to continue for the next four years, work which could truly be described as the basis of all further wartime biological developments of penicillin. The speed with which the Office of Scientific Research and Development initiated this research was a reflection of the importance in which the work was regarded by the government of the United States as part of its 'medical defence plans'.[120] Heatley found himself working closely with the chemist Andrew Moyer on the difficult task of finding answers to the problem of producing the new drug on an industrial and economical scale. The relationship between the two men was uneasy and exacerbated by the anti-British and isolationist stance taken by Moyer as war approached, not an uncommon attitude in the American heartlands at that time but one which did not make for good transatlantic co-operation. Yet despite these personal problems, they were able to find 'a greatly improved method for penicillin production whereby yields are increased twelve-fold over those previously reported'.[121] However, it soon became apparent that this new method using fermentation techniques was not well suited to Fleming's mould. The search was on for a faster-growing strain of *Penicillium*.

At first it had been thought that only the Fleming strain of *Penicillium notatum* actually produced penicillin, but then the researchers observed that most strains of the chrysogenum–notatum group of *penicillia* moulds produced it in greater or lesser quantities. Under the direction of Kenneth B. Raper, staff at the NRRL screened strains of the mould sought from around the world with the help of the Army Transport Command until they found one capable of producing sufficient penicillin in submerged culture. Raper believed that there might be an organism in soil which could produce larger quantities of penicillin. As a result, samples of soil were delivered daily to Peoria from all parts of the world in bottles, paper bags and paper cartons. Good penicillin-producing strains of the mould were found as far away as Cape Town, Chungkin and Bombay, but ironically the best of all was actually found in Peoria itself. Legend associates this with 'Mouldy Mary', a worker at the lab given the task of searching for moulds, one of which she found on a cantaloupe in a local market. The records actually show that the sample had been sent in by a local housewife doing her bit for the war effort.[122]

With the outbreak of the war, the United States Armed Forces wanted penicillin and did not care whether it was produced from a mould or was synthetic. Following a wartime precedent set by the United States Department of Justice which allowed chemical, rubber and petroleum companies to freely pool and exchange commercial information in the quest for alternatives to rubber supplies now cut off by the Japanese occupation of the Far East, the Attorney General exempted penicillin from the operation of the anti-trust laws on 7 December 1943, an exemption given to no other drug. Until this time, pharmaceutical firms had pooled information but only by violating the legislation with official connivance.[123] Moreover, the War Production Board was able to allocate some building materials, raw materials and manpower for penicillin production, and encouraged co-operation.[124] Tax relief was given to firms to offset the risk of plant being made obsolete by the advent of synthetic penicillin. An 85 per cent tax on excess profits also encouraged investment in research and development. However patriotic industrialists might have been, there was still a point at which it was better to retain as much profit as possible rather than lose it to government coffers even if it was to support the war effort.[125]

Wartime necessity led to industrial collaboration on an unprecedented scale that was to be the launch pad for the modern pharmaceutical industry. The big players initially were Merck, Squibb, Pfizer, Abbot and Winthrop. It was risky to invest so heavily in this new relatively untried drug, but it was a risk that was to pay handsome dividends in the future. Each company played its part, according to its own brand of expertise or previous production experience. Whilst the work of the Northern Regional Research Laboratory had conclusively shown that the future for large-scale production lay in the use of deep tank fermentation, most of the penicillin being produced in the United States continued to be produced in shallow layers in flasks, bottles and pans. Merck and Squibb indeed concentrated on the enlargement of their pilot plants, working from the assumption that the drug would soon be synthesised and fermentation plants proved to be unnecessary.[126] It was left to a new player in the drugs industry to take the necessary steps towards establishing a commercial-scale fermentation plant. Pfizer, pioneers of deep vat fermentation techniques for the production of citric acid for the food and drink industry, adapted these processes for penicillin production. By 1943 Pfizer was producing penicillin in fifty-gallon tanks and in 1943 at Brooklyn opened the first plant to produce penicillin in 7,000-gallon tanks on a mass scale by submerged culture. Unlike some of the more traditional pharmaceutical companies, there was more of an entrepreneurial spirit at Pfizer, a newcomer to the drugs industry anyway.[127] Smaller plants were started by 'amateurs who seemed to be doing it as much for fun as from patriotic or pecuniary motives'. One of these was a firetrap in a basement full of flammable liquids presided over by a cigar-chomping, gum-chewing chemist, whilst another businessman was re-using old whisky bottles in a derelict Brooklyn factory.[128] Yet patriotism and government direction did not entirely overcome normal commercial considerations as Albert Elder,

Co-ordinator of the Penicillin Program from 1943, acknowledged when he wrote that 'Progress could have been much more rapid with a free interchange of material. One industry man said that as he saw my job, I was to go from one plant to another collecting honey, but I was not to distribute pollen along the way.'[129]

By this time, the results of trials of penicillin on patients had aroused greater interest from British industry and the British government too. In September 1942, the General Penicillin Committee was set up with representatives from the Ministry of Supply, the Army Medical Directorate and representatives of the main pharmaceutical companies to 'ensure that all the available knowledge of the drug be pooled and concentration and extension of production facilitated, even to the extent of government assistance if required'.[130] Pooling knowledge and resources, British pharmaceutical companies were able to open penicillin plants some of them in converted rubber vulcanising, cheese and dairy products and even cattle feed factories, spread throughout the country so that production would be less vulnerable to air-raid activity.[131] There was some discussion in 1944 about putting penicillin on the secret list as a 'munition of war,' but it had been so well publicised, as to which firms were producing it and where, that such action would have been redundant.[132] There was also a suspicion that not all firms were fully pooling information. The firm of Kemble Bishop, which had a licence from Pfizer for citric acid production and which had supplied Florey with crude mould, came under intense official pressure because it was erroneously believed that it had knowledge from Pfizer about fermentation techniques in relation to penicillin production.[133] Yet some government departments were not giving penicillin the priority it might have merited. The Ministry of Labour did not consider penicillin production to be a reserved occupation and were not directing war workers to it.[134] Lactose, essential for growing the mould, was being used instead to make milk stout and in the manufacture of baby foods, the latter vital to maintaining the health of the next generation.[135]

Penicillin was now the wonder drug of its age and the results of trials on soldiers by the pathologist R.J. Pulvertaft in Egypt in July 1942 and by Florey and Hugh Cairns, Consulting Neurosurgeon to the army, in North Africa in 1943 showed that it could indeed make a contribution to fighting efficiency. Men who might once have lost limbs as a result of war wounds could walk again. Even the largest of war wounds healed completely when treated with penicillin.[136] The Allied invasion of Sicily in July 1943 intensified the demand for penicillin in the Italian theatre of war, but it was with the

Normandy landings of June 1944 that penicillin really came into its own for the treatment of war casualties. The photojournalist Lee Miller, reporting on the liberation of Europe for fashion magazine *Vogue*, marvelled that 'the magic life-savers in the war – Sulfa, Penicillin and Blood – were augmenting the skills of the surgeons'.[137] Now men who would once have died were injected with doses of penicillin on the invasion beaches of 6 June before being sent home 'to live'.[138] Such treatment, costing an average of £1,000 for each wounded man, was not cheap but in spending so much on the care of casualties the armed services showed awareness of what was owed to the citizen soldier in return for his sacrifices in combat.[139]

There was one unintended consequence of the speed with which penicillin could help the recovery of the serviceman. Soldiers felt aggrieved at missing out on what since the First World War they had termed a 'blighty wound'. Where once they would have been sent home, casualties now found themselves in convalescent depots with completely healed wounds within three or four weeks of being hit. The psychological result of such rapid healing was such that the Director of Medical Services of the Twenty-First Army Group ruled that all men who had been in hospital or a convalescent depot for a month after being wounded would be entitled to a week's sick leave in the United Kingdom. Even so, these men still returned to duty earlier than they would have done in pre-penicillin days, an outcome that 'led to a saving of manpower, a reduction in wound complications and an economy in hospitalisation, in supplies of drugs and equipment, in surgeons' and nurses' time which it is quite impossible either to compute or to appreciated fully'.[140]

Although primarily intended to be for the benefit of wounded soldiers, penicillin was sometimes available for the relief of injured or sick civilians from the countries rapidly being liberated as the Allied forces advanced towards Germany. John Hofmeyr, a South African medical student, volunteered to join a civilian relief team to the liberated Netherlands in spring 1945 only to find himself in the midst of a typhoid epidemic raging through an ill-nourished local population. Penicillin was begged from the military authorities to treat seventeen-year-old Cornelius Fuyschott, one of the patients in an emergency hospital set up in a former schoolroom, who was suffering not only from typhoid but also from a severe abscess in his leg. Once news of Fuyschott's almost miraculous cure from typhoid got abroad, the relief team was inundated with requests for help from doctors, each of them with 'a harrowing tale of how he could save a particular patient's life if only he could obtain penicillin'. The junior student Hofmeyr had the 'heartbreaking job' of refusing each request because there wasn't even enough penicillin for the relief doctors to use let alone anyone else.[141]

Undoubtedly, penicillin played its part in the liberation of Europe and would not have been developed so quickly had it not been for the war. Robert Coghill, who headed the fermentation division in Peoria, spoke truly when he said that 'Penicillin is a more or less direct ... by-product of the war. It has probably saved more lives and eased much more suffering than the whole war has cost us.'[142] Yet, why had the enemy not developed penicillin themselves? Fleming had sent samples of the mould to German laboratories before the Nazis came to power when there would have been no need to refuse a request for it.[143] There was an abundance of published literature available on penicillin, which could be obtained through neutral countries such as Sweden and Switzerland, yet Germany failed to develop the drug from the mould cultures it had and continued to rely on the profitable and Germanic sulphonamides.[144] Interest had been shown in penicillin as early as 1941 when Howard Florey was approached by the Swiss pharmaceutical company CIBA for a penicillin culture and suspected that the Germans were after it.[145] However, there was little concerted interest in pursuing its development and separate groups of researchers failed to share their information. It was not until October 1944 that a conference on penicillin was held at Potsdam under Professor Rostock, the Reich Minister of Health, but it was too late since raw materials were in short supply and government support was still unforthcoming.[146] It was left to companies such as Schering which was working on 'an old strain of penicillium' originally obtained from Fleming but it was so weak that they were unable to obtain any penicillin from it.[147] At the IG Farbenindustrie plant at Elberfeld, a strain of *Penicillium notatum* had been found in the local forests but, although penicillin had been produced from it, it was not sterile enough to be used clinically.[148] Meanwhile across occupied Europe there were attempts to develop penicillin without the knowledge of the Germans. In France, there were underground attempts to produce penicillin from cultures of the fungus acquired before the war.[149] At the University of Delft a drug named Bacinol, which was later shown to be identical to British-produced penicillin, was developed surreptitiously and tried out in the hunger winter of 1944–5 in the Netherlands.[150] In Prague, there were attempts to develop penicillin at the pharmaceutical company of Jiri Fragner which had offered refuge to scientists from the bacteriology department of Charles University which had been closed by the Germans in 1939.[151]

It was not until the beginning of 1944 that Japan took an interest in the strategic potential of penicillin, after the surgeon Katsuhiko Inagaki obtained copies of German articles on penicillin brought from Germany by submarine. He and his colleagues at the Tokyo Imperial University School of Medicine obtained permission from the Medical Affairs Bureau of the Ministry of War to prioritise research into penicillin production. Soon the Military Medical College in Tokyo was also involved in the research project and money was allocated by the Ministry of War. A few penicillin-producing moulds were found from the testing of 750 fungal strains, which reassured those sceptics who had believed that the whole story of penicillin was no more than a propaganda trick of the Allies. After nine months of work on penicillin, the Japanese were ready to begin production by November 1944. Two penicillin plants were set up in a milk and food factory and a former silk plant and Japan seemed to be on the verge of mass production as a result of a well-organised and concentrated approach. All that prevented it coming to fruition was the collapse of Japan after the atomic bombings of Hiroshima and Nagasaki.[152]

If war can ever be said to be 'good', the Second World War had been a good one for medicine. Advances had been made in the fields of burns, plastic surgery, psychiatry and, above all, antibiotics which would not have been so swiftly developed and brought into use had it not been for wartime pressures. Major Anthony Cotterell, writing in 1943, believed that the 'harvest of suffering would be infinitely reduced by the progress which medical science has made. The picture has not just been improved; it has been transformed. In some battles the badly wounded man's chances of recovery have been something like twenty-five times as good as in France in the last war'.[153] Moreover, experience on the battlefield had shown that there were strategic advantages in paying attention to hygiene and the health of the soldiers. Compared with the Western Allies, Nazi Germany had a poor record in the medical care of its soldiers however much it may have been efficient in strictly military terms. Even worse was the record of the Red Army, the great waster of manpower. Yet, it was important that due attention be paid to the health of the soldier, sailor and airman, not only to keep him at peak military efficiency but also to maintain morale. In the democracies, there was an unwritten pact that the citizen would defend the realm but in return could expect the best available treatment if wounded in service to his country, an agreement that was to be increasingly important not only on the battlefield but also on the Home Front.

6

Road to Utopia

No one in 1939 expected it to be business as usual on the Home Front as they had done a quarter of a century earlier. Indeed, it came as quite a surprise when the anticipated carnage of mass air raids did not follow hard on from the declaration of war. The conventional wisdom was that the bomber would always win through and the sirens that immediately followed Prime Minister Neville Chamberlain's radio broadcast effectively announcing the failure of his policy of appeasement seemed to confirm everyone's worst fears − only to prove a false alarm for now. For once, this was a war that had been planned for in advance. In the months since Munich, the British Government had been able to prepare for a modern war where the civilian at home would be as much in the front line as the serviceman in battle. Unlike in 1914, the health care needs of the man, woman and child left at home were not forgotten. Planning was the key with the State playing a more dominant role than it ever had in peacetime and providing a model for a system of state-provided healthcare that might actually work after the war.

It was recognized that the existing and competing patchwork of municipal hospitals and voluntary hospitals, run as independent charities, would not be up to the task of providing the 290,000 hospital beds thought likely to be needed for civilian air-raid casualties. Government co-ordination, re-organisation and funding were essential if Britain hoped to survive the onslaught. The Emergency Medical Service was set up to achieve this. England and Wales were divided into twelve EMS regions and Scotland into five.[1] The committees controlling each region were to be given powers to commandeer beds in hospitals for the reception of air-raid and military casualties and the funding to renovate old infirmaries, build new hospitals to be housed in Nissen huts and to set up such specialist treatment centres as might be needed.[2] Later, industrial war workers would also be eligible for treatment. It was a radical and new move into the state organisation of medical services which was not universally welcomed despite the advantages of a 'centrally directed organisation of all health services from Whitehall ... from the point of a view of preventative and curative medicine and of national efficiency'.[3] The challenge of bringing competing organizations together was only possible as a wartime expediency, but on the approach of war the Emergency Medical Service came into effect with few major problems even in London, where the brunt of any aerial bombardment was expected.[4]

Planning had begun as early as December 1937 into how best to deal with the expected casualties from the bombing of London when a survey began into the number of beds that would be available in voluntary hospitals and county council infirmaries in London and the surrounding area. Within a short time the results were in and it was agreed in May 1938 that any additional hospital beds needed should be dispersed among institutions in outlying areas close to the main roads out of the capital as 'there was the certainty that several of the London hospitals would be put out of action'.[5] A committee was set up, chaired by Sir Charles Wilson, soon to gain greater fame as Lord Moran and Winston Churchill's wartime physician, to consider the mechanics of evacuating air raid casualties to the outlying hospitals. It was known that 'Wilson ... is a man who will be impatient for what appear to be results'.[6] The Wilson Committee assumed that there would be 30,000 casualties each day for several weeks and that the priority should be to evacuate casualties from inner London as soon as possible. Even so it was estimated that 50,000 hospital beds would be needed in the heart of the capital.[7] For this an increase in the bed accommodation in 'the fully equipped hospitals in the central area is the only practicable beginning', even though the aim was to move as many of the injured out of central London as possible.[8] Plans were also made to construct a ring of hutted hospitals around the edge of London for the reception of casualties once they could safely be moved from the centre.[9] At Harefield County Sanatorium in Middlesex, the Chairman of the Middlesex County Council Public Health Committee, Mrs. F.M. Baker, was determined that the construction of thirteen prefabricated corrugated iron huts should not spoil the appearance of her newly built showpiece hospital and insisted that they be erected at a distance from the main hospital buildings despite the severe inconvenience this caused.[10]

The most important recommendation of the Wilson Committee was that London should be divided up into ten sectors radiating out from a centrally located teaching hospital at its apex. Casualties would first be taken to first aid posts and casualty clearing centres in the danger areas for emergency treatment before being moved out by ambulance to advanced base hospitals in safer areas where they could be operated on safely. In the safety of more rural areas would be located base hospitals where more advanced after care could be given. The whole evacuation chain was very reminiscent of the system in use for the treatment of wounded soldiers during the First World War.[11] London County Council was more than willing to place its hospitals and ambulance service at the disposal of the Emergency Medical Service but some of the voluntary hospitals, fearful that they might be brought under municipal control, were slower to respond.[12] The nascent power struggle between the voluntary sector and the London County Council was resolved in June 1939 in favour of the voluntary hospitals when it was decided that the medical officer of each sector would be a senior member of the honorary medical and surgical staff of the teaching hospital at its apex and that the house governor and matron would be the sector lay administrator and sector matron. The senior medical officer of a sector had direct access to the Ministry of Health, authority over EMS beds and facilities in the County Council hospitals and the power to allocate medical staff to particular hospitals according to specialty and skills.[13] Yet the payment of doctors for their work under the scheme raised concern that 'it would mean the end of the voluntary hospital system if doctors in voluntary hospitals were to be paid by the State' and that 'it was coming near a State medical service, which would be a very great departure in policy' for the British government.[14] The dominance of the voluntary hospitals within the Emergency Medical Service may have removed what could have been a great stumbling block to co-operation within the sectors but resulted in less co-ordination between the different sectors since each voluntary hospital traditionally prized its independence from the others. Nevertheless, 'the outstanding merit of the Emergency Medical Service is that it has begun a process which total war makes absolutely imperative – a pooling and reasonable distribution of medical resources and scientific skill.'[15]

The London Ambulance Service was also reorganised and expanded to deal with the transport of casualties since this was recognized as 'one of the main factors of success or failure' for the hospital scheme in the event of a national emergency. The existing ambulance services were chaotic and were supplied by a range of organizations including local authorities, individual hospitals, the British Red Cross, the Order of St John and even some private industrial firms. In addition to using the existing ambulances from all sources and increasing the number of available vehicles, plans were put into motion for the requisition of buses, coaches and private cars. There was a plan to organise units of 75–100 cars for the collection of casualties since 'experience during the great strike showed that there was a waste of time and labour in having too large a pool undivided into smaller units'.[16]

All the planning and preparation of many months swung into action on 31 August 1939 when the railway companies began to prepare thirty-four casualty evacuation trains and the Ministry of Health requisitioned a fleet of Green Line coaches for the evacuation of patients from London hospitals. Anyone well enough to go home was discharged and anyone in a fit enough condition to travel was got ready to be moved out to a sector hospital. Only those too ill to be moved were to be left where they were in hospital. Sandbags were filled and put in place to protect the hospital buildings against blast. Windows were blacked out and strengthened with tape or wire mesh as a protection against the dangers of flying glass. On Friday 1 September the great evacuation was ready to begin.[17] It was an emotional occasion for many of those involved. At the London Hospital in Whitechapel, the nursing staff assembled on 2 September to be evacuated by a long line of double and single-decker buses to hospitals out in the country. One nurse, Margaret Broadley, observed that 'as we rumbled down the street the excited chatter died away, as if the solemnity of the occasion had suddenly dawned on us all. We did not know whether we should ever see the familiar surroundings again'.[18] Archie Clarke-Kennedy, dean of the medical college, sent off his senior students to some thirty sector hospitals after addressing them on their future duties, then 'as they gathered up their things and went their ways, I could not help wondering when or if I would see them again'.[19] One of those students was much more sanguine about his chances. Ebbie Hoff, an American student, had prepared for the hardships to come by putting on his loudest checked suit and his tin hat and had set off with his suitcase, gas mask box and a basket containing cold chicken and salad, proclaiming his determination to 'never go to war on an empty stomach'.[20]

Such scenes were repeated all over London as the capital braced itself for the expected bombardment that failed to come. Doctors, nurses and medical students settled down in their sector hospitals with very little to do in the way of Emergency Medical Service duties, despite pre-war predictions that 'their service would be in conditions of just as great danger in the first months of a war in London as in service abroad'.[21] Instead many of them turned their attention to treating local civilian patients as a way of alleviating their boredom, though they were only supposed to be treating war casualties.[22] Even before the outbreak of the war, there had been official concern about how to retain doctors in the service which was seen as much less attractive to them than joining the Royal Army Medical Corps and a recognition of the need 'to put the Hospitals Service in a position in which it will be able to obtain its proper share of doctors who should not be placed at a disadvantage as compared with those who may join up for service with the Fighting Forces'. The intention had been to create an 'Emergency Medical Corps, not with a uniform, but with some sort of civilian ranks and under some sort of discipline in the way that doctors will have to go where they are ordered to go'.[23] In order to save money on wages and so as not to have more doctors on call than needed, it had been decided that 'at the outset only a nucleus would be called up'.[24] Even that was too many during the long months of the Phoney War.

Clinical medical students were especially disillusioned by 'the scandalous way in which [they] have been treated by the Emergency Medical Service and the Ministry of Health'. At the outbreak of war, they had been assigned to the various sector hospitals to assist in dealing with air-raid casualties and also continue with their studies as far as possible. Until January 1940, they were 'paid for their keep' with free accommodation though they received no other recompense, but then suddenly, without any warning, were charged thirty shillings a week for board and lodging. One disgruntled student complained that this was an unfair imposition and 'who knows that in the near future we may not be submitted to the great Blitzkrieg and be expected to uproot ourselves and more to give our valuable aid to the Emergency Medical Service, free gratis and for nothing – yes, for nothing, not even a little word of thanks for standing by as we have done these last six months'; he was aware that 'all this may indicate that I have a warped mind and am not showing the true spirit of National Service in wartime or something' but it was a grievance that had to be expressed.[25] Moreover, the conditions in which the students were accommodated varied from hospital to hospital. Lucky students at Harefield Hospital enjoyed rooms in a mansion house with its cosy log fire, while others less fortunate in their billets held a party to warm up their cold, leaking-roofed dormitory in a former patients' villa at Park Prewett Hospital, and female company sparked heat even among the most chaste whereby such upstanding students as 'our gramophone boy, "Big-Jaw" Phillips, under the constant gaze of admiring women, fell from his monastic pedestal', although the presence of senior members of staff and the fear of a raid by the matron and medical superintendent put a check on any excesses of youthful ardour.[26] Such youthful high spirits, aided by beer, card games and cigarettes, kept boredom at bay.

Despite this there were advantages for the students in being dispersed among the sector hospitals with the more senior staff of their teaching hospitals. They had a much closer relationship with the surgeons and physicians than they would have had at their own hospitals where the honorary staff had the distractions of their Harley Street practices and attendance as honorary consultants at other hospitals to stop them giving full attention to the medical students. They were no longer being taught in large classes and received more personal attention, even though they perhaps saw less variety of medical cases. Charles Wilson praised such a set up where 'the teacher is always in the hospital and the student shares his day. And when the work is done student and teacher go to the same building, they talk and play together, they live together with incalculable gain to both'.[27]

Unlike the situation in the First World War, every encouragement was given to medical students to complete their courses and qualify before being called up in the Second World War. Just as the call-up of young men to serve their country was more orderly and calm than it had been in the last war, so was the position of the medical student now clear. His duty was to qualify as a doctor as soon as possible to meet the country's needs for medical services. There was no conflict of conscience as to whether it was better to be a doctor or soldier: both were needed. In Germany, medical students were exempted from military service although their university courses were shortened. This offered young men a way of avoiding military service and it was observed by the authorities at the University of Marburg that many students 'who earlier on would never have thought of becoming a doctor' were now entering medicine.[28] British medical students too were exempted from conscription until they had qualified and served as a house officer for up to a year. However, this exemption was not unlimited and no longer could a medical student take over a decade to qualify, idling his time away with games of rugby, card playing and heavy drinking so long as his fees were paid. Now, if his academic performance was unsatisfactory and he repeatedly failed his examinations, he would be de-registered and be liable for call-up. Medical practitioners were removed from the category of reserved occupations in June 1940, but attempts were made to minimise the disruption this would have meant to civilian services. The War Office was required to inform the Central Medical War Committee of the British Medical Association of the need of the armed forces for doctors. The Central Medical War Committee then decided upon a quota of doctors to be called up from each part of the country and local committees would then chose those most suitable for military service.[29] Inevitably there were disagreements between the British Medical Association and War Office over the degree of priority that should be accorded to military and civil needs and in 1943 an outbreak of influenza in Britain created a crisis and disagreement that was in danger of overshadowing the needs of the armed forces overseas. Politicians too had to balance the medical needs of the army and the much more visible population at home, not always to the interests of the military services.[30] For young doctors languishing in hospitals at home and awaiting their call-up, this was not the best use of manpower.

The frustrated sense of idle waiting was felt not only by those staffing the emergency hospitals. It was a common feature of the life of the naval surgeon, described by one young surgeon, Peter McRae, as being 'as good as it can when one hasn't a job to do'[31] and where 'the staple food, nourishment, business, hobby and relaxation of all the officers is gin'.[32] McRae was to see action when his destroyer HMS *Mahratta* was hit by a torpedo while escorting a convoy to Russia in 1944. Finding himself on an overcrowded raft with seventeen other men, he is said to have jumped back into the sea with the words 'I seem to be in the way here'.[33] In the popular wartime morale-boosting film *In Which We Serve*, the frustrations of the ship's doctor are summed up by the elegantly languid ship's surgeon played by James Donald when he remarks on 'years of expensive training resulting in complete atrophy: the doctor is very bored'.[34] In most ships, the doctor's duties were centred on them acting as wine steward in the wardroom, messing, acting as a cipher officer and censoring mail, except when treating battle casualties or minor ailments when the priority was to return the sailor to duty.[35] Yet even the non-medical duties could have a value since 'the doctor … can make himself very useful and busy in his capacity of being an officer, yet not bound by the same rigid code of his executive colleagues … responsible for doing all he can for their mental as well as their physical health'.[36] Moreover, the battleships did have large, well appointed sick bays with isolation wards, operating theatres, X-ray apparatus and dispensaries which would have been the envy of less well-equipped hospitals at home.[37]

With medical and nursing staff dispersed throughout the various Emergency Medical Service hospitals and beds kept empty in readiness for air-raid casualties, there was a shortage of hospital beds for the ordinary needs of the civilian population of the big cities. The younger staff at Guy's Hospital in Southwark avoided tedium by holding noisy parties once the evacuation of the hospital's patients had left them with little to do, though one member of staff, Dr Bishop, remarked that 'we who remained looked upon ourselves as a doomed garrison'.[38] At St Mary's Hospital, Paddington, only 105 beds were available for ordinary patients and 200 were reserved for air-raid casualties in 1939, a great reduction in the peacetime complement of 480, despite the Board of Management's policy of 'affording the widest possible facilities for the treatment of the civilian sick' so that the hospital might 'maintain without interruption and without serious modification the beneficent work for the sick and suffering which has been carried out within its walls for nearly 100 years'.[39] As the war went on, the Ministry of Health agreed to the provision of more civilian beds and by the end of 1944 St Mary's was providing 270 beds for the civilian sick, 100 EMS beds reserved for air-raid casualties and servicemen and sixty-six private beds, although civilian facilities were always liable to be curtailed during periods of heavy bombardment or when military demands peaked as during the Normandy landings.[40] Hospitals had little choice but to do as the Ministry of Health decreed. There was also far more interference from other outside authorities than would once have been tolerated since 'the L[ondon] C[ounty] C[ouncil] can dump on St Mary's at short notice two separate convoys of aged and infirm from bombed hospitals of their own. One of these convoys consisted of over eighty people who remained under our roof during one of the worst nights we ever had'.[41] Old rivalries and snobberies died hard even in time of total war.

The people of the larger towns and cities were not only suffering from greatly reduced levels of hospital care: other medical services for them were also reduced. Planning for wartime medical services in London had been made around the assumption that the capital would be emptied of its non-essential population and that all school age children would be evacuated to the safety of the country. Civil servants and the BBC were evacuated to spa towns and seaside resorts and many private businesses evacuated themselves and their employees to safer parts of the country, but the most visible sign of evacuation was the exodus of schoolchildren from London and the other big cities under a well-rehearsed government scheme. However less than half the number of expected evacuees turned up at their evacuation points. Whereas between sixty-one and seventy-six per cent of the schoolchildren of northern cities such as Manchester, Salford, Newcastle, Gateshead and Liverpool were evacuated, under half of the children of London, 393,700 in total, left the capital. Many parents were reluctant to send off their children to the care of strangers in unknown destinations for an indefinite period of time even if they might be safer. When the expected bombing did not materialise, a number of parents chose to bring them home and to reunite their families.[42] However, there were no schools open since the teachers had been evacuated with their pupils, no school meals or milk and greatly reduced health services. Dorothy Bannon, Matron in Chief of the London County Council Nursing Service had reassigned school nurses to other duties in the belief that they would not be needed.[43]

Evacuation also revealed the social disparities in the pre-war provision of health care. Host families complained about the 'dirty, diseased or ill-mannered children' they had taken into their homes.[44] Such criticisms were bitterly resented by working class families who had made financial sacrifices to ensure that their children were sent off adequately clothed and with everything they needed, as well as by middle class families whose children were billeted in 'poor dirty houses where they have to do any housework that gets done'.[45] In many cases the billeting officers compounded the problem of a social class mismatch by a lack of imagination in the placing of evacuees in unsuitable accommodation, such as placing five 'mental defectives' with a retiring seventy-year-old antiquarian who was forced to evacuate his collections of china and first editions to safety.[46] Many families were shocked to find that their evacuees suffered from ringworm, impetigo and nits, traditionally associated with dirt and neglect. In one Scottish town, all evacuees had their hair shorn regardless of whether or not they actually had lice. The London County Council claimed that only 10 per cent of evacuees from London were verminous, an underestimate of the scale of the problem, and the Ministry of Health put the high infestation rate down to evacuation having taken place at the end of the school holidays when children had not been medically inspected by school nurses for many weeks. Most people saw the infestation by nits as an indictment of school medical services.[47] Bedwetting was even more prevalent and was blamed on poor parenting and hygiene rather than the trauma of separation from family and home.[48] For the pacifist and socialist Vera Brittain, the health and hygiene differences between social classes would 'not disappear until the West End really knows and cares how the East End lives'.[49]

Pregnant women suffered the traumas of evacuation just as much as children. By the outbreak of war, three quarters of London midwives had been reassigned to casualty work and two thirds of hospital maternity beds had been allocated for the reception of air-raid victims. There remained few facilities for expectant mothers who wished to stay at home in the large cities. The arrangements for their evacuation by train and accompanied by midwives were efficient enough, but less thought had been given in the early days of the war to provide adequate maternity beds in the reception areas. Boys clubs, local authority offices, country houses and even the trades union sponsored Ruskin College in Oxford were hurriedly converted to childbirth and infant welfare facilities.[50] However, restful and comfortable the rural maternity hospitals may have been, they proved too quiet for many mothers-to-be, who missed the support of their families and the bustle of city life. Despite the dangers and lack of midwives, some of them would return home to have their children in familiar settings with their mothers and other family members in attendance.[51]

Back in the cities, the blackout was more of a menace during the early days of the war than the bombing it was meant to protect against. One of the earliest casualties of the war was a London policeman who fell to his death from a drainpipe he was shinning up to put out a third floor light showing in a doctor's Harley Street house.[52] Much more common were the minor injuries that came from people tripping up, falling off the curb or bumping into obstacles such as lampposts in the darkened streets, especially when it was forbidden even to carry a torch in the first few days of the war.[53] Fluorescent paint was applied to keyholes, debonair men tucked white handkerchiefs into the breast pockets of their suits and soigné women carried white handbags or wore corsages of artificial white flowers in vain attempts to increase visibility. Despite such artifices, road deaths increased as a result of the blackout. Over 400 pedestrians were killed on London streets in the last four months of 1939, twice as many as a year earlier.[54] For prostitutes, the darkness of the blackout offered opportunities to ply their trade unmolested by the police, their clients enjoying an added frisson from the risk of death by bombing as well as that of contracting a venereal disease.[55]

The ubiquitous fashion accessory in the blackout was the gas mask, first issued during the Munich Crisis when it was expected that gas attacks would be a feature of air raids. Babies and infants under the age of two were supplied with metal-framed rubber hoods, tied at the waist, which covered their head, chest and arms, and children up to the age of five were fitted with 'Mickey Mouse' masks held in place by harnesses. The clatter of a rattle sounding a gas attack was dreaded and decontamination teams were equipped with supplies of chloride of lime to neutralise the poison gas.[56] Air-raid precautions workers organised lectures warning of the dangers of 'phosgene that fills your lungs with water and produces gangrene of the extremities', of mustard gas 'that had hardly any odour but blinds you and eats your flesh away' and other gases that 'smell of geraniums, one whiff and you're a goner'.[57] Such lectures frightened nervous members of the public who imagined that they had been gassed; in Glasgow, an air-raid warden lost all sense of proportion after studying the effects of gas and, when he and others began to cough after the all-clear had sounded, assumed that he had been gassed.[58] Nevertheless before long, people became blasé about the dangers of gas attacks and stopped carrying their respirators everywhere with them. A popular song sung by the film star and singer George Formby, 'I Did What I Could With My Gas Mask', suggested alternative uses for them, including service as a child's potty.

Fears of gas attacks may never have materialised, but the realities of modern warfare became apparent when the first casualties returned from France as Western Europe fell to the Nazis in the summer of 1940. Virginia Woolf was moved when 'I saw my first hospital train – laden, not funereal, but weighty as if not to shake bones' and struggled for the correct words, 'grieving and tender and heavy-laden and private', to describe the vehicles 'bringing our wounded back carefully through the green fields at which I suppose some of them looked'.[59] The men arriving at the Emergency Medical Services hospitals from the evacuation at Dunkirk all looked as if they had come straight from the battlefield to a field dressing station rather than to a base hospital. Many of them had lost their uniforms in the sea and arrived at Ashridge Hospital in Hertfordshire dressed in an array of once smart business suits, black striped trousers, women's blouses and even draped in the Belgian flag, which they had acquired by various means, not all of them legal, on their way to the hospital. What remained of their uniforms had to be cut off. Men who should have been stretcher cases were coming in as the walking wounded and the stench of blood was pervasive.[60] The psychologist William Sargant was shocked at the number of Dunkirk escapees in states of 'total and abject neurotic collapse'. After not sleeping for five days and nights, they swarmed into the hospitals cursing the officers who they believed to have let them down and vowing that they would never fight again: 'so complete a loss of morale in some was scaring to behold'.[61]

The hospital system was soon to be even more severely tested as the Spitfire summer of 1940 gave way to the autumn Blitz. Not only were the London hospitals treating casualties at long last but they were also targets themselves. The attitude of their staff was resolute: 'we are bound to be hit tonight; but taking it by and large, we would not miss it for the world'.[62] It seemed as if 'we never see civilian cases other than raid casualties now.'[63] Medical students formed Home Guard companies to defend their hospitals and the adjacent area against enemy attack, an excuse for high jinks amidst the military exercises, undertook fire-watching duties on the hospital roofs and acted as stretcher-bearers during raids.[64] At Clayponds Hospital, two young doctors, Daniel Crawford Logan and Mustapha Kamill came on duty one morning to find an unexploded bomb in a ward. Coolly and calmly, they carried it out to a nearby field, wrapped in blankets and placed it in a tin bath, where properly trained bomb disposal squads could deal with it. It was valour enough to earn them the George Cross, though for Dr Kamill 'the day the bomb fell was probably the most exciting day of his life. He qualified that day'.[65]

The London Hospital in Whitechapel bore the brunt of casualties from the bombing of the East End. During the zeppelin raids of the First World War, the hospital had offered shelter in its basements to the local East Enders; now, despite being hit by enemy bombs, it never stopped treating patients throughout the war. A routine was soon established. Each evening during the Blitz, doctors, nurses and other staff would don their tin helmets and make their way to their posts. The house governor Henry Brierley toured the hospital during every raid; the doctors manned the receiving room, resuscitation room and the operating theatres; and the sisters and nurses attended their patients in the wards. The acting matron, Alice Burgess, was on one occasion knocked down by the force of a bomb blast and cut by flying glass while doing her ward rounds. The war could not stop the London Hospital from celebrating its bi-centenary in September 1940 with a visit from the King and Queen, who inspected the bomb damage and attempted to raise morale. That evening, after staff had enjoyed a 'rather better dinner than usual' to mark the occasion, a delayed action bomb fell in the garden at the centre of the hospital next to a statue of Queen Alexandra; it was left for six days before being covered with soil and detonated.[66] Throughout the Blitz, the 'old night scrubbers', many of them aged over seventy, always arrived punctually at six o'clock in the morning to clean the hospital floors, even if it meant walking from their ruined homes when the bombing had disrupted public transport, and only stopped 'to argue from time to time with their scrubber friends as to who had had the biggest bomb dropped near her during the night'.[67]

The same spirit was abroad at St Thomas's Hospital, whose Thames-side location opposite the Houses of Parliament made it an easy target for the German bombers. The hospital had spent the Phoney War perfecting its air raid precautions, but when the bombs came nothing went according to plan. The first bomb fell in the early hours of 9 September 1940, demolishing three floors and crushing two nurses and four masseuses beneath the masonry. The water supply failed and most of the patients had to be transferred to the sector hospitals. A week later on 15 September, after many other raids and heavy damage to the hospital, the air-raid sirens sounded as theatre staff were preparing to operate on a policeman suffering from acute appendicitis. Almost immediately after the sirens had been sounded, a bomb crashed into the basement of St Thomas's, killing three staff and injuring fifty-two others. The staff in the theatre, located in a former linen room in another part of the basement, heard nothing but felt the vibration of the blast and decided that it might be safer to move their emergency theatre further along in the basement when steam and gas began to leak from the huge pipes in the ceiling above them. The dispensary was completely wrecked with the contents of the instrument cupboards strewn among the broken glass and rubble, compelling the theatre sister to search in the dark for the instruments needed to continue with the operation as soon as possible. Meanwhile the alcohol and acids from the dispensary stores had caught fire. H.E. Frewer, the assistant clerk of works, formed a rescue party with assistant physician H.R.B. Norman and medical student P.B. Maling to find anyone trapped in the debris, administer morphia to them to deaden the pain and extricate them from the rubble. The following day, all of the patients were again evacuated. By 1941, the hospital buildings were so badly damaged that the governors of St Thomas's decided to lease the emergency hospital at Hydestile, Godalming, next to the King George V Sanatorium, to house its inpatients, though outpatient services continued to be provided on the original site amidst the rubble and dust.[68]

During the destruction of Coventry in November 1940, the Royal Warwickshire Hospital was bombed but it was impossible to move many of the expectant women from the wards to places of safety and babies were delivered while incendiary bombs hit the hospital and windows were shattered.[69] Similarly, during the destruction of Dresden in the firestorm bombing of 13 February 1945, some of the expectant mothers from the Johannstadt Hospital could not be moved to shelter in the basement of the Rudolph Hess Clinic but as soon as their babies were born they were carried to safety by the nurses, wrapped up to protect them from the drifting smoke, though many of the mothers and babies in the cellars were doomed to be buried alive in the rubble of the hospital.[70]

Only with the intensification of Allied air raids on Germany from 1942 onwards had German hospitals faced a serious risk of destruction from bombing. A belief that Germany would be safe from the air attacks that the Luftwaffe was inflicting on enemy cities meant that not only were air defences seriously neglected but there was nothing equivalent to the British evacuation of inner city hospital facilities to the safety of the countryside. During the firebombing of Hamburg in July and August 1943, when about 50,000 people were killed, most of the city's hospitals were put out of action. As the saturation bombing of Germany continued, the university clinics of Leipzig, Münster and Düsseldorf were almost totally destroyed and the municipal hospital system in Stuttgart collapsed. By the end of the war, most German hospitals had been reduced to piles of rubble.[71] During a raid on Leipzig on the night of 3 December 1943 the paediatrician Werner Catel and his colleagues tried to save their patients by carrying them piggyback through the inferno while other children lay moaning and bleeding on the frozen pavements. He was shocked to come across the head of one of his best nurses sticking out of the ruins of a tuberculosis clinic, her face 'frozen in fear of death and despair'.[72] Such scenes were to be repeated in hospitals all over Europe. The hospitals were not themselves the primary targets but were the victims of the indiscriminate bombings of cities and towns with prominent industrial targets.

Within the bomb-struck hospitals, the matron played a pivotal role in maintaining morale and providing leadership. At St George's Hospital at Hyde Park Corner, Miss Hanks, the matron and an ardent spiritualist, believed that the hospital was protected by 'a green light of safety hovering over the building' and urged her nurses to wear pink underwear that would radiate happiness, though this did not save the hospital from being bombed in 1940 even if the bomb did not go off on that occasion.[73] Across Hyde Park at St Mary's Hospital, the matron Mary Milne offered a much more robust leadership by which she came to personify the hospital in wartime. Combining great efficiency with a deep sense of humanity, Milne would visit each of the wards during an air raid and reassure the patients and nurses on duty that all was well.[74] It did not escape her notice that when she asked the student nurses if they had a torch and matches in case of emergency, most of them would produce a cigarette lighter.[75] Wartime conditions enabled her to encourage previously prohibited social contact between her nurses and medical students; she overcame opposition with the argument that if her nurses had to work with the medical students, they should be allowed to play with them too. If nurses were to be recruited in wartime London, it was necessary to relax some of the strict peacetime rules. She instituted a matron's ball and supported joint musical and dramatic societies. Her own fiancé having died in action during the First World War, she encouraged romances and marriages between her nurses and the medical students. On finding male students in the nurses' home she is said to have commented, with a strategic blind eye, 'I suppose you are all busy fire watching, gentlemen'.[76]

The problem of nurse recruitment was highlighted in the 1943 film *The Lamp Still Burns*, where the petty restrictions imposed on nurses by the more conservative and autocratic of matrons are shown as deterring new recruits and driving many trained nurses from the system. In the film an architect played by Rosamund John retrains as a nurse but fights against the strict and sometimes pointless rules imposed on her, yet the heroic nature of the nursing tradition begun by Florence Nightingale is still highlighted.[77] Recruitment posters for nursing stressed the valiant image of 'the women of today' who had kept the flame lit at Scutari 'burning brightly not only in France, Egypt and Greece but in Poplar, Portsmouth, Liverpool, Hull and all other battlefields of the Home Front.'[78] Nurse recruitment was indeed a matter of great concern throughout the war. The recruitment of trained nurses into the military nursing services caused severe staff shortages in many civilian hospitals, especially when the more experienced of the senior nurses joined up. In the fields of midwifery, tuberculosis and mental health nursing, such shortages were particularly acute. As a result of this more and more assistant nurses were being employed to fill in the gaps. The public needed to be reassured that these assistants were proper nurses even if they had not passed their state registration examinations. The 1943 Nurses Act established a new grade of state enrolled nurse, less academically qualified than the state registered nurses but who could be relied upon to provide sound, practical nursing.[79] State enrolment was resisted by many members of the nursing profession, who saw it as a dilution of labour and an erosion of their hard-won professional status.[80] The feeling that the status of the nurse was threatened was reinforced by the establishment of nursing cadets for girls aged over fifteen but below the age of eighteen, when they could start nurse training. This was one of the recommendations of the McCorquodale National Advisory Council for the Recruitment and Distribution of Nurses and Midwives aimed at relieving the nursing shortage.[81] Much more popular were the recommendations of the Rushcliffe Committee on Nurse's Salaries, which called for a national pay structure for all nurses. The grants made to the voluntary hospitals were to be conditional on acceptance of a state imposed salary level.[82] Improved conditions and wages, coupled with the new grades of nurse, helped to ease the problem of recruiting nurses but there still remained an unresolved conflict between civil and military needs.

A different solution had been found to the nursing shortage in the United States with the establishment of a Cadet Nurse Corps by the Bolton Act of Congress in June 1943. Students enrolled in the Cadet Corps received an accelerated training programme and had their fees, text books and wages paid for them by the federal government in return for agreeing to serve in the army or vital nursing services for the duration of the war. In many hospitals student nurses in the military style uniforms and berets of the Corps outnumbered those in 'starch and stripes'. Their military bearing complemented the equally visible presence of soldiers and sailors in training. In Chicago, student cadet nurses formed 'dates committees' to request uniformed escorts from the Great Lakes Naval Base to take them to dances.[83] Civilian hospitals also relied heavily upon volunteers to supplement their depleted nursing and medical staff. At Wesley Memorial Hospital in Chicago, a plethora of voluntary groups kept the hospital going during the war. The American Red Cross supplied members of the Nurse Aide Corps, all of whom could boast eighty hours of training, to carry out basic ancillary nursing tasks in order to free nurses for more specialised, professional duties. The Men's Volunteer Corps assisted nurses in the operating rooms and on the male wards. The Junior Army and Navy Guild Organization, made up of the wives, daughters and sisters of military and naval officers donned patriotic red, white and blue uniforms to serve in wards set aside for military patients. The American Women's Voluntary Services supplied volunteers to work in the pharmacy and laboratories as well as to undertake clerical work, roll bandages and make dressings.. Meanwhile, a group styling themselves the 'Victory Volunteers' did whatever else needed to be done. Undoubtedly 'many hospitals would have had to close their doors were it not for the Victory Volunteers', as Wesley Memorial's superintendent Edgar Blake admitted at the end of the war.[84] At nearby Passavant Memorial Hospital, Dr Irving S. Cutter in July 1942 complained that the call-up of staff 'leaves us stripped to the bare ribs. Without exception every available man is gone. The balance are either cripples or must be considered indispensable'.[85] Acute as this staffing shortage was in the United States, far removed from the theatres of war, it was front line Britain that had suffered more.

Not only were nurses in Britain needed to treat the casualties of the Blitz, but also vital was blood for transfusion. Just as the armed forces had set up a blood transfusion service so did the Emergency Medical Service. At first the Emergency Blood Transfusion Service, the forerunner of the modern National Blood Transfusion Service, was small-scale and concerned with maintaining lists of volunteer blood donors, but in July 1938 the Medical Research Council set up four depots in London for the collection, storage and supply of blood. The scheme was extended to the rest of the country in July 1940 with the formation of a regional blood transfusion service with centres in every civil defence region.[86] Although primarily intended 'to meet civilian casualty requirements', there was 'closer liaison with the Fighting Services' as the war progressed.[87] Great demands were made by the armed forces in the aftermath of Dunkirk, but the demand for transfusions for civilians rose considerably once the air raids on London began. Paradoxically though, 'since air raids have become more frequent the response has not been so good' from donors, presumably on account of the difficulties of attending donor sessions in the midst of competing demands on the individual.[88] Transfusion was vital for the treatment of cases of shock among air raid casualties.[89]

Walking air-raid casualties preferred to attend first aid posts set up in the hospitals rather than ones set up in schools or civic buildings because they expected to get more immediate and better medical treatment.[90] They had a point as many doctors were themselves concerned that 'there was too much first aid being done without reference to a doctor', including one case where a first-aider was 'using the arm of a casualty like a pump, looking for a fracture, because he had been taught to look out for crepitus[91] as a sign of a fracture'.[92] Generally, the first treatment a casualty received on arrival at such first aid posts was a cup of tea and a cigarette, often accompanied by a painkiller.[93] Afterwards all that could be done was to apply simple dressings, treat the patient for shock, administer morphia and send him or her off to a hospital. Where there were no suitable buildings available, mobile first-aid units actually treated the casualties in their vehicles. One mobile unit operating in Newport was called to rescue 'a small child whose voice only could be heard' until 'sufficient debris was removed to expose an arm'. The child's pulse was weak and the doctor, Wade Thomas, was uncertain about how much morphia to inject into such a small child, but took the risk of guessing and was rewarded by the casualty making an excellent recovery.[94]

Civilians caught up in the air raids and confronting 'war in its most brutal savagery' often felt powerless in the authoritative presence of Air Raid Precautions Workers and nurses, many of whom barked out instructions in 'a concise, firm business-like voice, as if she was talking to a Mother's meeting'.[95] When eighteen-year-old city clerk Colin Perry, incongruously clad in his well-tailored office suit and conscious of lacking the protection of a steel helmet, came across casualties during a night time raid near his home in South London in October 1940 he felt inadequate because 'I knew no first aid, and I had never before so much wanted to be a doctor'.[96] Faced with an injured child crying for his mother, a young woman with blood oozing from her scalp and an old lady with a two-inch long red mark where a piece of shrapnel had become embedded in her leg, there was little that Perry could do but watch the professionals at work. The difficulties facing these doctors, nurses and ARP workers was not helped by the growing tendency for people to treat the first-aid posts as outpatient departments and seek treatment for such conditions as diabetes or 'the first stage of labour which commenced in a public shelter'.[97]

The air-raid shelters were themselves becoming matters of concern about public health. The journalist Ritchie Calder declared that 'the foetid atmosphere of most of them was like the germ incubation rooms of a bacteriological laboratory; only the germs were not in sealed flasks, but hit you in the face in a mixed barrage'.[98] Doctors were afraid of outbreaks of lice-born typhoid, cerebro-spinal meningitis and influenza, but fortunately these fears were not realized. Measures were put in place to counteract some of the effects of gross overcrowding in the shelters, with regular cleaning and inspection of them. By October 1940, chemical toilets had been installed in almost all the large London shelters, but these were easily knocked over, spreading excrement over the floors. Some local authorities began to install waterborne sanitation in the larger shelters, but the lack of washing facilities remained a problem for the shelterers who had to find public baths in which to wash and shave if they did not have time to make the trek home before setting off to work again.[99] Medical Aid Posts, staffed by unpaid auxiliary nurses, were also established in some of the deep tunnel shelters to act as 'watching posts for the outbreak of disease' and provide 'treatment for cases of sudden illness or accident' among the shelterers.[100] It was recognised that allocating space for first-aid facilities would mean that fewer people could take shelter from the bombs, but the benefit of offering medical aid outweighed the reduction in capacity.[101] However, the Medical Aid Posts could not solve all problems, since 'access to these tubes will be somewhat difficult and tedious and should they become infested with vermin the difficulties are going to be very great'.[102] It was little wonder that Colin Perry, working in the heart of the blitzed City of London, preferred to take his chances in the open rather than risk the chance of catching something in the airless, stuffy, stifling 'tunnel of disease' that Bank underground station and the other public shelters represented.[103]

Before the war it had been assumed that the stresses of wartime life would produce 'one vast raving Bedlam' among the civilian population, but to the surprise of the psychiatrists most people proved more resilient. One young woman aged seventeen was the only survivor, except for her friend who had had an epileptic fit during the ordeal, of a direct hit on a public house. She suffered from headaches for weeks afterwards until an injection of the drug evipan enabled her to relive the horror she was suppressing: 'there is a man's head under the piano. It's horrible. I'm going mad'. Yet, having described what she had witnessed, she 'recovered well'.[104] Casualties, showing signs of disturbance, were told that 'their reaction was due to fear' shared by everyone else and that it was their duty to 'return to their normal work and resist the temptation to exaggerate the experiences through which they had passed'.[105] Little encouragement was given to people to come forward with psychiatric problems since the emphasis was on 'carrying on normally'. After a big raid, the main psychiatric problem tended to be that of 'coping with the early senile cases who had become maladjusted and mental defectives who should long ago have been institutionalised'.[106] For most people, the greatest problem was 'the utter dreariness of war on the home front' and the difficulty of maintaining good spirits amidst the frustrations and privations of daily life and the fears of what a raid could bring.[107] Morale was further maintained through the indefatigable bomb site and hospital visiting of George VI and Queen Elizabeth, though St Mary's Hospital went overboard in 1940 when its annual report expressed 'deep sympathy with Her Majesty the Queen, as President of the Hospital, in the ordeal through which the Royal Family are passing, together with so many of their subjects, during the intense bombardment of London'.[108] For many of those subjects who lost all their possessions and family in the bombing, it was the loss of home that angered and bewildered them more than the loss of friends or relations according to a secret government report, because they had lost all sense of individual identity.[109]

As more homes suffered from war damage and a lack of maintenance due to the shortage of building materials and labourers, more people faced the problem of 'rheumatism, coughs, colds and all kinds of ailment, due to dampness and draughts, while he waits for his claim to be paid and a licence for further essential work ... it is a blessing ... that those responsible for the strategy of the war are gifted with more drive and initiative than those whose job is to care for the bombed and blasted homes of the civil population'.[110] The Chief Medical Officer of the Department of Health in 1943 calculated 'the vast loss of hours of work to the national war effort' from influenza and the common cold 'as equivalent to the loss of 3,500 tanks, 1,000 bombers and 1,000,000 rifles in one year'.[111] It was not even as if extra clothing was always available to keep the civilian warm. When clothes rationing was first introduced in 1941, a man had enough coupons in one year to replace the suit, shirt, tie, shoes and underwear in which he stood, but this allocation was reduced in 1942 so drastically that it would have taken two years to replenish such a wardrobe and even longer if he needed a new winter overcoat. Women found it even harder to manage with their clothing ration and had to make do and mend if they wanted to eke out an inadequate allocation, blankets being refashioned as overcoats and the better quality pre-war suits of many husbands now in military uniform being turned into tailored frocks, skirts and winter outfits for their wives 'if you are quite sure he won't want them again after the war'.[112] Shabbiness may have been patriotic, but what really mattered was being sufficiently clad to stay healthy.

Poor living conditions were exacerbated by food shortages, though attempts were made to overcome dietary deficiencies through the rationing system and campaigns to encourage the housewife to make the most of what foodstuffs were available. Digging for Victory became a duty. When industrial workers complained about the lack of meat in their diet, Elsie and Doris Waters, in character as the popular radio cockney charladies Gert and Daisy, gave cookery tips on how to use leftovers and vegetables as alternatives to meat, while Dr Charles Hill in his role as the 'Radio Doctor' dispensed slightly more professional dietary advice.[113] However, for those wealthy enough to eat at restaurants food was unrationed except by price; and less prosperous sections of the population resented the society figures, affluent businessmen and slick traders in noticeably expensive new suits seen emerging from the smart restaurants.[114] For the less well off in the cities, cheap off-ration meals were available in the British Restaurants, first set up in 1940 to provide hot meals for the victims of the bombing but soon extended throughout the country.[115] Vulnerable members of society in need of extra vitamins to maintain their health were given special rations. Pregnant women were given extra rations of dried eggs, milk and vitamin supplements and had priority entitlement to such luxuries as oranges and bananas if they were ever available 'to ensure your health and that of your child'. Children were given milk at school and were also dosed with orange juice and cod liver oil to keep them healthy.[116]

Medicines, as well as foodstuffs, were in short supply, with priority being given to the armed forces. In Germany there were restrictions on the use of imported drugs and directives on the economical use of bandages from the beginning of the war. Insulin, chloroform and morphine were to be used sparingly in the absence of synthetics and became almost unavailable for civilian use while military needs for them were heavy during the siege of Stalingrad. There was a greater emphasis on the use of herbal medicines that tied in with Nazi beliefs in natural folk medicine. By 1942 glass was in short supply with the result that thermometers, syringes, bottles and test tubes were difficult to obtain.[117] In Britain the new wonder drug penicillin was for a long time denied to civilians: so long as there was not enough of it available for military use, civilians would have to wait. Even by 1944 when production made it possible to use the drug widely on casualties from the liberation of Europe, it was only possible to release it for use in cases that would extend knowledge of its use. It was not to be used to save lives or for any humanitarian use, but only for clinical trials.[118] When it was used to treat as prominent a patient as Sir Montagu Norman, Governor of the Bank of England, who was suffering from pneumococcal meningitis, great pains were taken to stress that he was acting as 'a human assay' and had not been given it because of his influential friends.[119] In the United States, the redoubtable Eleanor Roosevelt attempted to obtain it to save the life of the dying sweetheart of a serving American soldier, even though it would have had little effect.[120]

For most doctors and nurses on the Home Front, their first experience of the new drug about which they had heard so much came when the casualties from the Normandy landings flooded into the Emergency Medical Service hospitals after D-Day, 6 June 1944. At the base hospital at Basingstoke, the wounded were treated in a hectic atmosphere, where 'arms were sent upstairs and legs downstairs'. Intra-muscular injections of penicillin were given by medical students at three-hourly intervals, duties later taken over by the nurses. The results were 'miraculous'.[121] At Queen Alexandra's Hospital, Portsmouth, one badly burned soldier from the Normandy beaches told the nurse that 'I'm quite good-looking really' and asked her for a kiss and although it was against all the rules 'I bent down and kissed him on his horribly burned lips with the awful smell coming off his burns'.[122] For this soldier penicillin would be a lifesaver. So long as it remained in short supply, there was something of a penicillin mania with talk of such wonders to come with the peace as penicillin toothpaste and penicillin lipstick to be marketed for 'that hygienic kiss' and the possibility to 'kiss whom you like, when you like, how you like and avoid all the consequences except matrimony'.[123]

For the disabled soldier, the post-war world did not always appear so rosy. The charities set up to look after the needs of the disabled serviceman in the First World War, such as St Dunstan's and the Star and Garter Home, continued to deal with the needs of a new generation of disabled. Nevertheless, the trauma of adjustment to physical disabilities remained, allied to the general psychological stress for the ex-serviceman of adjusting to 'Civvie Street'. One of the most popular films of 1946 dealt with just this very problem in the United States. *The Best Years of Our Lives* told the story of three war veterans returning to small-town America. One of them, Homer Parrish, played by a real-life amputee Harold Russell, has lost his hands in a naval battle and is embarrassed and angry when he can not control his hooks as well as he could have done his own hands. He mistakes the love of his pre-war sweetheart for pity and a misplaced sensed of duty but it is her determination to marry him despite his disability which finally makes him accept the loss of his hands. The other two demobilised soldiers have less severe adjustments to make, in their cases psychological ones. The banker Al Stephenson played by Frederic March turns to drink in the face of the independence shown by his wife and children in the years he was away at the war, though it is again the common sense of his wife, portrayed by Myrna Loy as the humorous, wise and practical help-mate, that is his

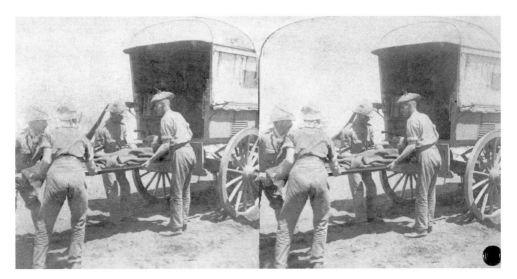

1 A stereoscopic photograph of Boer War casualties who, after fighting on the Modder River, are lifted by stretcher bearers into an ambulance. (Australian War Memorial, P00044.023)

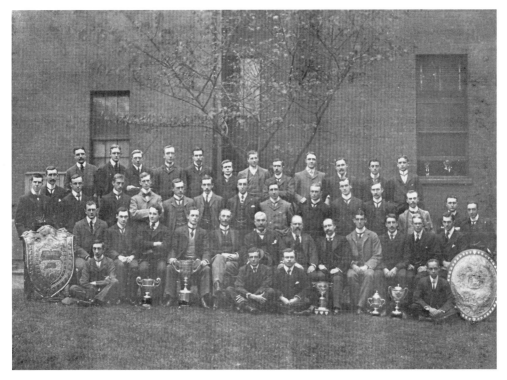

2 In the wake of the Boer War sporting activity was essential in promoting manliness for national efficiency: the fresh-faced young doctors and students of St Mary's Hospital Medical School, celebrating their success on the sports field in 1900, were all to be hardened tending the wounded on the First World War battlefields. (St Mary's Hospital Archives)

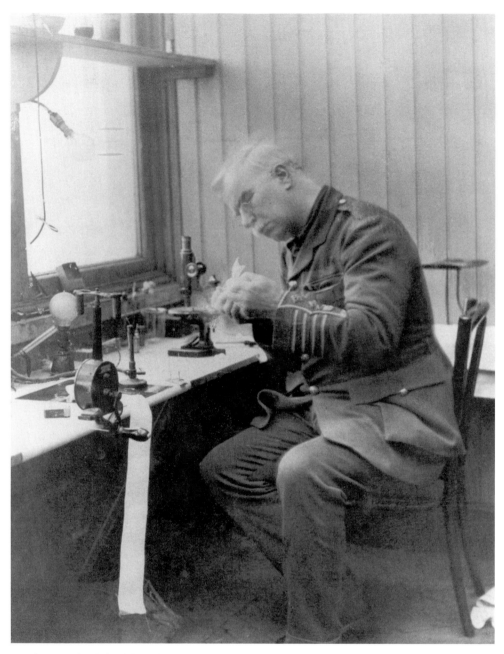

3 A thorn in the flesh of the military commanders and doctors, in both the Boer War and First World War: Sir Almroth Wright. (Alexander Fleming Laboratory Museum)

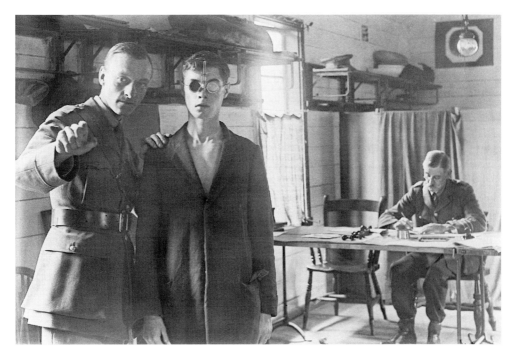

4 Selecting the fittest to fight, the medical inspection of recruits in 1914 included eyesight tests. (Imperial War Museum, Q 30067)

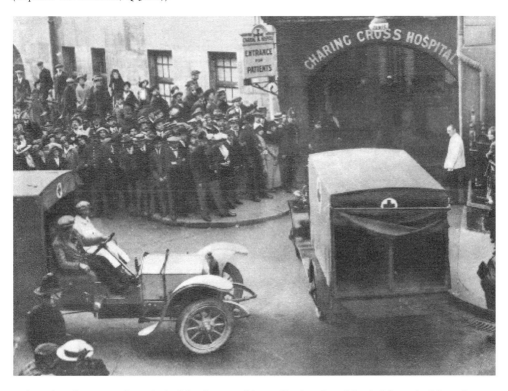

5 Crowds gather to see the arrival of the first casualties at Charing Cross Hospital from the Marne in 1914. (St Mary's Hospital Archives)

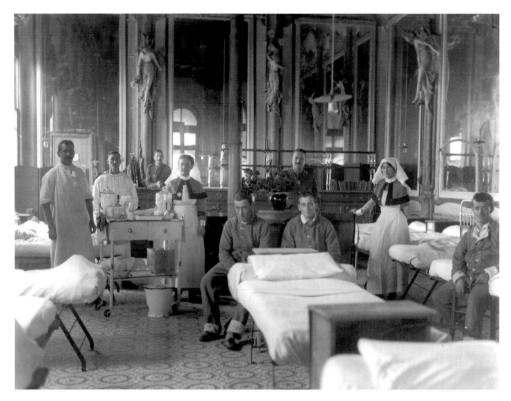

6 The Casino at Boulogne transformed into No. 14 General Hospital, October 1916. (Imperial War Museum, Q 29142)

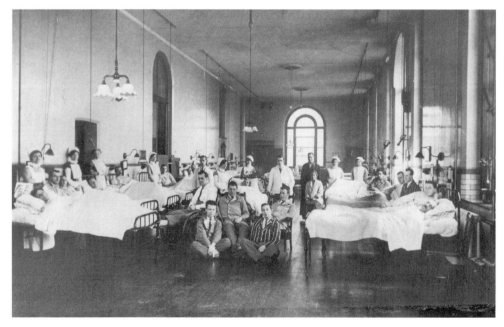

7 Blue coated wounded soldiers fill the wards set aside for military use in the civilian hospitals and are often tended by senior students acting as unqualified house officers, 1917. (St Mary's Hospital Archives)

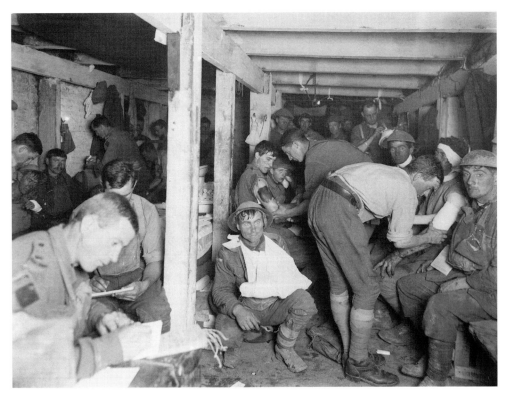

8 All action on the Western Front; the wounded are treated at an Advanced Dressing Station near Ypres, 20 September 1917. (Australian War Memorial, E00715)

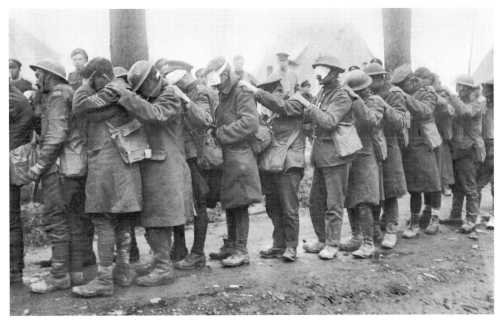

9 Troops, blinded by tear gas during the Battle of Estaires, line up outside an Advanced Dressing Station near Bethune in a scene reminiscent of John Singer Sargent's painting *Gassed*, 10 April 1918. (Imperial War Museum, Q 11586)

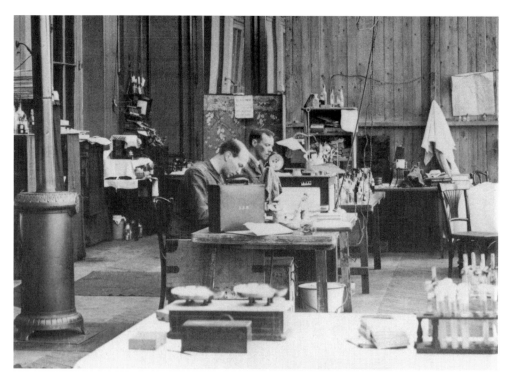

10 A makeshift laboratory, without running water or gas in the Fencing School at the Casino at Boulogne, was the scene of important work on war wounds in the First World War. (Alexander Fleming Laboratory Museum)

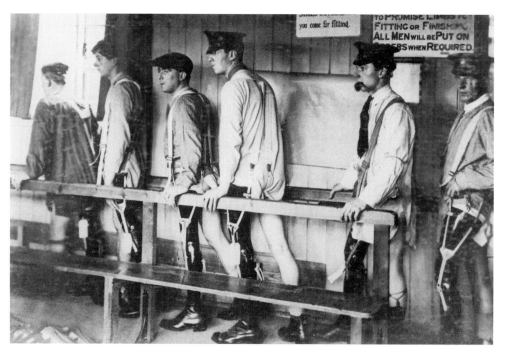

11 Rehabilitation: limbless First World War soldiers learn to walk with artificial legs at the workshops of J.E. Hanger at Roehampton. (Imperial War Museum, Q 33693)

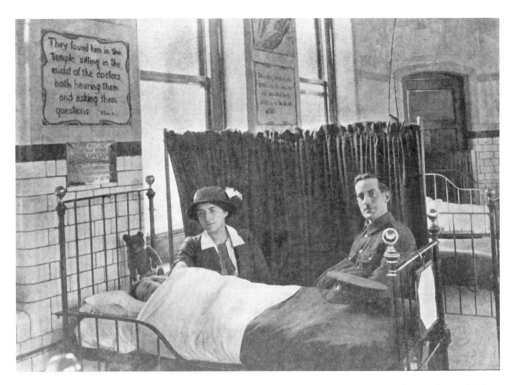

12 The health of the soldiers' child represented the imperial assets of the future and was safeguarded by Paddington Green Children's Hospital, while the welfare of children was a concern on the Home Front in the First World War. (St Mary's Hospital Archives)

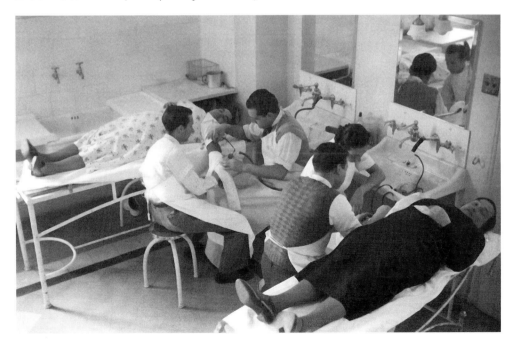

13 Spanish Civil War blood transfusion pioneer Frederic Duran i Jordà collects blood from donors at Hospital 18 in Barcelona, 1936. (Duran family and Miguel Lozano, Barcelona)

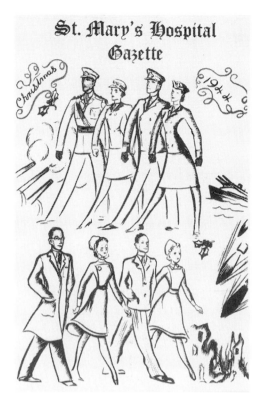

14 Civilian doctors and nurses were as much on the battle lines in the Second World War as those serving in uniform. (St Mary's Hospital Archives)

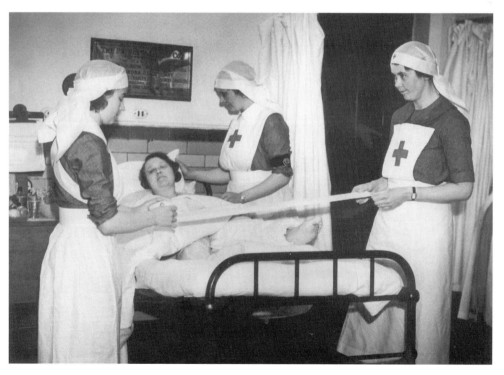

15 VAD (Voluntary Aid Detachment) take on the duties of nurses during the Second World War just as they had done during the Great War. (St Mary's Hospital Archives)

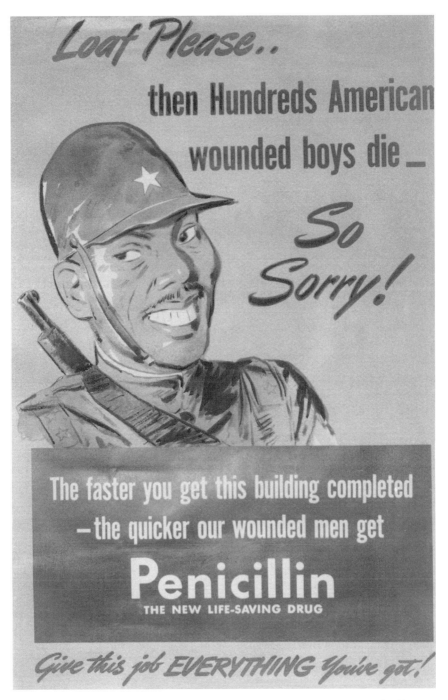

16 An exhortation with racist overtones urging workmen not to slacken when building a penicillin plant, a reflection of the strategic importance of the new miracle cure during the Second World War. (Alexander Fleming Laboratory Museum)

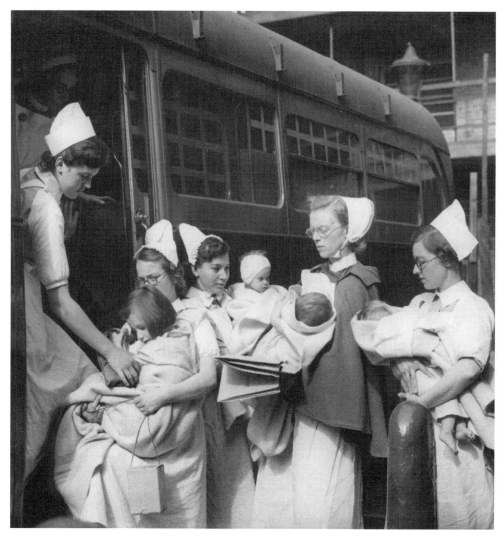

17 Nurses and babies leave Great Ormond Street Children's Hospital during the great evacuation of 1939. (Great Ormond Street Children's Hospital Archives and Museum)

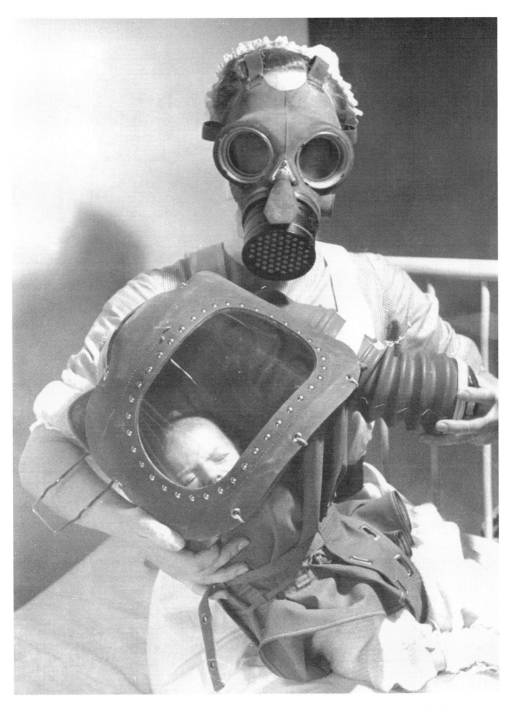

18 A nurse and infant at Great Ormond Street Children's Hospital do what they can with their gas masks, 1940. (Great Ormond Street Children's Hospital Archives and Museum)

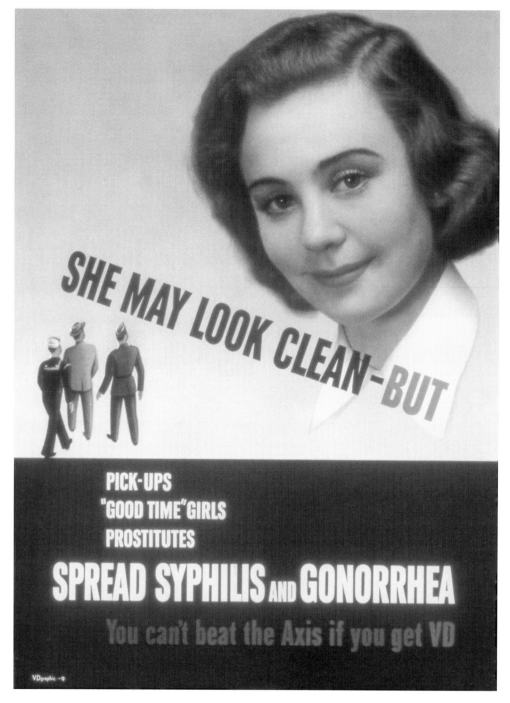

19 During the Second World War soldiers are exhorted to stay clean and avoid the temptations that might reduce their fighting capacities. (United States National Library of Medicine)

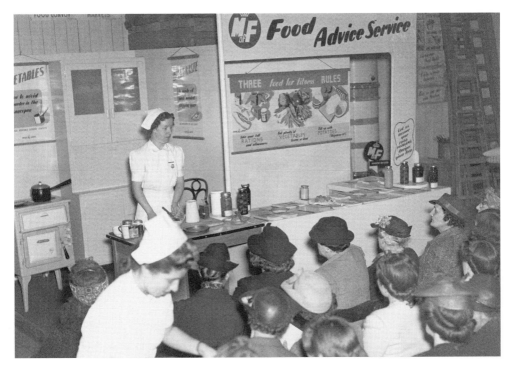

20 A wartime cookery demonstration to remind housewives of the importance of eating healthily, despite rationing, in order to keep fit for the war effort. (St Mary's Hospital Archives, SM/PH 32/2)

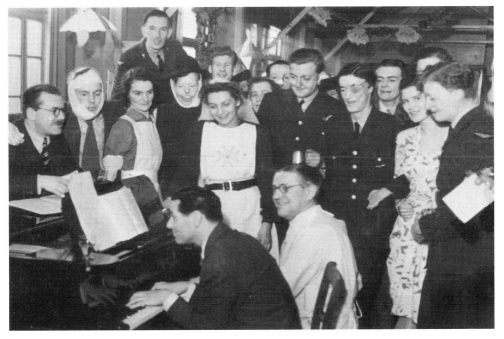

21 Archibald McIndoe encourages members of the Guinea Pig Club to enjoy themselves as part of his treatment of Second World War RAF burns victims at East Grinstead, Christmas 1944. (Queen Victoria Hospital Museum, East Grinstead)

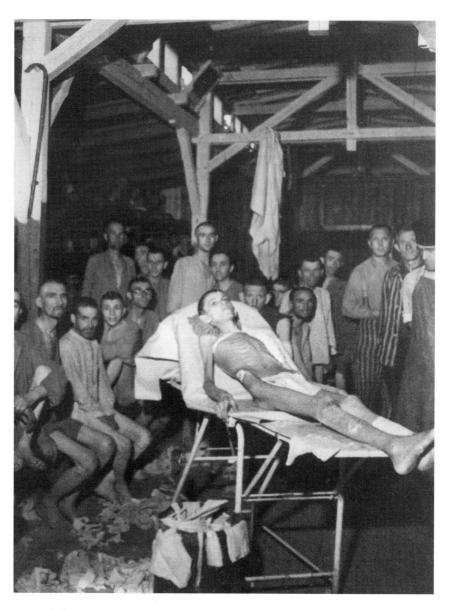

22 Amid 'the very abomination of desolation', Hungarian, Polish and Russian inmates await treatment by British medical students in the emergency hospital set up after the liberation of Buchenwald Concentration Camp, 1945. (St Mary's Hospital Archives, SM/ PH 99/7)

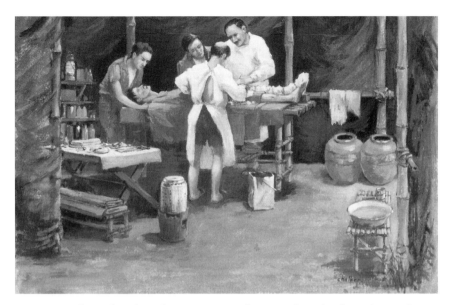

23 Weary Dunlop and Jacob Markowitz never actually operated together, but prisoner of war and artist Jack Chalker paid tribute to both of them in 1946 when he depicted them amputating a thigh in the prisoner of war camp at Chungkai. (Australian War Memorial, ART91848)

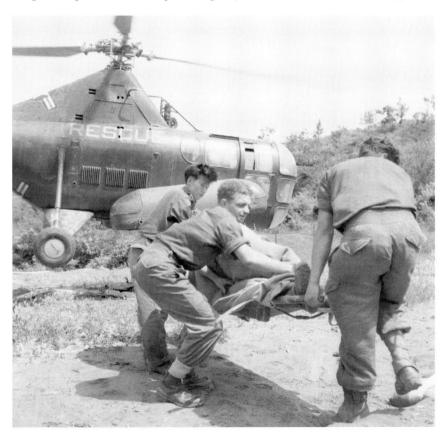

24 A quick evacuation by Sikorsky S–51 Dragonfly helicopter to a US Mobile Army Surgical Hospital (MASH) in Korea, 26 June 1953. (Australian War Memorial, HOBJ4348)

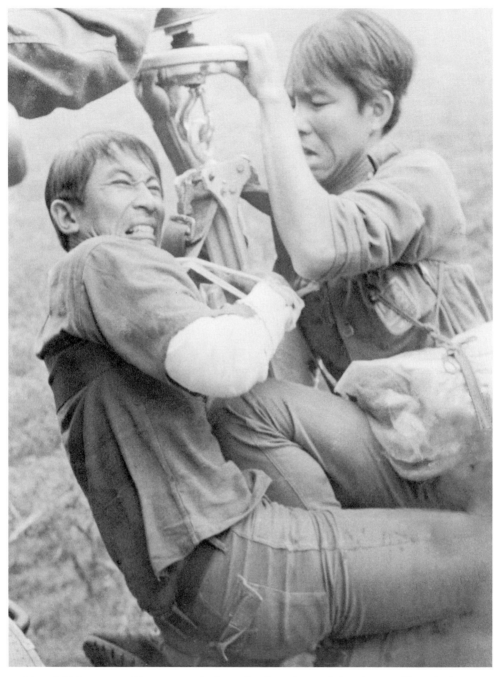

25 Wounded Vietnamese soldiers are winched to safety from the jungle by a 'Dust Off' (medical evacuation helicopter), April 1970. (Australian War Memorial, CAM/70/0174/VN)

salvation. The third of the trio, Fred Derry, played as the sensitive tough guy by Dana Andrews, has risen from a working-class origin on the wrong side of the tracks to become an officer in the air force, but lacks the self-confidence to find a post-war job that matches his wartime status and is dragged down by an unfaithful wife until he finds a new love with Al's daughter, acted by Teresa Wright as a younger version of her mother. The problems of psychological health of all three men are cured by the common sense and loyalty of a good woman. The tensions of the film struck a chord with audiences who were themselves coming to terms with the emotional, psychological and practical problems of demobilisation, but ultimately *The Best Years of Our Lives* represents the yearning for a better post-war world and the healing process of domestic security after the traumas of war.[124]

Planning for post-war reconstruction had begun in Britain early in the war and improved health services were to be an important part of building the New Jerusalem. There had been discussion since the end of the First World War of the possibilities that could be offered by a state health service, but to the physician Lord Dawson it seemed that this would be 'a state medical service by instalments, almost by stealth'.[125] Indeed, in the twenty years following the establishment of the Ministry of Health in 1919 there had been a stream of legislation that had increased the responsibilities of local authorities in the area of health. The formation of the Emergency Medical Service had been a further step in the direction of a national health service. *The Lancet* commented that Hitler and the Ministry of Health had achieved in a few months what would have otherwise taken twenty years to accomplish.[126] The voluntary and municipal hospitals learned how to work together despite their ingrained mistrust. Doctors realised that a salary did not turn them into civil servants or compromise their professional independence. A Blood Transfusion Service and Public Health Laboratory Service were both lasting legacies of the Emergency Medical Service. Above, all there was a move away from the pre-war system of local health services to a more centralised model that would become the basis of the National Health Service. To some commentators this 'assumes almost the proportions of a revolution'.[127] Younger doctors and medical students who had seen the wartime expedient in action accepted that 'the time is now ripe for organising a more complete and comprehensive Medical Service, to be used not only as a weapon of war, but as a means of conveying more equally and fully the benefits of medical service to the populace'.[128]

There was a determination that an uncoordinated, haphazard system of healthcare must become a thing of the past. Since 1934 the Labour Party had been committed to a free and comprehensive health service with a full-time salaried staff, local control of hospitals and a network of health centres that could spearhead preventative health campaigns as well as provide primary care. The Trades Union Congress criticised the 'frantic endeavours' of the voluntary hospitals to raise funds through flag days, bazaars, charity matinees and collecting boxes and stressed that 'it cannot be in the interests of the nation that such a vital thing as the health of the people should be subject to such haphazard methods'.[129] The voluntary hospitals themselves were not averse to anything that might provide the income to guarantee their survival in what were expected to be financially difficult post-war years. The British Medical Association too accepted the need to 'render available to every individual all necessary medical services, both general and specialist, and both domiciliary and institutional'.[130] Public pressure prompted the Ministry of Health to make a commitment to a government-provided comprehensive service for everyone who needed medical care after the war. It was assumed that any such system would retain 'the best features of the old voluntary system ... side by side with public health and other public medical services' organised by the local authorities.[131]

In December 1942, the publication of the best-selling Beveridge Report on *Social Security and Allied Services* sparked further debate on the form that would be taken by post-war health services. The report was the result of the deliberations of an interdepartmental committee but was very much shaped by its chairman Sir William Beveridge for whom it took on the character of a personal mission.[132] He identified 'Disease' as one of the 'Five Giants' which stood in the way of post-war reconstruction and which could be felled by a health service ensuring 'that the best that science can do is available for the treatment of every citizen at home and in institutions, irrespective of his personal means'. The free service would not only provide primary and specialist medical and surgical care but would also supply nursing and midwifery services, dental, ophthalmic and surgical appliances, and rehabilitation after accidents.[133] Churchill warned against giving people 'false hopes and airy visions of Utopia and El Dorado'[134] but the momentum for change was too great for expectations to be contained. A White Paper on Health was published in February 1944 declaring the Government's commitment to providing a comprehensive health service. This was to be both all-inclusive and free but would be based on the existing plethora of local authorities and voluntary efforts.[135] The Labour Party did not think it went far enough and many local authorities felt it gave to much power to doctors, whereas the 'radio doctor' Charles Hill portrayed it as a form of 'creeping state control'.[136] Political discussion rambled on to the end of the war, without any positive outcome and it was left to the Labour government of 1945, elected in a landslide victory that gave it the mandate to build the long desired land fit for heroes, to frame proposals for, and finally implement, a National Health Service on 5 July 1948 that would nationalise the hospitals, set up regional boards of administration and provide free and comprehensive medical treatment. It was to be the jewel in the post-war crown that seemed to fulfil the expectations raised by the war.

Although the hopes of post-war reconstruction and of a better post-war world were high throughout the world it was only in Britain that the war was followed by a dramatic reorganisation of civilian health services. The United States had been far enough away from the war arenas and had emerged unscathed and suspicious of anything that might be considered 'un-American', including state intervention in welfare. Much of continental Europe was in a state of collapse and in no position to implement such far-reaching plans. West Germany preferred to carry on with its tried and tested Bismarckian system of health insurance rather than try out anything new as it strove to rebuild. France continued to rely on state welfare benefits by which the patients were reimbursed for their medical expenditure. Britain, though, had been unoccupied and was one of the victors, albeit on the verge of bankruptcy. It was committed to building a better world for its people after the war and the health of the people was central to that vision. It was also part of the informal, unspoken pact that in return for sacrifices for national survival in wartime the people would be looked after in peace. The demands of wartime in maintaining national fitness had shown that a state provided system could work and offered a model for the future. Utopian in vision it may have been, but it was practicable and although the response to war it served the nation well in peace.

Behind the Wire

'The very abomination of desolation' permeated with 'the smell of burning filth' was how Belsen appeared to the 100-strong group of British medical students who had answered a call for volunteers to help with relief work in liberated Europe in April 1945. When they arrived at Belsen, a fortnight after the concentration camp's liberation, they found the camp itself in a superficially 'fairly orderly state' but 'the state of the sick in the huts was appalling'. The sick were lying in three-tiered wooden bunks and sprawled on the floor on piles of dirty rags, between 200 and 300 crowded into a space that would have been cramped for eighty people. Nearby were 'the mounds of the common graves containing the bodies of thousands of all the nations of Europe'. Typhus, starvation and diarrhoea raged unchecked. By the middle of May, the typhus epidemic was under control thanks to a liberal use of DDT, but tuberculosis was rife. Former prisoners who were well enough over-ate and suffered from diarrhoea as a result of the unaccustomed richness of their diet. Those too weak to claim their share of the food now available starved. People speaking different languages found it difficult to communicate with each other or with the doctors, nurses and medical students trying to help them. German, Russian and Polish ex-prisoners quarrelled. Meanwhile, 'amongst the fit, even doctors and nurses, there was at first, an almost complete indifference to the fate of the sick'. Janet Vaughan, a haematologist working with a Medical Research Council team of doctors, developed a new diet for gradually increasing the amount of food given to the starving, feeding them 100cc of skimmed milk, glucose and vitamin solution either as a drink or, controversially, administered intravenously every fifteen minutes; she was later to be criticised for trying this out as an experiment on ex-prisoners who had already suffered enough without now becoming the subjects of further experimentation. As soon as feasible, the sick were showered and cleaned up in what was termed the 'human laundry' and transferred to hospitals sent up in a part of Belsen that had been disinfected, deloused and cleaned or to a German military hospital. A patient was considered fit when 'capable of collecting his own food and maintaining himself'. As they left Belsen, their role now taken over by fully qualified medical teams, the students 'thought of the thousands of survivors, many maimed and ruined in body and mind; we thought of … the pathetic photographs of happy family groups, now with a sole survivor'. Only once their mission was over did they have the time to reflect on the dreadfulness and pathos of what they had witnessed but vowed that 'we will remember the terrible end of a wrong political idea'.[1]

War unleashes monsters, both real and imagined. The propaganda of the First World War dwelt on the brutal Hun bayoneting Belgian babies and nuns and turned Wilhelm II into a figure of menace leading to popular cries of 'Hang the Kaiser!'. In the Second World War, Hitler and Hirohito were demonised. Posters warning of the dangers of venereal disease depicted the Axis leaders hand in hand with a diseased woman who was declared to be 'the worst of the three' since the spread of syphilis and gonorrhoea was helping the enemy.[2] In medicine, though, the demons realised by war were only too real, even though it was not until after the end of the war that the full horror of the atrocities was revealed. During this war, with memories of some of the untrue horror propaganda of enemy brutality from the First World War, many people were cynical about reports of inhumanity. They were all the more shocked, like the medical students who helped at Belsen but without the first-hand experience, when they saw the conditions in the liberated Nazi concentration camps on newsreels in the cinemas and read newspaper reports of atrocities in the Far East. Medicine had become perverted in war conditions.

In Europe, this perversion of medicine had its origins in Fascist ideology and the closely linked doctrine of the eugenics movement. The German eugenic movement had been concerned with the protection of the blood purity of the German people and Nordic race against contamination from races thought to be genetically inferior. By keeping the unfit alive and able to reproduce, modern medicine and the costly public welfare programmes of the Weimar Republic interfered with natural selection. At the same time as inferior stock was multiplying, members of the fittest, educated classes were marrying later and using birth control to limit their family sizes. The Nazi ideology of Aryan supremacy rose directly from such eugenic concerns. It also fed on resentment about the economic and human costs of defeat in the First World War, seen as catastrophic in wiping out nearly 2 million young German heroes. In the immediate aftermath of the war, Karl Binding, a lawyer, and Alfred Hoche, both as a psychiatrist notorious for his experiments on the spinal cords of guillotined criminals and also as a father who had lost his son at Langemarck during the war, urged their fellow countrymen to imagine 'a battlefield covered with thousands of dead youths ... and then our institutions for idiots and their care' only to be 'most appalled by ... the sacrifice of the best of humanity while the best care is lavished on life of negative worth'.[3] They raised the question as to whether the unproductive inmates of the asylums ought to be allowed to live as a drain on society. It was a question that was debated throughout the interwar years. Some of the opponents of euthanasia for the inmates of asylums were strong supporters of the sterilisation of the unfit on the grounds that, whilst it was wrong to kill people once they lived, it was vital to prevent the birth of 'life unworthy of life'.[4]

Under the Nazi regime after 1933, racial hygiene became an important element in the policies of the German state. Joseph Goebbels declared that 'our starting point is not the individual and we do not subscribe to the view that one should feed the hungry, give drink to the thirsty, or clothe the naked ... we must have a healthy people in order to prevail in the world'.[5] This ideology had an impact on the role of the doctor in the fascist state. No longer was the doctor primarily concerned with the care of his individual patient: now his priority was the racial well being of the German nation. During the twelve years of the Nazi dictatorship, almost half of the German medical profession joined the National Socialists, a higher rate of affiliation than any other profession,[6] and the swastika was paired with the medical symbol of the caduceus on the cover of a leading medical journal in 1933.[7] Jewish doctors, considered as alien and polluting to national racial purity, however deeply integrated they may have been into German society, were progressively hounded from the profession until in 1938 they had their licences revoked and their status reduced to 'treaters of the sick' and were prohibited from treating anyone but fellow Jews. Many went into exile and had to retrain, however eminent they may have been in their own specialties, if they wanted to qualify and practise in their host countries; others were to perish in the concentration camps. Their practices were taken over by unemployed but ambitious young doctors with impeccable Aryan credentials.[8]

It was not only public and professional life that the Nazis hoped to purify. They also tried to reverse the falling birth rate. Adolph Hitler laid it down that the state 'must declare the child to be the most precious treasure of the people ... must see to it that only the healthy beget children ... must put the most modern medical means in the service of this knowledge'.[9] First of all, the Blood Protection Law of September 1935 banned marriage between German Jews and non-Jewish Germans. Then the Marital Health Law of October 1935 banned marriages between those deemed to be 'hereditarily healthy' and the genetically unfit. Both acts were aimed at the prevention of undesired offspring, but something also had to be done to encourage desirable births through marriage loans, tax rebates for husbands and fathers, child allowances and a rigid anti-abortion policy.[10] In 1936 the Reich Central Office for Combating Homosexuality and Abortion was set up to target antisocial activities that were obstructing reproduction policies. Getting married and having children was a national duty for the 'racially fit'. A medal, the 'Honour Cross of German Motherhood', was awarded for courage in fertility: bronze for mothers of four or five children, silver for six or seven, and gold for eight or more. It represented in a tangible form Hitler's claim that 'in my state, the mother is the most important citizen'. Yet such positive eugenic policies were not a great success. Among the elite *Schutz-Staffel* (SS), sixty-one per cent remained unmarried in 1939 and the average family size was 1.1 children.[11]

Samuel Beckett, the Irish dramatist, pointed out the irony of Nazi policies aimed at producing a tall, blond, blue-eyed master race: 'he must be blond like Hitler, thin like Göring, handsome like Goebbels, virile like Röhme – and he can be called Rosenberg.'[12] Like their German counterparts, the Italian fascists did not live up to the ideal images they promoted among their people whether in terms of physical fitness or moral purity. The leader of the Balilla, the fascist youth movement, and a manly, upright role model for all Italian boys was the tall, handsome, athletic, soldierly Renato Ricci. In physical appearance he was the perfect figurehead at a parade or assembly able to inspire even the youngest of his boys to see himself as a soldier in the making, though in reality he was little more than a ruthless businessman and corrupt politician.[13] Mussolini's son-in-law Galeazzo Ciano was also promoted as a fascist pin-up and tried to live up to the image of the dashing, honed hero by having an exercise bicycle publicly installed in his office at the Palazzo Chigi when he became Minister of Foreign Affairs, though this, coupled with his insatiable passion for golf and an active extramarital sex life, did not save him from the increasing portliness that went with his liking for high society, bespoke tailoring, good food and beautiful women, and all despite the fact that he abstained from tobacco and alcohol in a nod towards the purity of the fascist health ideal.[14] Propaganda, ideology and reality rarely coincide, though the chiselled, physically perfect images on posters invariably look impressive enough.

The fascist leaders may have been far from being physical exemplars for fitness and racial purity, but fascist ideology in Germany extolled the ideal of Aryan masculinity and feminine beauty, and promoted strength through joy and the cult of physical fitness. Healthy diet and lifestyles were promoted. Subsidised bathing and hiking holidays, discounted admission to golf courses, sailing clubs and tennis clubs, and the building of new athletic and sports facilities were all intended for the revitalisation of bodies and minds tired by routine. They were also vehicles for making men vigorous as future soldiers and making women healthy for motherhood and the production of the next generation.[15] The Hitler Youth Movement and League of German Maidens aimed at keeping the youth of Germany fit, healthy and ready to march to war as well as at inculcating Nazi ideology. In the elite Adolph Hitler Schools, in which the future Nazi leaders were trained, military drill was given more prominence than in the Hitler Youth but this was intended as a mere preliminary to the Order Castles for the training of those selected to be the new 'aristocracy of the nation'. Here, they were indoctrinated in the ideals of racial hygiene and toughened by mountain climbing, shooting, parachuting and mountain combat. The training of the elite would then climax at Marienburg, the reconstructed castle of the Teutonic knights that epitomised German expansion eastwards, after which these young men would be physically and mentally the idealisation of the healthy Nazi warrior.[16] Meanwhile in Italy the Balilla and Gioventi Fascisti brought the cult of physical fitness to young Italians. Sports for girls were to strengthen them for motherhood and were not to be competitive for that was unfeminine. At the same time, Renato Ricci insisted that every gymnasium for boys aged from eight to thirteen should contain weapons since exercising them made children into men.[17]

In Germany, the aim of creating an effective nation in arms also resulted in positive health initiatives aimed at eliminating 'genetic poisons' linked with birth defects and genetic damage. Research was sponsored into the medical effects of alcohol, tobacco and syphilis, which were seen as the major health threats to the German people. Research by Fritz Lickint begun in the days of the Weimar Republic had first established a statistical link between smoking and lung cancer and an epidemiological study by Franz Müller had confirmed this relationship by 1939. Smoking was banned in government offices, hospitals and rest homes and tobacco ration coupons were held back from pregnant women during the war to prevent harm to the foetus. No one was allowed to pollute with tobacco the presence of the non-smoking Führer. There were campaigns to encourage healthy diets and exercise and to improve public and occupational health. Citizens were reminded that it was their duty to be as fit and healthy as possible for the good of the nation.[18]

Yet, there still remained the fear of what would happen if those people with genetic diseases were allowed to reproduce without restriction and continue to impose ever-increasing burdens on the genetically healthy. In July 1933 the Law for the Prevention of Genetically Diseased Offspring was passed, based on a voluntary scheme drafted by Prussian health officials the previous year before the Nazi seizure of power. Men and women suffering from nine medical conditions believed to be hereditary were to be sterilised: feeblemindedness, schizophrenia, manic-depressive disorders, epilepsy, Huntington's chorea, blindness, deafness, severe physical deformities and chronic alcoholism. All cases went before special hereditary courts, but the decisions reached were routine. Men would be given a vasectomy and women would have their tubes tied in a procedure that resulted in the deaths of hundreds of women. They were given no choice in the matter and might be forcibly carried to the operating table.[19] Abroad there were mixed reactions to the sterilisation law. In the United States, where there were already sterilisation laws, many eugenicists saw it as a logical and welcome development of earlier thinking, but there was some concern about its possible extension to Jews and the political opponents of the Nazis. Finland, Norway and Sweden passed their own sterilisation laws, which were whole-heartedly endorsed by liberals committed to a scientifically planned, progressive, social democratic welfare state.[20]

The outbreak of the Second World War provided the opportunity and excuse for moving on from sterilising burdens on society to eliminating them completely. In a national emergency it was easier to implement policies in secrecy and mobilise support for what would have otherwise been unthinkable using a wartime rhetoric of self-sacrifice and acting for the 'good of the Fatherland'. Karl Brandt, Hitler's physician, was later to admit that in regard to euthanasia 'the Führer was of the opinion that it would be easier and smoother to carry out in wartime, since the public resistance from the churches would not play such a prominent role amidst the events of wartime as it otherwise would'.[21] Yet, the first steps towards euthanasia had been taken on 18 August 1939, even before the outbreak of war, when the Reich Ministry of the Interior had instructed all midwives and obstetricians to report all babies born with such severe birth defects as mental deficiency, hydrocephaly, missing limbs, cleavages of the head or spinal cord and paralysis. These reports were reviewed by three paediatricians who selected those children deemed unworthy to survive. The infants were then injected with morphine or given overdoses of the sedatives Luminal or Veronal mixed in their food.[22] In October 1939, mercy killing was extended from the newly born to 'incurable' adults under Operation T-4[23] which targeted patients in mental hospitals and mental deficiency institutions. These people were considered to be unproductive members of society and to be a drain on the national resources at a time when these were most needed to fight the war. Six mercy killing centres were set up in remote areas near good road or railway links throughout Germany and patients selected for euthanasia were transferred to them.[24] After a few weeks their relatives received notification of their deaths from natural causes, mainly blood poisoning, in their new institutions and were sent their ashes. In reality, they had died of carbon monoxide poisoning in gas chambers disguised as showers and had been cremated to avoid any possibility of an autopsy revealing their true causes of death.[25] The centres were staffed by specially selected doctors and nurses, who were vetted for their willingness to kill for 'the good of the State'. Many of them showed concern about the comfort of their dying charges and justified their role in the euthanasia programme on the grounds that it was for the ultimate good of their patients and society as a whole, though there were some who failed to question their actions either then or later. A number of the nurses subsequently excused themselves on the grounds that 'from the time when I was a nursing student, I learned to show unquestioning obedience towards the superior and older nurses' or that they were only following the instructions of the doctors as they had been taught.[26] The involvement of doctors and nurses was more to give the whole process the appearance of medical respectability than because their healthcare skills were needed other than to reassure their unwitting victims. It did not require a medical or nursing qualification to turn on a gas valve.[27]

Murder on such a scale could not be covered up and on 3 August 1941 Clemens August von Galen, Bishop of Münster, denounced the euthanasia programme from the pulpit and warned that 'if you establish and apply the principle that you can kill unproductive fellow human beings then woe betide all of us when we become old and frail!'[28] The Lutheran pastor Gerhard Braune publicly asked how it was that more than 2,000 people could have died in a forty-day period at Grafeneck Asylum which only contained 100 beds. When Lothar Kreyssig, a provincial judge in Brandenburg, threatened to prosecute T-4 officials for murder, he was removed from office by early retirement. The Royal Air Force dropped fliers on German towns warning that the next step might be euthanasia for the most severely war wounded. The Nazi propaganda machine too brought the issue into the open in 1941 with a feature film *Ich lage an* ('I accuse') which skilfully confused voluntary euthanasia, through the story of a young woman with multiple sclerosis who wishes her husband to help her to die, with the issue of killing the weak without their consent. Public opinion was not convinced and Hitler decided to halt the gassing programme, though deaths continued from starvation diets and overdoses of medication in the hospitals and mental institutions of the Third Reich, partly to release beds for the overwhelming casualties returning from the Eastern Front. Among the victims were the severely traumatised air-raid casualties as Germany was pounded by Allied bombing raids.[29]

The comparative success of the T-4 euthanasia programme by gassing offered a way of eliminating other biological threats to the racial health of the German people. Eastern Europe offered space for German expansion but only at the expense of the existing Slavic populations that were considered inferior to the Aryan race represented by the conquering Reich. The occupation of Poland had from the start been more brutal than anything experienced in the West. In pursuit of the aim of reducing Poland to a nation of manual labourers fit for nothing but to serve their German masters, the occupying power had systematically imprisoned or executed the Polish political and intellectual leaders. However, many Poles were tall, blonde and blue-eyed, far more Aryan in appearance than most of the leading Nazis. Obviously then these Poles must actually be German by racial origin but were being corrupted by Polish ways. Just as inferior blood had to be destroyed, good stock had to be saved and added to the Aryan gene pool for the future health of the race. As a result, suitable Polish children were abducted from orphanages and from their homes and sent to Germany for adoption by German families or to one of the SS Lebensborn children's homes for the propagation of the master race where they could be Aryanised.[30]

However, even lower racially than Poles were the Jews of Eastern Europe. In Polish cities, they were segregated into ghettos by the occupying forces. German public health officials justified this segregation as helping to prevent the spread of typhus and other infectious diseases.[31] However, the German invasion of the Soviet Union on 22 June 1941 unleashed new levels of savagery against perceived inferior races. The 'Final Solution to the Jewish Question' began with special squads of SS following the German Army into the Soviet Union and murdering more than a million Jews in open-air shooting. The psychological stress on his men of the face to face shooting of men, women and children led Heinrich Himmler, chief of the SS, to find a cleaner and more efficient way of killing. Mass shootings were also too public. The euthanasia programme offered an answer, and T-4 staff was redeployed to the gas chambers and crematoria of the death camps in the East such as Chelmno, Sobibor, Treblinka, Belzec, Majdanek and Auschwitz-Birkenau. Once again, the gas chambers were disguised as showers to reassure the victims before their hygienic murder.[32] At Auschwitz, the SS improved upon the T-4 methods of killing by combining the gas chambers and crematoria in one building and replacing carbon monoxide by the faster acting hydrogen cyanide or Zyklon B, which was already in use as a pesticide in their barracks.[33]

The process of murder in the concentration camps was medicalised just as it had been in the euthanasia killing centres. SS doctors were involved in every aspect of the killing process in the camps. SS-Obersturmführer Paul Kremer, a doctor at Auschwitz, said that by comparison with the 'special actions' he was involved with, 'Dante's *Inferno* seems almost a comedy'.[34] When a convoy of prisoners was brought to the camp, it was doctors who made the selection of who was fit for work and who should be sent to the gas chambers. When each transport arrived, men and women were separated into two rows and passed in front of a doctor who spent no more than a few seconds in deciding who should live or not. At Treblinka, a death camp, they arrived at a railway station designed to give an impression of normality with fake timetables. Lulled into a false sense of security, they were all the more shocked to be given five minutes to disembark from the train and, when divided up into separate rows of men, women and children, forced to undress, while camp workers collected up their clothes to take to a store hidden behind the façade of the station restaurant. The sick and elderly were taken to a compound known as the Lazarett with a Red Cross flag on its gates that promised them hoped-for medical treatment. There they were shot. Everyone else was marched naked to the gas chambers.[35] At Auschwitz, which was both a labour camp and a death camp, the new arrivals received their perfunctory medical inspection and selection fully clothed. The assumption was that doctors could see at a glance who was most capable of standing up to the rigours of work in the camp, but in reality selections were usually totally arbitrary. What could make the difference was whether someone wore glasses, stood up straight or stooped or looked physically strong. Yet the doctors were involved to give the impression that the whole process was nothing less than scientific, as did their presence when the gas was turned on. Indeed at Auschwitz, the Zyklon B was transported to the gas chambers in a van made up to look like an ambulance and marked with a red cross.[36] At Chelmno, deportees from the Łódz ghetto about to be gassed in mobile vans were reassured at seeing men in white coats with stethoscopes; what they did not know was that the white coats and stethoscopes had been stolen from the luggage of Jewish doctors, who had themselves already been murdered.[37] Doctors gave legitimacy to the whole process for both the killers and the killed.

It was not only prisoners judged suitable for hard labour who survived the selections at the Auschwitz-Birkenau concentration camp complex. Many of the medical personnel there were engaged in medical research and were looking for suitable subjects for their experiments. Foremost among them was Josef Mengele, a specialist in hereditary biology from the University of Frankfurt who was interested in the subject of twins. Aged only thirty-two when he arrived at Auschwitz in March 1943, Mengele was the holder of the Iron Cross won for bravery after rescuing soldiers from a blazing tank while serving in combat on the Eastern Front. Always immaculately dressed in his SS uniform, the handsome doctor, known as 'the angel of death', could exert considerable charm when he wished but was equally capable of shooting a mother and child on the selection ramp when they caused him trouble. Towards the children selected for his experiments, he would show superficial benevolence by giving them chocolates and kindly words, yet when they returned to their barracks block from a visit to their 'kind uncle' they would be screaming with pain. His main research interest was in the relationship between genetic inheritance and behaviour and development, though he varied his studies of twins with experiments on dwarves, the reactions of the blood of different races to infectious diseases and studies of facial gangrene, known as noma, common among the gypsies imprisoned at Birkenau. He was also interested in fertility and how multiple births could be encouraged, but his main, almost sadistic, interest remained in investigating hereditary traits. Children were deliberately infected with typhoid and tuberculosis and then killed to see what the effects on them were and if they differed between twins. If one twin died as the result of an experiment, Mengele would kill the other so that he could perform a comparative autopsy. Myklos Nyiszli, a Jewish prison doctor working closely with Mengele, commented that 'this phenomenon was unique in world medical history. Two brothers died together and it was possible to perform autopsies on both. Where, under normal circumstances, can one find twin brothers who die at the same place at the same time?'[38] The opportunity to do so brought out the dark side of Mengele and turned him into one of the worst monsters of Auschwitz.

He was not the only one. Sterilisation was the main research interest of the gynaecologist Carl Clauberg, who earlier in his career had been interested in helping infertile women to conceive. Now his aim was to find a more effective and safe way of sterilizing a woman during a regular gynaecological examination that could be used by any doctor. Using 700 camp inmates at Auschwitz as his guinea pigs, he injected toxins into the uterus and experimented with irradiation from huge X-ray machines. Other doctors did experiments on the functioning of the cervix even if it meant abusing the women in their care. Men too were castrated by irradiation while they stood at counters to fill in forms. Like Mengele's experiments with twins, this research was solely motivated by the ideological eugenic interests of German society and medicine performed on unwilling subjects deemed to be members of an inferior racial group and thus fitting material for research for the benefit of the genetically fit.[39]

Some of the concentration camp experiments were the result of military problems facing the German war effort. At Dachau, high altitude experiments were conducted by the schizophrenic doctor

Sigmund Rascher and his wife on prisoners to investigate the limits of human endurance and existence using low pressure chambers in which many of the victims died. As a result of these experiments, Rascher concluded that an airman could safely leave his aircraft at 68,000ft, but the Luftwaffe wisely ignored these findings and instead developed a parachute which would open automatically when the pilot was more than 10,000ft above the ground, an altitude at which all but Rascher believed the airman abandoning his plane would lose consciousness. In a further series of experiments conducted at Dachau on behalf of the Luftwaffe, victims were left in tanks of freezing water for up to three hours and then revived to investigate the most effective means of treating airmen with hypothermia. Some of them were dressed in their camp rags and others in flying suits. Many prisoners were kept naked outdoors in temperatures below freezing as part of the same experiment; some of 'the victims screamed with pain as parts of their bodies froze'. Hot baths were found to be the most effective means of reheating men though the use of women was one of the most notorious aspects of this work; it was believed that temperatures would rise rapidly during the excitement of sexual intercourse. Other prisoners were deprived of food and drink and given only chemically processed sea-water to see whether it could be made drinkable for shipwrecked sailors and airmen brought down at sea. At Ravensbruck, sections of the bones, muscles and nerves of prisoners were removed so that the doctors could investigate body tissue regeneration and experiment with bone transplantation. The survivors of the experiments suffered intense agony, mutilation and permanent disability.[40]

Drugs trials were also carried out using concentration camp prisoners. The effects of sulphanilamide on war wounds were tested in 1943 at Ravensbruck in conjunction with the Bayer pharmaceutical company, part of the chemical giant I.G. Farbenindustrie. Wounds were deliberately inflicted and infected with streptococcus, gas gangrene and tetanus. The circulation of the blood of the subject was then interrupted by tying the blood vessels at both ends to simulate battlefield wounds. The infection was further aggravated by doctors and nurses forcing wood shavings and ground glass into the wounds. These particular experiments had been inspired by arguments over whether sulphonamide should have been used to treat Reinhardt Heydrich, Himmler's deputy, after he was fatally shot in Prague. At Buchenwald and Natzweiler-Struthof, healthy inmates were infected with spotted fever to keep the virus alive while other inmates had various vaccines and chemicals tested on them. Similar experiments were carried out on jaundice, yellow fever, smallpox, typhus, cholera and diphtheria. At Dachau, healthy camp inmates were infected with malaria by mosquitoes and then treated with vaccines to test the efficacy of vaccination. At Buchenwald, burns were deliberately inflicted with phosphorous taken from incendiary bombs to test the effects of various pharmaceuticals on them.[41]

Selected Jewish skeletons were sent to the University of Strasbourg where the anatomist August Hirt was establishing an anthropological anatomic collection of what was expected to be a vanished race. The University of Strasbourg had been evacuated to Clermont Ferrand at the beginning of the Second World War when the entire population of Alsace had been evacuated from the war zone. When Alsace was reincorporated into the German Reich after the fall of France, the Germans established the Nazi Reichsuniversität Strassburg which became a centre of studies on physical anthropology and racial biology under Hirt who was appointed head of the Institute of Anatomy. Among his collection of Jewish skeletons were the bodies of eighty-six prisoners from nearby Natzweiler-Struthof concentration camp whom he had conducted medical experiments upon before having them gassed and their bodies transferred to Strasbourg for further research. The suffering caused was justified on the specious grounds that in the long term it would produce a healthy race through understanding of human anatomy and physiology. The invasion of Russia offered Hirt the opportunity of obtaining more Jewish skulls for his collection and he especially requested from Heinrich Himmler those of Jewish-Bolshevik Commissars who to him represented 'the prototype of the repulsive, but characteristic sub-human'.[42]

Medicine in the concentration camps was not just concerned with research or with eliminating the unfit, but was also aimed at keeping prisoners well enough to work since most of the camps were vital to the war economy though their workforce was ultimately expendable. Any patient too sick to work would be admitted to one of the camp hospital huts staffed by prisoner doctors and nurses with grubby white coats over their striped camp uniforms. Anthony Faramus, a Jersey-born prisoner, described the operating theatre at Mauthausen as being like the shop of 'a squalid backstreet barber-abortionist from the dark ages'.[43] If the patient could not be cured and returned to work within a few weeks, a selection by the SS doctors would take place, and death and the crematorium were inevitable.

Even in the hospital, patients were squashed two to a bunk and had to rise for the 4a.m. reveille, but, except for the medical inspection of patients filing past the doctor, it was 'a life in limbo' with no work to do. Yet it was in the hospital that camp inmates like the Italian chemist Primo Levi began to 'speak of other things than hunger and work and one begins to consider what they have made us become, how much they have taken away from us, what this life is'.[44] Primo Levi was lucky to catch scarlet fever in January 1945 when the Germans abandoned Auschwitz, leaving behind the sick to fend for themselves. His friend Alberto was one of many comparatively healthier prisoners to perish on the forced march from the camp in the height of winter.[45]

Conditions were just as bad in the Russian camps in which many Poles found themselves if they were spared the German camps. In some of these, 'the prisoners' one dream is to get to hospital' and 'a prisoner willingly chopped off his finger in the hope of getting admitted'.[46] Gustav Herling, arrested in 1940 by the Soviet forces while trying to escape from Poland to join the Free Polish Forces in the West, considered the camp hospital to be 'something like a refuge for the shipwrecked'.[47] It represented a dream of being looked after by a kind nurse and polite doctor in conditions that restored to the prisoner a sense of his humanity and human dignity. Nevertheless sick prisoners still had to lie on the passage floor for several days while awaiting a bed. The dispensary was poorly supplied and most prisoners were so familiar with the uses of what was available that they would ask for a particular medicine even before the doctor had diagnosed them. Doctors erred on the side of strictness in admitting and discharging patients for fear that they might be denounced for helping a prisoner to shirk work. Herling found 'something incomprehensible' in the contrast between the 'human atmosphere' of the camp hospital and the brutality shown to prisoners outside it.[48] Yet in some of these camps, there was little or no medical care at all.[49]

Lack of medical facilities was a situation only too familiar to prisoners of the Japanese in the Far East where defeated soldiers were considered to have lost their honour and with it many rights under a martial code that looked on surrender as shameful. Nor was the health of interned civilians given much consideration either. The brutality of the Japanese towards doctors, nurses and the sick during the fall of the European colonies before the Japanese advance at the end of 1941 and in early 1942 gave a warning of what was to come. At Hong Kong, a Royal Army Medical Corps Unit from the Shaukiwan Medical Store was captured early during the fighting on 19 December and forced to strip down to their underclothes by their captors and surrender their rings and watches before being butchered with bayonets and swords. Anyone who survived this was finished off with a revolver. Two men survived. Lieutenant Thomas from a Field Ambulance was shot in the back but managed to crawl away after being left for dead. Corporal Norman Leath survived by feigning death after being hit on the back of the neck with a sword, falling 'to the ground face downwards … with blood pouring into my eyes, ear and mouth'. He managed to roll down into a gully and managed to survive in hiding for over a week until his injuries left him no choice but to surrender at an internment camp at North Point in the hope of receiving some treatment.[50] Worse was to come on Christmas Day at the hospital set up at St Stephen's College when the Japanese disrupted a Christmas service being celebrated by the hospital padre at dawn. The commander of the hospital, Lieutenant-Colonel George Black, and a medical officer, Captain John Whitney, were shot in the head and bayoneted when they tried to protect their patients and staff from the intruders, their bodies being left in the lavatory and sitting room. One survivor, Sergeant Anderson, recalled that 'there were sounds of shouting and shooting as the Japanese ran down the main hall amongst the patients and any patients who were too slow in getting up out of bed, or who could not move owing to wounds, were bayoneted or shot'. St John's Ambulance Brigade men were taken aside and systematically butchered. The eighty-six surviving staff and patients were herded into a small room, only for men to be dragged out at random and tortured.[51] The female nurses were kept separately and repeatedly raped before being killed; nurses at the Jockey Club Hospital were also 'outraged'.[52] One of the VAD nurses at St Stephen's, Mrs Begg, was found with her 'head almost severed from her body'.[53] What made Mrs Begg's death particularly poignant was that her husband was one of the wounded in the hospital and, after their capture, 'they consoled each other with the fact that although they had lost everything they still had each other'.[54] Luckier was an 'elderly woman' in charge of the wounded at the Repulse Bay Hotel who confronted the Japanese when the soldiers started 'their usual practice of ripping the bandages off the patients. Wearing her uniform and medals from her nursing days during the First World War, she 'resisted so strongly and continuously that in the end the Japanese left them alone', although usually resistance to their orders provoked violence.[55]

The atrocities in Hong Kong prompted the authorities in Singapore to begin to evacuate female nurses from the hospitals there when it became obvious that the city would fall. It was a wise move as the fall of Singapore was marked by further massacres of wounded soldiers. Nevertheless there was criticism that more had not been done to evacuate the 'many hundreds of wounded and sick men, who obviously would not have been fit for many months'. Among those left behind to become prisoners 'if still alive', was an officer who had been diagnosed with cancer before the war and another young man who had been wounded with shrapnel in his lung.[56] At the Alexandra Military Hospital, patients were fired at and a surgeon was bayoneted with his patient in the operating theatre. A medical officer surrendering the hospital and claiming protection for it under the Geneva Convention was also bayoneted as a sign of contempt for the defeated.[57]

In the Philippines, 80,000 American and Filipino troops, together with 25,000 civilian refugees, retreated into the Bataan peninsula. Lacking fresh food, medicines, clean drinking water and the most elementary of sanitary facilities, they soon succumbed to scurvy, beriberi, malaria and dysentery. The invading Japanese, unprepared for a long siege, suffered from the same diseases. American surrender was inevitable. The Bataan contingent did so on 9 April 1942 but it was 6 May before the troops on Corregidor, with thousands of sick and wounded men crammed into the dank 826ft shaft of the Malinta Tunnel finally conceded. The Japanese, contemptuous of their captives and themselves suffering high sickness rates, herded their prisoners along the infamous 'Bataan Death March' to primitive prisoner of war camps hurriedly established at the base of the Bataan peninsula. En route, stragglers were clubbed and bayoneted and water was denied to the thirsty. Almost 10,000 Filipinos and 600 American prisoners died as a result of the cruelty of their Japanese and Korean guards. There was to be no relief for them when they finally reached the camps near Manila.[58]

The regime in the prisoner of war camps was brutal. Beatings were common, diet was meagre and overcrowding and poor sanitation spread infectious disease among the men. At North Point Camp in Hong Kong, 120 men were crowded into huts built for no more than forty. Sanitary conditions were bad, since the camp was located in an area that had previously been used as a rubbish dump and as stabling for horses. A shortage of building materials made it difficult to do anything to improve sanitation or fly proofing of the quarters in which the men lived.

It was little wonder that dysentery and diarrhoea were 'practically endemic'[59] and that men were 'dying like flies'.[60] The Sultan of Johore would visit the camps on Singapore Island in his Rolls Royce and throw obsolete bank notes over the fence to the prisoners of war. These were practically worthless at that time but, since everyone was suffering from dysentery, had an immediate value as toilet paper.[61] A military camp at Changi at the eastern end of Singapore, which normally accommodated 3,000 men, was used to house 50,000 prisoners of war with the result that sanitary hygiene broke down completely. Attempts to control the outbreak of dysentery by opening a separate ward for dysentery patients were thwarted at first by the Japanese who insisted that all the sick should be centralised in one small barrack area even if it did encourage the spread of infectious diseases.[62] At the Argyle Street camp in Hong Kong, the Japanese even refused to allow facilities for a camp hospital to be set up until fears of a cholera outbreak prompted a change of heart.[63] Hospital conditions in camps in Japan were no better and at Shinagowa Prisoner of War Camp, 'the Japanese, apart from admitting that the place was dirty, seemed incapable of conceiving or supplying anything better'.[64]

After the poor sanitary conditions, the main medical problem was the lack of drugs and medical supplies. It meant that doctors had to be very creative. Prisoners of war improvised artificial legs[65] and spectacle frames[66] from whatever materials they had to hand. Captain Bill Frankland, conscious that while drugs might have been in short supply in Singapore there was plenty of sea water, like many of his fellow doctors, reverted to Almroth Wright's ideas about saline dressings on wounds. One of his patients had attempted to escape but had been immediately recaptured and slashed with a bayonet. He also suffered from beriberi and had ulcers all over his body. Frankland treated him using the saline method and within two months he was able to walk again only to be executed for his escape attempt.[67]

The only drugs that were available were what the medical officers had brought to the camps with them, although later some supplies came from Red Cross parcels.[68] On many occasions, though, the Japanese stole drugs from Red Cross parcels and diverted them for their own use. Other supplies were obtained by bribing the guards to buy them in such towns as Singapore and Hong Kong.[69] When five prisoners escaped from the camp at Cabanutan in the Philippines on the day that medical supplies had been brought into the camp, the guards emptied cartons of pills and broke open vials of serum in the search for messages that might give a clue to the escape, even though these medicines had cost thousands of pesos and were badly needed by the sick and dying internees for whom they had been obtained; ten messages were found from the wives and friends of the men interned in that camp.[70] All medical supplies had to be used where they could do the most good. Frankland had a patient suffering from beriberi, tropical ulcers and diphtheria. At that time there were only six anti-diphtheria sera available in the entire camp. Frankland's superior officer refused to release any for his patient, a private, but insisted that it be given to an officer who, apart from his diphtheria, was otherwise relatively fit. At first Frankland was indignant that an officer should be given preference over a private until he realised that the decision had been made on the medical grounds that the officer was more likely to survive if he received the serum whereas the private might die anyway from his other ailments.[71] Such dilemmas were faced on a daily basis.

The recovery of the sick was further held back by the malnutrition that lowered the health of all the prisoners. Rations of twelve ounces of rice a day were totally inadequate for the maintenance of the health of the prisoners, and deficiency diseases such as beriberi, pellagra and ariboflavinosis were widespread. Many men suffered from scrotal dermatitis as a result of a lack of vitamins. Known to its sufferers as 'Changi balls' or 'rice balls', this was marked by the skin of a man's genitals splitting and peeling off to leave the scrotum sticky, raw and painful.[72] Another result of malnutrition was that a quarter of the prisoners began to suffer from poor vision. Red Cross parcels when they actually reached the men helped, as did illicit trading with local people outside the camps, but only to a very limited extent and 'shortage of food and nutritional diseases remained our most serious problem and constituted the most serious and sustained threat to life and health'.[73] It was observed that those officers who took reasonable exercise enjoyed the best health. Captain Warrack, imprisoned in Hong Kong, also observed that 'the short stocky type of individual was more adaptable, both mentally and physically to the diet' whereas 'tall, bulky men seemed to take longer to become acclimatised and suffered more from general debility and weakness in suffering from diarrhoea.'[74]

The health problems of the prisoners of war were similar to those suffered by civilian internees, who were used to a comfortable expatriate lifestyle attended by native servants and so were unaccustomed to the primitive conditions in which they now found themselves. Even a garage manager such as the thirty-one-year-old Czech motor engineer Val Kobouky, one of the last Europeans to escape before the fall of Singapore in February 1942, could afford to live in a fine house with servants, dress stylishly, entertain lavishly and was able to run two cars. He described the people of Singapore as the 'modern Pompeiians' for the insouciant way in which the colony had continued its sybaritic luxury even as the Japanese advanced on it. In keeping with the Singapore tradition, colonial society had held parties at the Raffles Hotel and had consumed vast quantities of alcohol at the Cricket Club, albeit to prevent liquor stocks falling into enemy hands, even as hospitals for the wounded were being set up in the Singapore Club and the vestry of the cathedral was turned into an operating theatre.[75] Internment had come as a shock, but the internees had to adapt quickly if they were to survive. They had an advantage over military prisoners in that many of them still had contacts with other nationalities outside the camps with whom they could trade money and valuables for food and medicine. At Stanley internment camp in Hong Kong, 'there can not have been more than a dozen wedding rings left in the camp by the time we were released'.[76] The only medical equipment and supplies were those brought into the camps by interned doctors. The Japanese refused requests for drugs and a single bale of cotton wool was the only medical supply they provided in Singapore. There in the camp hospital there was a serious shortage of medical instruments, bandages, anaesthetics, sedatives and drugs for stomach complaints, trusses for patients with hernias and even mattresses, pillows, sheets and towels.[77] In Hong Kong, Dean Smith, a colonial medical officer before the war, found that 'although most doctors, pharmacists and nurses took in a few medicines with them … the dispensary cupboard was often bare and prayer and fasting the order of the day'. As for his captors, 'the Japanese were not helpful. A favourite response to any appeal for drugs or medicines was "Any fool can cure people with medicines – you are a doctor – you should be able to cure them without medicines" – to which I do not know the answer.'[78]

Not all Western doctors were interned. Some were allowed to continue to work in hospitals outside the camps. Dr P.S. Selwyn-Clarke, the Director of Medical Services in Hong Kong was allowed to continue in his role, though with reduced staffing, to ensure that public health standards were maintained in the occupied colony as a precaution against epidemic disease. From this position he was able to smuggle medicines and clothing into the camps for the internees on his weekly visits of inspection. On such occasions he was forbidden to pass on any war news but could discuss only medical and relief matters. Then suddenly in the summer of 1942 he was arrested by the Japanese on a charge of treason and his usefulness was at an end.[79] The American writer Agnes Keith, interned in a camp in Borneo by the Japanese, was sent to the native ward of the Sandakan Civil Hospital with her two-year-old son when they contracted malaria. This hospital was run by an Australian and a Scottish doctor who had been released from internment and worked on the 'principle that a doctor's first duty is to the sick of a country, regardless of the race or politics of its administrators'.[80] Their position of freedom allowed them to smuggle drugs and powdered milk to the prisoners of war and civilian internees until they too were once again interned.

The harsh conditions in which the internees lived and worked took their toll on their health. Food was always in short supply, often consisting of 'rice and water only and occasional scraps of other food'.[81] In Hong Kong, a shortage of clothing was a serious health problem in the winter months but in the tropical climate of Singapore this was not such a problem except in so far as 'the exposure of the body to the sun for four to six hours daily was a contributory cause of certain skin affections and tended to lower vitality' whereas the lack of decent footwear often led to the development of tropical ulcers on the feet of the ill-nourished internees. There were too few latrines and long queues for the ones that existed. Ulcers, dysentery, pellagra, dermatitis and malaria were rife. At Changi prison between internment in 1942 and May 1944, the average weight of young men, aged between twenty-five and thirty-four, fell from 161 to 125lb, and of older men, aged between forty-five and fifty-nine, fell from 173 to 123lb. Yet, despite this the average annual death rate was low at 18.1 deaths per 1,000 in Changi during the three-and-a-half years of internment. Many of the men formerly working as government officials or planters in Malaya had had to pass stringent medical tests before their appointment so could be presumed to be fit when they entered the camps. Moreover, they now no longer had the opportunity to overeat, smoke heavily or drink alcohol to excess and there were 100 doctors in the camp from all branches of medicine to treat them, even if operations were performed without anaesthetics.[82] This was no consolation to the internees whose death was a result of their incarceration in appalling conditions with the most primitive care, such as thirty-nine-year-old business manager Alexander Mitchell who died before his time of acute cardiac failure and bronchial asthma in Sime Road Internment Camp, Singapore, in December 1944.[83]

Conditions for the prisoners of war sent to work on the infamous Burma-Siam Railway were dire and almost half of them died before returning to Changi as a result of the hard labour, the inadequate ration of rice and the lack of facilities for the sick. Dysentry, diarrhoea and ulcerated feet were commonplace. Cholera and malaria were rife. If a man was too sick to work, he was often not fed. Yet, epidemic disease was a greater fear for the men than starvation. Henry Traill, a thirty-two-year-old former rubber plantation manager serving in the Royal Ordnance Corps, considered that 'all the beatings and insults, the weariness, discomforts and hunger' were as nothing compared with the outbreak of a cholera epidemic. One of his tent mates was one of the first fatal victims and within a few hours of his first trips backwards and forwards to the latrine 'the flesh seems to turn to water and the body becomes wasted as through from weeks of starvation.' As more men in the tent were struck down with cholera, the remaining occupants were sprayed with disinfectant and their possessions burned before being moved into isolation; so fearful were the Japanese of an epidemic that they were happy for once to follow the advice of the British medical officers.[84]

Surgeons had to work in atrocious conditions in the jungle and find new ways of treating the sick. Weary Dunlop, an Australian surgeon, became a hero to his men through his dedication in dealing with what he called a 'medical tragedy'. He was not above digging sanitary trenches when the only men available for such essential duties were too sick to work. One of the strangest operations he ever performed in the jungle was at night in February 1943 on Private Jones, an Australian soldier whose perforated peptic ulcer had almost certainly condemned him to a painful death. Patients with dysentery were moved out of the hospital tent to give Dunlop and his colleagues Arthur Moon and Ewan Corlette space in which to work. An operating table was improvised from bamboo. Light and warmth were provided by fires and candles, while water was sprinkled on the floor to keep the dust down. A stretcher was used as an instruments table and a bamboo mask was made for the anaesthetist. A Japanese corporal 'became excited about the patient being exposed' when Jones was being prepared for the operation and tried to cover him up with a blanket, only to be 'restrained'. The operation lasted for two hours and at the end of it the patient was left on the table wrapped in a blanket with hot water bottles to keep him warm. Despite his condition deteriorating immediately after the operation, Jones rallied and five days later was much improved.[85] Dunlop was to prove himself the master of understatement when summing up his wartime achievements after he had been liberated: 'owing to the sub-human brutality of the Japanese, mass starvation, squalid conditions of living and the prevalence of tropical diseases of all sorts, medical organisation was fantastically difficult, but we did achieve a good deal'.[86]

Whereas Dunlop used whatever he could find in the jungle as substitutes for conventional medical supplies, such as a pocket knife or razor instead of a scalpel, cotton or parachute silk for catgut and bamboo for splints, the Dutch doctor Henri Hecking used traditional folk remedies learned during his childhood in Java, including forest herbs for the treatment of malaria and fungi from pomelo trees for application to wounds. He was also a proponent of the use of placebos such as concoctions of boiled ipecacuanha that had no medical effect other than reassuring his patients that they had been given some medicine. If there were no medicines or treatments available, it was better to suggest that something was being done to relieve pain and alleviate medical problems if only to reassure the patient that he was being treated in some way. As well as reinforcing the professional mystique of the medic, the psychological effect of believing in a treatment could raise morale and relieve the patient. At the very least, no harm was being done and perhaps much spiritual good.[87]

Prisoners of war were also the subject of medical experimentation by Unit 731, otherwise innocuously known as the Epidemic Prevention and Water Supply Unit. Under Shiro Ishii, this unit had been set up in 1936 at Pingfan in northern Manchuria to work on bacterial warfare. Disease bombs, containing anthrax, dysentery, cholera, typhoid or bubonic plague, were dropped on the Chinese during the Sino–Japanese War that had begun in 1931. Infection patterns and the amount of lethal bacteria needed to engineer epidemics were tested on human guinea pigs or *marutas*. These unfortunate prisoners were also shot in ballistic tests, frozen to investigate frostbite, electrocuted, boiled alive, exposed to lethal radiation and vivisected. When the war ended, the survivors were gassed or poisoned and the facilities at Pingfan destroyed. Ishii and his team of doctors and scientists then traded their iniquitously acquired medical information to the American authorities, in return for immunity from prosecution as war criminals.[88]

The victorious allies were not themselves innocent of experiments into biological warfare. The United States had manufactured anthrax and botulin bombs during the war, though these were never trialled let alone used in warfare. They had subjected their own unwitting troops to secret radiation tests as part of the programme to develop the atom bomb. In Britain Paul Fildes established the Biology Department at the Chemical Defence Experimental Station at Porton Down in Dorset in 1940 to study the possibilities of biological warfare and establish ways of retaliation if Germany resorted to such weapons. Anthrax tests were carried out on the Scottish island of Gruinard and at Penclawdd in Wales where the effects of a proposed cluster bomb, the 'N' bomb, were investigated by releasing bursts of the bacteria, which had been produced on a culture medium made up of marmite, molasses and simple salts, to infect and kill sheep through inhalation. The bomb was never developed but a simpler method of using anthrax in biological warfare was developed through the manufacture of cattle cakes that could be dropped by aircraft over pastures where grazing cattle might eat them. By 1943, an operational stockpile of 5 million cattle cakes had been built up, but they were all destroyed at the end of the war apart from two boxes that were kept until 1972 as curiosities.[89] Compared with the German and Japanese medical experiments on prisoners, this was small beer.

Across the globe, the catalogue of atrocities committed as a result of the Second World War can become an unrelenting litany of inhumanity. But who had the force to speak out against and prevent these violations against mankind? The International Red Cross had been established in 1863 to provide relief for wounded soldiers irrespective of nationality as a result of the experiences of the Geneva businessman Henri Dunant in the aftermath of the 1859 Battle of Solferino. The first Geneva Convention of 1864 had granted neutral status to soldiers wounded in battle and to military hospitals and ambulances, and civilian doctors and nurses serving in national Red Cross Societies to aid the wounded. A red cross on a white background was recognised as a protective emblem for medical personnel and civilians aiding them under the provisions of the Convention. Rapidly adopted by many countries throughout the world, it came through its first major tests in the Austro-Prussian War of 1866 and during the Franco-Prussian War of 1870. During the First World War, the International Committee of the Red Cross had extended its work into the protection of the rights of prisoners of war, though these were not actually covered by the Geneva Convention until 1929.[90] During the Second World War, Germany, Italy, Britain and the United States complied with the Geneva Convention. Although hospitals and ambulances might occasionally be deliberately targeted, most attacks on them were the result of accidents of war. Often such facilities were located close to fuel depots, railways and other legitimate military targets. Conditions in some prisoner of war camps might be harsh, especially in German camps where Russian and Eastern European prisoners of war were classed among the racially inferior, but they were generally in compliance with the Geneva Convention and were regularly inspected by neutral monitors sent by the International Committee of the Red Cross.

However, things were very different in the Far East. The Japanese, with their own warrior code and a tradition of brutality within their armed forces, were prone to showing a callous disregard for the wounded and for the rights of medical personnel. The atrocities committed against the wounded at the fall of Hong Kong and Singapore were symptomatic of a contempt for the defeated and a lack of recognition of the non-combatant role of the doctor and nurse; no respect was shown to the Red Cross emblem. Permission was refused to the defeated troops to even collect the 'European dead' for decent burial and so prevent the spread of disease.[91] Generally, though, the Japanese were 'guilty of neglect rather than actual misuse of prisoners'.[92] The Red Cross had no right to visit the civilian internment camps or to represent the interests of the internees[93] and was often refused permission to send its representatives to inspect the military camps. The International Red Cross admitted that 'the ICRC's greatest worry was the absence of permission to visit prisoner of war camps'.[94] Even when Red Cross delegates were granted rights of access to the camps, they were not always allowed to see the prisoners. Marcel Junod was only allowed two hours in which to visit a camp and most of this time was taken up with a meeting with the Japanese commandant; even when he was able to enter the camp, it was only to find that most of the prisoners were away on labour detachments.[95]

The failure of the International Red Cross Committee to be effective in the Far East can be understood through the problems faced by their delegates in Hong Kong. Rudolf Zindel, a successful Swiss businessman who had lived in Hong Kong before the war, and Edward Egle, an International Red Cross official based in Shanghai, sent back positive reports on the conditions they found in Argyle Street, North Point and Shamsuipo camps after managing to obtain permission to visit them in July 1942.[96] Zindel's excuse for sending misleading reports was that the

Japanese were 'extremely sensitive to anything implying criticism' and that it was difficult to talk to the prisoners let alone see how haggard and ill-looking they actually were:'I could study and admire at leisure every piece of poultry or cattle on the camp farms, but it required a special effort on my part to get close even to a comparatively small proportion of POWs in the camps'. One prisoner of war boldly walked up to Zindel in front of the Japanese and shook his hand, slipping him a note about the true conditions hidden in a hollow bamboo tube that Zindel 'succeeded in getting into my trouser pocket without arousing suspicion'. The note gave him 'valuable information' but it was not passed on to Geneva. He had to be cautious in his dealings with them and 'one of my greatest disappointments ... was my failure to induce the POW camp authorities to disclose to me information concerning the whereabouts and welfare of prisoners of war believed to have been in Hong Kong camps'.[97] He was working under strain since 'the Japanese would not recognise him as having any status', his reports were censored and withheld by Japanese censors, his flat and office were regularly searched by the police and he was worried about the safety of his wife and children living with him in Hong Kong. One civilian internee believed that 'Mr Zindel was working to the best of his ability, but he was young and inexperienced and was afraid of the Japanese'.[98] Nevertheless he did succeed in seeing the civilian internees and providing some help for them, including selling the watches, jewellery and clothing of internees so they could buy food or medicine and also obtaining supplies of insulin for five diabetics in Stanley camp.[99]

Where the Red Cross did miserably fail was in doing anything for the civilian victims in the Nazi concentration camps. The Geneva Convention did not cover the protection of civilians. The International Committee of the Red Cross did attempt to persuade the German government that it should accord civilians the same rights as combatants but failed to insist for fear that taking too intransigent a stance might endanger the relief being given to prisoners of war. However, from November 1943, it was given the concession of sending relief parcels to any detainees in the concentration camps whose names were known. The parcels sent to Dachau, Buchenwald, Ravensbruck and Oranienburg-Sachsenhausen may have been symbolic rather than affording widespread relief but a much greater achievement came in March 1945 when Carl Burckhardt, president of the International Committee, received permission for ten delegates to enter the camps 'on condition that none of them leaves before the end of the war'.

The delegates, among them Louis Haefliger at Mathausen, Paul Dunant at Theresienstadt and Victor Maurer at Dachau, were thus able to give succour to the survivors of these camps and help at their liberation at great personal risk to themselves.[100]

However, there was little that the Red Cross could do to help those persecuted civilians who had gone into hiding or even were under threat of deportation to the concentration camps. Courageous doctors such as Roger Leforestier and Juliet Usach provided essential medical care to Jews in hiding in the Le Chambon area of south central France. Leforestier had formerly worked with Albert Schweitzer at his leper hospital in Africa and was to be executed in August 1944 for using his medical skills to help Jews and the resistance movement.[101] The Swedish businessman Raoul Wallenberg bought medicines and organised infirmaries for the sick among the Jews he had taken under the protection of the Royal Swedish Legation in Budapest to save them from deportation after the occupation of Hungary by the Germans, and on occasion even gave up his own bed to an expectant mother about to go into labour.[102] His efforts were not the sole ones. Giorgio Perlasca, the Italian placed in charge of the Spanish Embassy's safe houses for Jews in Budapest, also had to organise medical care for the sick under his care although without the resources enjoyed by his Swedish counterpart. Wallenberg planned to use the fear of a typhus epidemic to protect his safe houses from raids by the fascist Arrow Cross gangs by persuading Barna Yaron, a young Jew sheltering in one of the houses to have an injection to produce the symptoms of the disease but abandoned the plans when it appeared that the scheme might actually trigger off a real epidemic.[103] He also coordinated the relief efforts of the other neutral powers and in doing so Wallenberg appeared to put the Red Cross to shame.

The 1949 Geneva Convention set out to rectify the limitations to its relief powers revealed by the impotency of the International Red Cross in the face of the fate of those people deported to Nazi concentration and deportation camps. The new protocols, which remain the basis of current international humanitarian law, now protected civilians in time of war as well as the wounded and sick in armed forces on land and at sea and prisoners of war. However, they did not apply to victims of civil war or direct attacks on civil populations, though some protection in these areas was given by additional protocols added in 1977. Curbs were placed on medical experimentation and a code of practice drawn up to ensure that the wartime abuses of medical research would not be repeated. This Nuremberg Code was drawn up after the Nuremberg trials of the Nazi war criminals and attempted to give ethical guidance for future medical research. It laid down the principle that 'the voluntary consent of the subject is essential'.[104] However, nothing was done to prevent the continued use of the research data that had come out of the wartime experiments on concentration camp inmates without their consent. Many of the doctors concerned would have justified this on the grounds that they had merely been doing what they could to contribute to medical advance, national survival and for the ultimate benefit of mankind whatever the short-term pain. If the data exists, however unethically it may have been obtained, it could be argued by some that it is valid to use it. Many others would dispute that any use of iniquitously acquired data could ever be ethically justifiable.

Trauma and Terror

The dropping of the atom bomb on Hiroshima and Nagasaki in August 1945 brought the Second World War to an end but ushered in a new age of fear and fresh problems for medicine. Winston Churchill used a medical metaphor to justify the use of 'Little Boy' and 'Fat Man' as the first atom bombs were innocuously dubbed: 'to avert a vast, indefinite butchery, to bring the war to an end, to give peace to the world, to lay healing hands upon its tortured peoples by a manifestation of overwhelming power at the cost of a few explosions, seemed, after all our toils and perils, a miracle of deliverance'.[1] For eyewitnesses of the effects of the atomic bomb, the issues were not so simple. One British doctor who visited the ruins of Nagasaki observed that 'the great majority of the buildings ... were just charred ashes, and amongst these I was able to identify, to the gruesome interest of my companions, skeletal remains of their quondam inhabitants'. The dreadfulness of the scene was 'indescribable' and he was convinced that 'any gentleman who is in future desirous of making war should pay a visit to Nagasaki to ensure his recognition of the horror that may be loosed'.[2]

That horror was even more apparent to the survivors of the atom bomb and to the doctors treating them in the immediate aftermath of the bombing of the two Japanese towns. Yoko Ota remembered that 'there was a fearful silence which made one feel that all people and all the trees and vegetation were dead'.[3] The lucky ones were those who died at once. At a first-aid station 'there were so many burned that the odour was like drying squid' and the survivors seeking treatment 'looked like boiled octopuses'. One man stood there with his eye resting in his palm, which disturbed the physician Michihiko Hachiya since 'what made my blood run cold was that it looked like the eye was staring at me'.[4] In the river were the corpses of victims who had tried to escape the firestorm but had then drowned.

Even more horrific were the corpses of soldiers 'burned from the hips up; where the skin had peeled, their flesh was wet and mushy … they had no faces. Their eyes, noses and mouths had been burned away and it looked like their ears had melted off. It was hard to tell front from back'.[5] The victims who had not died at once seemed to improve but then they 'began to notice in themselves and others a strange form of illness', consisting of nausea, vomiting, diarrhoea, fever, ulceration of the mouth, throat and gums, hair loss and low white blood cell counts.[6] What they were suffering from was radiation sickness, which caused the destruction of the body tissues, haemorrhaging and infection that ultimately killed many of those suffering from it. At the Hiroshima crematorium, the bodies of those who died from radiation sickness were 'black in colour … most of them had a peculiar smell, and everyone thought this was from the bomb … the smell was caused by the fact that these bodies were decayed – some of them having their internal organs decay even while the person was living'.[7] For the victims it was 'the misery of being thrown into a new world of terror and fear, a world more unknown than that of people sick with cancer'.[8]

Medical planning for a nuclear war was to dominate civil defence plans for the next forty-five years until in 1989 the ending of the Cold War, marked by the fall of the Berlin Wall and the end of communist regimes in central and Eastern Europe, briefly ushered in hopes of a better world. There was something old fashioned about such plans which in many ways harked back to the Second World War but with a more chilling edge in the light of the destruction that could be wreaked by nuclear weapons and chemical and biological warfare. Civilians were warned that 'at the first indication of an atomic attack, e.g. a blinding flash in the sky, the individual caught in the open should immediately drop flat on the ground face downwards … a quick reaction in dropping flat within the first second may well save him becoming a casualty'.[9] So great was the fear of biological warfare that in the late 1940s Britain and America refused to allow the export to Eastern Europe of fermentation equipment for the manufacture of penicillin because it could be used for the development of biological weapons, especially anthrax.[10] Bombs and bugs were most likely to be targeted on the centres of population where they would have the greatest impact on the most people. Evacuation of casualties on a greater scale even than in 1939 was accordingly envisaged. London was again organised into sectors with central hospitals acting as 'casualty transit sectors' from which the injured could be moved to 'recovery units', 'cushion hospitals' and base hospitals to be set up in existing country hospitals, requisitioned schools and public buildings and tented hospitals. Essential medical equipment and supplies would be evacuated from the large towns that were expected to be the main targets and the epicentre of any nuclear fallout.[11] Civil Defence planners simulated the likely effects of a bomb falling on Trafalgar Square to assess whether the system would work and logically and, not unexpectedly. concluded that transport might be a problem so there would need to be 'arrangements made ... for the temporary care of casualties pending their removal by ambulance to cushion hospitals'. First aid workers would be concerned with the decontamination of victims of a nuclear blast, emergency treatment for those who were slightly wounded so that they would not overburden the hospitals and 'such primary treatment to casualties as may be necessary to save life before sending patients to hospital'.[12] Such plans ignored what many military planners now realised, that 'it is essential in thermo-nuclear warfare [to] take account ... what is happening in, or is likely to happen, not only in forward areas but also in the rearward area ... on occasion the distraction, the confusion and the incidence of casualties may well be much greater in the rearward than the forward areas'. Some people tended to assume, based on their experience of the Second World War, that all would be 'plain sailing' once casualties had been evacuated.[13] One acknowledged difference from the Second World War, as well as the need for decontamination facilities, was that there would be no distinction made between the supply of blood for transfusion for service personnel and civilians.[14] In the event of a nuclear attack everyone would be in it together. Thankfully, Armageddon did not come.

However, nuclear weapons continued to be tested and both observers and others who unwittingly found themselves in the path of the fallout were to suffer the health effects as a consequence. The explosion of the world's first hydrogen bomb at Bikini Atoll on 1 March 1954 may have given a name to a 'red hot' bathing costume, but the force of the blast exceeded the expectations of the scientists and proved 750 times more powerful than the atom bomb dropped on Hiroshima. Radioactive ash spread across distant islands in the Pacific. The crew of a Japanese fishing boat no more than ninety miles away from the blast were alarmed when their skin turned darker and sores broke out on their fingers and necks. Some of them lost their appetites and displayed all the signs of radiation sickness, yet the American authorities initially refused to acknowledge that any of it was connected with their nuclear tests.[15] The Russians were also conducting their own experiments in the Ural Mountains in 1954, with few safety precautions, to see whether their troops could continue to fight after the explosion of an atom bomb similar in size to the ones that had resulted in the capitulation of Japan nine years earlier. Despite the intense heat, smoke and dust, many soldiers managed to complete their manoeuvres within two miles of the centre of the blast. They wore little in the way of protective clothing and were reassured that it was merely a simulation of a nuclear explosion. Local villagers were not even given that information. Soon both soldiers and civilians were falling sick, lost their sight or developed cancers as a result of their exposure to radiation.[16] The United States, Britain, France and the Soviet Union all conducted nuclear tests throughout the 1950s and early 1960s which recklessly exposed the civilian and military personnel involved in them, the people involved in the subsequent clean-up operations and anyone caught down-wind of the blast to the long-term health effects of radioactivity.[17]

Human guinea pigs were rarely given full information when they participated in research projects to study the effects of nuclear, chemical and biological warfare during the Cold War. Many of the servicemen who volunteered to take part in such experiments at Porton Down in the 1950s thought that they were being paid and given extra leave to take part in a project to find a cure for the common cold. Once at Porton Down, they were asked to volunteer to participate in experiments crucial for national defence. They were assured that there was no danger to them and that everything would be done under constant medical supervision. They were then exposed to such nerve gases as sarin, mustard gas, tabun and soman, which they either inhaled or had dripped on to their skin in liquid form. These tests were used to assess the efficacy of respirators and protective clothing against gas warfare. They also showed that the best way of decontaminating men exposed to nerve gases was to use Fuller's Earth, aluminium silicate hitherto used for cleaning cloth, rather than the liquid bleach and anti-gas ointments that had been in use since the First World War. The research was defensive in aim rather than being concerned with the development of new forms of chemical warfare.[18] This was no consolation for the subjects of these experiments, many of whom were to suffer lasting ill health as a result of their participation in medical research projects connected with predictions of new forms of waging warfare.[19]

The Korean War, which began in June 1950, was a much more conventional conflict. President Harry Truman was adamant that nuclear weapons should only be used as a last resort and declared 'I don't want to see it used. It is a terrible weapon and it should not be used on innocent men, women and children who have nothing to do with this military aggression'.[20] Ground operations, though, were always expected to be difficult on the rugged and mountainous terrain of the Korean peninsula with its poor roads and lack of railways. It was not only military action that was to be made trickier by the inhospitable environment in which the fighting took place. The evacuation of casualties posed an enormous challenge. Although rapid evacuation to a hospital was critical to the survival chances of a wounded soldier, only forty per cent of the casualties were reaching a hospital on the day that they were wounded, transported by army motor ambulances and gasoline-powered Korean railway carriages nicknamed 'doodlebugs'. Not surprisingly, casualties often went into shock as they were jolted on the long journeys and valuable time was lost before they could receive their necessary treatment.[21] However, a solution was found in the small number of Second World War helicopters being used to rescue pilots downed in the sea or behind enemy lines. The Third Air Rescue Squadron of the United States Air Force started off by answering calls to evacuate casualties from especially difficult terrain. Very soon it found itself acting as a full-time medical evacuation service. However, there had to be limits on what could be done. Requests for air evacuation would only be considered in urgent cases involving head, chest, and abdominal wounds, multiple fractures, and great loss of blood where an ambulance could not reach the patient or he would be seriously injured by a rough ambulance ride.[22]

Air medical evacuation, having started almost by accident as a result of requests for help in airlifting patients in need of rapid treatment, soon received official sanction and four helicopter detachments were assigned to 'medevac' or combat medical aero-evacuation. The helicopters were modified to make the patient more comfortable, though the litters were attached to the external skids of the helicopter. Stretchers were fitted with removable covers with Plexiglas windows to protect the patient's head and warm air was piped from the engine manifold to keep him warm. Plasma bottle holders were fitted to the exterior of the cabin doors to aid blood transfusions while airborne.[23] Nevertheless, the journey could be uncomfortable and even frightening for many of the wounded soldiers. For one frightened South Korean soldier who vainly tried to climb into the helicopter from his litter, 'his eyes got as big as silver dollars and he withdrew back into the litter. He rode the rest of the way with his hands firmly attached to the sides of the litter.'[24] Some patients even froze to death in the harsh winter months. For other patients, however, such as Fred Wolf, wounded in the arms, legs and stomach, the contrast with 'the four agonizing hours of being carried down a ridge, first in a raincoat, then in a litter, and then in a bumpy jeep' was so great that the helicopter journey was a relief with 'the take-off ... so gentle he didn't know when it left the ground and the ride was so soothing that he dozed off and didn't even notice the landing at the Mobile Army Surgical Hospital'.[25] Nevertheless by the end of hostilities in July 1953, army helicopters had evacuated 21,658 casualties and made a substantial contribution towards achieving, at 2.4 per cent, the lowest mortality rate for wounded in any war until that time.[26]

The lessons of American airborne evacuation were not lost on Britain and it was reported that 'it is considered in Korea that the prime value of the helicopter is in its ability to rush patients to better medical facilities preferably within the first three hours due to the shock factor'.[27] The Director-General of the Army Medical Services during the Malaya Emergency had been convinced as early as 1948 that 'a helicopter would be invaluable for the evacuation of casualties in the type of country' in which the British forces were 'clearing-up the Communists', although 'helicopters on this side of the Atlantic are still in their infancy, and so far as casualty evacuation is concerned at present do not exist'[28] and was interested in American discussions about air evacuation.[29] In low-lying Malaya, helicopters could easily land to pick up casualties though the jungle sometimes made it difficult to locate the wounded. It took one helicopter pilot, the best part of a day to locate a group of wounded men. Once they had been found in a small clearing, they were able to mark a landing space for him with towels and he was able to pick up two walking wounded and two stretcher cases, all of them National Servicemen whose 'patience and uncomplaining cheerful attitudes were a credit to their regiment', and get them to base within 105 minutes of take-off.[30] A few years later in Kenya during the Emergency there in 1955 the forest clearings were so dense that 'the helicopter could not hover nor could it ascend or descend vertically at altitudes at which it was to operate with a casualty on board', although it had 'proved to be a big lifesaver and as such has been and is still a big morale-booster'.[31]

It was to the mobile army surgical hospital, better known by its acronym of MASH, that the helicopters brought the casualties in Korea. The definitive image of what is often now a forgotten war is of the helicopter bringing in casualties to the MASH, a symbol of hope and an enduring emblem of the war. These mobile-tented units had first been established shortly after the end of the Second World War in order to bring emergency surgery closer to critically wounded casualties than was possible with the field hospitals and casualty clearing stations of that conflict. Mobile sixty-bedded, fully staffed and equipped, truck-borne hospitals were to travel with each military division and set up medical facilities in forward locations just out of the range of enemy artillery fire. Patients could then be evacuated to hospitals in the rear when they were fit to travel. The Korean War was the first time the system was tested in action and it worked. It was difficult to set up effective evacuation hospitals in Korea because of the transport problems, so the MASH units were expanded to first 150 and then 200 beds and began to take medical as well as critical surgical cases. Over 400 patients might pass through the MASH each day.[32]

Each unit had to be ready and able to move at six hours notice. Once the MASH had arrived at its new location, it was expected to be operational within four hours. Five tables were in use at any one time in the operating tent. Once a patient had recovered after the operation, he was made ready for evacuation to the rear of the combat area, often by helicopter. Air transports evacuated many patients to Japan for further treatment by the army medical units stationed there, and serious injuries were flown back to the United States for more specialised care and rehabilitation. The level of activity in these hospitals varied according to the time of year. When fighting was at its peak in the winter and early spring, the hospitals would be crowded with United States, United Nations and enemy wounded, and the operating tent would be working non-stop. Military activity slackened in the summer and the number of wounded accordingly fell. The influx of casualties reflected the pattern of the war.[33] In the first year of the conflict, the 8076th MASH moved every three weeks.[34] As the war progressed through 1952, the fighting became more static and the units were spared the constant upheaval of moving in synchronisation with troop advances and retreats. Tents were replaced with prefabricated buildings as the hospitals settled down to a semi-permanent existence in a fixed location. Newer doctors, such as Mel Horwitz attached to the 8225th MASH, never saw the mobile units to which they were attached actually move location and were used to working with new and decent equipment.[35]

The fresh-faced young doctors, many of them straight out of medical school, who manned the MASH units, were often unprepared for what they were to find on their arrival at their postings. Otto Apel received no training at all for dealing with military medicine in the field and had to figure out for himself how to establish a defensive perimeter and how to appreciate tactics without even a manual to consult.[36] Mel Horwitz, a year later, received eight weeks of training before his posting to Korea but experience remained the best teacher of all in the field itself.[37] They were given no time to settle in to the strange and unfamiliar situation in which they now found themselves and were unaccustomed to military life and discipline, though their medical training had given them a respect for hierarchies of competence and experience. As soon as he arrived at his unit, Otto Apel had no choice but to start operating immediately and worked with hardly any respite for the next eighty hours. His feet were so swollen that he had to cut his boots off at the end of this mammoth shift and baptism under fire. Very little warning was given that casualties were on their way, so the doctors always felt that they were on call and dared go no further than three minutes away from the tents in case they were needed to operate for another twelve-hour shift.[38] Not surprisingly, Hollywood seized upon the dramatic life and death potential of life in a front-line medical unit with the release in 1952 of the film *Battle Circus*, in which a nurse, cutely played by June Allyson, falls in love with Humphrey Bogart's tough, wise-cracking army surgeon against a life and death backcloth of emergency surgery.[39] The reality was that there was carnage in the operating tents, which reeked with the stench of blood. There might be the traces of the blood of people from between ten and fifteen different countries on the boots of the doctors as they operated amidst these chaotic scenes.[40]

It was in these unpropitious circumstances that several advances were made in emergency medicine.[41] New drugs were used on the troops. The newer antibiotics, such as aureomycin, chloramphenicol, streptomycin and teramycin, were now brought into use as well as penicillin. Chloroquine and primaquine were used to combat malaria. Sodium pentobarbital, also known as Nembutal, was used as a sedative. Heparin was used as an anti-coagulant and serum albumin and whole blood were used to treat shock.[42] Anti-tetanus injections were now routinely given to the wounded and it was realised that antibiotics alone would be insufficient unless accompanied by removal of the dead tissue of the wound. Artificial kidneys were used to perform dialysis on patients with Korean haemorrhagic fever and with renal failure due to septic shock. A more effective blood programme was devised to meet the needs of this particular war. Blood was brought in by air from

Tokyo to medical supply depots from which it was then distributed to the hospitals. Then at the MASH, most men who needed them would receive blood transfusions before they were evacuated. Elsewhere there was very little blood available for any form of transfusion. Fortunately in the freezing Korean winters the intense cold inhibited bleeding so blood loss was less of a problem than had been expected, though frostbite was a greater danger than Chinese bullets.[43] Severe arterial injuries from gun wounds that usually resulted in the amputation of limbs inspired advances in vascular surgery. Veins and arteries from the patient would be grafted to repair damaged blood vessels, thus restoring blood circulation and thereby saving many limbs. Such vascular injuries could be treated in the crucial nine to fourteen hours after injury, with the result that there were fewer amputations than with similar injuries in the Second World War.[44]

The soldiers were expected to maintain high levels of fitness that would be honed in combat. Many of the British servicemen in Korea were doing their National Service and it was important that they should lose the flabbiness of civilian life as soon as possible after they were called up and before they saw battle. Physical training courses were 'closely allied to the work and tasks which the doctor may be called upon to perform in the course of his duties'. Nevertheless, after a number of deaths of young soldiers during endurance tests from such causes as infection, heat stroke and 'the impaction of an undigested pea in the larynx', Lord Moran, Winston Churchill's physician, spoke out against the severity of the endurance marches of two hours' duration in which the soldiers were in battle dress and carrying the equipment and arms that they would have to bear in action. He considered these tests to have 'no scientific basis' and to be unsuitable for boys of eighteen years of age. Most military doctors disagreed and argued that the physical training and endurance tests were far from exacting and not too strenuous if the soldiers were properly trained.[45] They would have to cope with far greater strains, both physical and mental, when called upon to fight.

There was a high rate of psychiatric illness, running at about 250,000 men a year, during the opening stages of the Korean War when the first troops sent into Korea from the comforts of their bases in Japan found themselves in battle with inadequate winter clothing, insufficient weapons and very little training.[46] Most of these men, at the rate of about twenty a week, were evacuated to Japan or the United States for treatment until the hospitals there became overwhelmed by the numbers of men coming in 'with face drawn and expressionless or full of terror. Tremulousness, voice difficulty, dilated pupils, rapid pulse, profuse sweating, tremors and sometimes tearfulness'.[47] When the military psychologist Al Glass was sent out as theatre consultant in October 1950, he decided that the only answer to the problem was to return to the Second World War idea of the advance treatment of psychiatric casualties close to the battlefield with the aim of returning them to action as quickly as possible. While there was a possibility of evacuation to the comforts of hospital and the nightlife of Tokyo and Hawaii, there was little incentive to recover if it meant being sent back to the cold of the combat zone. A high incidence of frostbite and other accidental injuries was believed to be because 'the unhappy and dispirited soldier may become apathetic to an injury that may possibly rebound to his personal benefit and remove him from a traumatic environment'. After March 1951, soldiers psychologically unfit for battle were reassigned to support functions. There was no lasting bolthole for anyone in Korea.[48] The principle of proximity, immediacy, expectancy, otherwise known as 'PIE', was adopted: casualties should be treated near the line, as soon as possible and in circumstances that encouraged them to return to their units. Moreover, importance was now given to ensuring that the men had adequate periods of rest away from the fighting. However, a new problem in military psychiatry was to arise with the return of brainwashed prisoners of war after the armistice had brought hostilities to a close. Suffering from diarrhoea, respiratory infections and vitamin deficiencies, the prisoners of the North Koreans and Chinese were lucky to survive their imprisonment and psychiatrists concluded that 'the individual's fighting spirit had to be maintained at a high level for him to survive any illness'.[49] Confused and disoriented, many had been persuaded to make statements in support of their captors. They were treated less sympathetically than the other psychiatric casualties of the war, though in the long term there was to be more understanding of the effects of such extreme stress.

All of these new developments ultimately were to have an impact on emergency civilian medicine in casualty departments, though it would take time for these ideas to filter through into the treatment of trauma. Helicopter evacuation, the use of paramedics and shock treatment were to become the staples of accident and emergency centres. MASH methods had become the standard for emergency medicine throughout the world.[50] The MASH units themselves continued in use wherever American forces saw action until they were superseded by smaller Combat Support Hospitals that could get even closer to the front line and the last MASH was converted to one of these units in 2006.[51]

The MASH units of the Korean War were immortalised in the 1970 film *M*A*S*H*, directed by Robert Altman and based on a novel by Richard Hooker, who under his real-name of Richard Hornberger had served as a MASH doctor in Korea.[52] His book was not an anti-war novel but rather juxtaposed the grimness of war with the outrageous behaviour of the doctors witnessing it. The film, by contrast, is a subversive anti-war comedy in which the Korean War serves as little more than a cover for an attack on the Vietnam War. Altman minimised all references to Korea in the movie and it was very easy for the film's first audiences to assume that it was actually about Vietnam. Servicemen went AWOL to see the zany antics of Hawkeye and Trapper John, played by Donald Sutherland and Elliot Gould, and their 'laughs and loves between amputation and penicillin'. Anti-war protestors relished the message that the only way to maintain sanity in war is through laughter and took Nurse 'Hotlips' Houlihan's complaint that 'this isn't a hospital: it's an insane asylum' to be a reference to the madness of war itself. *M*A*S*H* as a film tells us more about Vietnam than Korea.[53]

Guerrilla warfare was the dominant new feature of the Vietnam War, which lasted from 1959 until 1975 although the United States only got heavily involved in the conflict in 1964. This meant that the battlefront was much less obvious than in previous wars. In such a situation, fully mobile hospitals were no longer seen as essential to the rapid treatment of casualties. Many of the American hospitals in Vietnam had become semi-permanent with the introduction of Medical Unit Self-Contained Transportable (MUST) facilities. The MUST hospitals were expandable, mobile shelters with inflatable ward sections.[54] Despite the static nature of most of the hospital units, it was proudly boasted by the American forces that no casualty was more than ten minutes away from hospital treatment thanks to the efficient system of aeromedical evacuation.[55] This was an exaggeration although developments in the design of helicopters made the system much more efficient and swifter. It was now possible for between six and nine patients to be transported at a time. Patrol leaders would radio for 'Dust Off', as the evacuation helicopters were known, and arrange a suitable pick-up point in a jungle clearing. The helicopters were often vulnerable to enemy fire as they collected the casualties since the Vietcong rarely respected the Red Cross markings on them or on the hospitals. Most patients would be evacuated by this means within thirty-five minutes of being wounded and few had to wait more than two hours. Once airborne, they might indeed have the ten-minute flight to hospital.[56] Vietnam doctor Ronald Glasser was optimistic when he declared that 'If you're going to die in Nam, you'll die straight out, right where it happens. If you don't die right out you've got a pretty good chance; the evac and surgical hospitals do anything and everything'.[57] Between January 1965 and December 1970, 97,659 wounded men were admitted to army hospitals. The overall mortality rate of 2.6 per cent was higher than that of 2.5 per cent in Korea, but this was because the greater efficiency of helicopter evacuation meant that more mortally wounded men were reaching hospital rather than dying on the battlefield.[58]

Improvements in the evacuation times and developments in vascular surgery reduced the amputation rate in Vietnam to 8 per cent.[59] Amputations, when absolutely necessary, were carried out at base whenever possible but often had to be carried out on the spot when shattered limbs were left hanging by nothing more than tissue and mangled flesh. Don Rion, wounded on the Razorback ridge in December 1966, attempted to 'get up on two stubs of legs severed at mid thigh' but was more concerned at 'the prospect that he might have lost his means of procreation' than he was by the amputation of his legs. He was reassured that he would still be able to have children, though his case was indeed hopeless.[60] The high velocity firearms in use, such as the Soviet AK-47 and the American M-16, were deadly. Deep disabling wounds were caused by the punji stakes, sharpened bamboo sticks often smeared with excrement by the Vietcong guerrillas, hidden in dense foliage as booby traps. Many men suffered horrendous injuries from the hidden landmines, containing ten pounds of explosives and three pounds of metal fragments. These caused 'frag wounds', the American term for shrapnel wounds. It might take the surgeons up to six hours to remove as much as sixty fragments from the chest or abdomen of one casualty. In cases where it would have been more harmful to remove debris from the body, it would be left as a lasting souvenir of the man's service in Vietnam.[61]

Burns were a major medical problem in the Vietnam War. Many were caused when helicopters were shot down, but others were the result of the mishandling of flamethrowers or exposure to napalm and the toxic chemical Agent Orange used to clear the jungle in which the guerrillas were hiding. What many of the victims found most distressing was that all their hair, including eyebrows and eyelashes, were burned away, but at least they had survived. Men with 90 per cent of burns on their body were expected to die but even where they only had 60 per cent burns, skin grafts were difficult. Patients with severe burns were placed between the two metal arches of Stryker frames, devised so that they could be turned over without too much pain. The drug Sulfamyalon and fluid resuscitation techniques were developed for use on burns, resulting in a 50 per cent reduction in mortality since the Korean War.[62]

As great an achievement was the development of an organized military blood programme. The collection, processing, shipment and distribution of blood and plasma were orchestrated by the Military Blood Programme Agency. The supply of blood to American forces in Vietnam rose from 100 units each month in 1965 to 38,000 units a month in 1969.[63] Technical advances, such as the use of adenine to preserve blood cells, the use of lightweight Styrofoam containers and improved refrigeration methods increased the shelf-life of blood and blood products from twenty-one to forty days.[64] Often the wounded man had such a weak pulse that it was difficult to take blood for cross-matching in the hospitals as the blood would not flow.[65]

The greatest threat to health in Vietnam, though, did not come from wounds but from tropical diseases, which were responsible for 70 per cent of all admissions to American military hospitals. Virulent strains of malaria could hospitalise a soldier for five weeks or more. In the wet monsoon season, skin diseases and immersion foot, also known as paddy foot, were prevalent. Michael Holladay, a Marine Corps commander, complained that his clothing was 'wet damn near all the time' and 'because we went through the old tiger grass, which had a razor edge to it, the crotch of the utilities wore out'. Groin infections and boils were common in such conditions.[66] Preventive measures and military hygiene could only do so much in such conditions and men continued to suffer from the unpleasant conditions in which they fought.

Military doctors and nurses have inevitably been drawn into providing civilian healthcare in the areas in which war is being waged down the ages, driven by the humanitarian motive to relieve suffering especially where existing healthcare facilities are inadequate and the climate unhealthy. In the twentieth century, such care has become part of an official campaign to win over the support of the population of the country in which a foreign army is based. Such was the motivation behind American medical aid in Vietnam when it set up the Medical Civil Action Program (MEDCAP) to provide healthcare to Vietnamese civilians during the Vietnam War, and spent between 500 million and 750 million dollars on the treatment of Vietnamese civilians. In 1965, the Military Provincial Health Assistance Program (MILHAP) provided hospital care for civilians and was meant to train civilian Vietnamese doctors in modern techniques. Then in 1967 the Civilian War Casualty Program (CWCP) set up field hospitals for wounded civilians. Army doctors immunised patients, deloused them and treated their illnesses. Skin diseases, dysentery, intestinal parasites and trachoma were widespread. MEDCAP personnel made periodic visits to the hamlets, displaced person's refugee camps and orphanages which otherwise would have received no medical care at all. They had very little in the way of equipment or modern facilities, but when the charge was made that eighteenth-century care was being delivered to the people of South Vietnam, Dr Tom Dooley replied that if all they had had until now was fifteenth- or sixteenth-century medicine then this must be considered great progress. Unfortunately, with the withdrawal of American troops, medical aid, which had been so closely linked with military medical services, also came to an end. Undoubtedly it had provided good care at the time but left no lasting legacy in Vietnam, unlike in Korea where a continued American presence after the end of the Korean War together with the training of Korean doctors did have lasting effects on the civilian health care system. In Vietnam, even the battle for hearts and minds was lost.[67]

Some soldiers found relief in alcohol and others in sexual intercourse, seeking their rest and recreation not in Japan as in the Korean War but instead in the fleshpots of Saigon with its burgeoning sex industry. The draft meant that it was a young man's war in which 'only the eighteen-, nineteen- and twenty-year-olds need to worry, and since no one listens to them it doesn't matter'.[68] With a mixture of naivety, strong sexual impulses and the fear of death or disfigurement constantly with them, these young men were willingly lured into the local brothels. The availability of antibiotics lulled men into a false sense of security that, if they were unlucky enough to go with a Vietnamese prostitute who was not clean, the resultant infection could easily be cleared up. Venereologists, though, were concerned about the increasing prevalence of antibiotic-resistant strains of gonorrhoea.[69] Unless something could be done about the problem, 'the capability of the overseas command to fulfil its mission could be jeopardized without adequate indoctrination and education in health subjects'.[70] One way of doing this was the release in 1969 of a short film, *Where the Girls Are: VD in South East*

Asia, which emphasised prevention rather than cure. In the film, a clean-cut, all-American air force sergeant, Pete, is persuaded by his comrades to visit a massage parlour where he fails to use a condom and catches gonorrhoea. A relationship with another Asian prostitute when he is lonely during a rest and recuperation leave gives him a dose of syphilis which is only revealed when he later undergoes a premarital test for syphilis after he has proposed to the loyal sweetheart he left at home. Pete is then faced with the possibility that he might have also infected his girlfriend and 'sure they give you shots and tell you you're okay, but you can't promise a girl like Julie you'll be true to her and show up with a case of syphilis'.[71]

Not only sex and alcohol were widely available in Vietnam: drug taking became a major problem among bored and disturbed servicemen. With the drug-culture of the 1960s already beginning to establish itself in the United States, it was little wonder that American soldiers should smoke marijuana when it was so freely available in Vietnam. The heaviest users were support troops but it was also smoked by combat units in lulls in the fighting since its 'sedative and tranquilizing properties helped reduce anxiety and blunt the hyper-arousal state so frequently seen between periods of combat'. In a world where 'peer group ties assumed heightened importance', it seemed as if 'marijuana often became the sacrament which bound a group together. Its tranquilizing and euphorgenic properties allowed combat losses to be temporarily forgotten while new relationships were solidified'.[72] Just as cigarette smoking had been universal during the two World Wars, not just as an antidote to stress but because most of the smokers enjoyed it, recreational drug taking became popular in this war; the difference was that the drugs now being taken were illegal. Cocaine, popularly known as 'crack', was also used, but by 1970 heroin or 'skag', once associated in the United States with poor urban African Americans, had become popular with white troops because of its 'potency, availability and difficulty of detection'. By 1972, more soldiers were being evacuated from Vietnam because of narcotic drug abuse than for wounds.[73] The politicians were alarmed and President Richard Nixon launched an ineffective war on drug abuse. Under 'Operation Golden Flow', servicemen had their urine tested at the end of a tour of duty and were not allowed on the plane if they had 'dirty urine'. Few of the returning servicemen considered themselves to be addicts and, with misplaced confidence, they expected to leave their drug habit behind on their return home.[74] Many were to have problems in adapting when they returned home from a war that had become deeply unpopular back in the States.

Whatever, post-war problems the Vietnam veterans may have had, their psychiatric health during the war remained good and there were fewer psychiatric casualties than in any previous war of the twentieth century. This may seem surprising considering the stresses of dealing with guerrilla warfare. Jim Tolomay came very close to 'breaking point' while on patrol when a marine stepped on a landmine and was cut in half. So disturbed was he by this that 'I thought I was going to lose my mind' but 'I regained my composure only because of the mental toughness of the marines around me and their support'.[75] Such group self-help and hardness may have kept men from weakening, but it could also produce callousness towards death and the enemy. William Broyles, a marine lieutenant, later said that his unit 'disposed of the enemy dead like so much garbage. We stuck cigarettes in the mouths of the corpses, put *Playboy* magazines in their hands, cut off their ears to wear around our necks'.[76] Yet, there was not the combat exhaustion of previous wars. Tours of duty were limited to a year and there were plenty of rest and recreation periods within that time. Battles tended to be short and there were few major artillery barrages. Morale remained high. It was even claimed that 'psychiatric casualties need never again become a major cause of attrition in the United States military in a combat zone'.[77]

This success did not appear so spectacular once the Vietnam War had been lost and the maladjusted young man returning from Vietnam was perceived not as a hero but as a social problem. Now the very reasons previously given for the low rate of psychiatric illness among servicemen during the war were used to explain the post-war alienation of a very visible group of veterans. Short tours of duty had prevented the growth of solidarity among the soldiers and contact with home had lowered morale by revealing that public opinion was turning against the war. Substance abuse may also have concealed psychiatric disorders. The term 'post-traumatic stress disorder' was coined in 1980 to describe the condition of the veteran alienated from the society to which he had returned. Drug rehabilitation programmes and improved benefits for ex-servicemen were attempts to solve the problem. Yet, the majority of Vietnam veterans were actually successful in their return to civilian life and the prominence given to those men who did not make the transition to civilian life so well may be the result of America's attempts to come to terms with the aftermath of a controversial and divisive war.[78]

Whereas the conflict in Vietnam had been long-drawn out and exposed deep-seated tensions in American society, the 1982 Falklands Campaign was short and seemed more like a throwback for the United Kingdom to the colonial wars of the nineteenth century. The greatest military challenge, one with repercussions for the provision of medical services, was of maintaining a sea and air supply line stretching for 8,000 miles in order to retake the distant Falklands Islands in the South Atlantic after their invasion by Argentine forces. The luxury cruise liner *Canberra* was pressed into service alongside regular vessels of the Royal Navy, such as the aircraft carriers *Hermes* and *Invincible*, to carry troops, and sick bays were set up on board these ships. The SS *Uganda*, another cruise liner specialising in educational cruises for schoolchildren, was requisitioned specifically as a hospital ship. The need for a fully equipped hospital ship was more than justified after the bombing of the landing ships *Sir Galahad* and *Sir Tristram* at Bluff Cove on 8 June 1982. The attack killed fifty-six Welsh Guards and over 100 others were severely wounded or burned. They were evacuated swiftly to the hospital ship for immediate treatment. For the most severely burned, plastic surgery awaited them at home. The badly burned face of Guardsman Simon Weston became an emblematic image of the survivors. Others of his colleagues were treated for post traumatic stress disorder. Meanwhile, a 'buddy system' was instituted for survival in the harsh climate of the Falklands. Men were paired up and ordered to watch their partners for any signs of drowsiness, lassitude or pallor that could indicate frostbite or exposure; the afflicted man would then be placed in his survival bag, a transparent plastic bag which trapped his body heat and thus warmed him up.[79]

Just as short in its duration as the Falklands was the First Gulf War of 1991, fought to liberate Kuwait after its occupation by the Iraqi forces of Saddam Hussein. During the months of preparation before the launch of the brief but bloody and violent Operation Desert Shield and Operation Desert Storm, there had been fears of biological and chemical warfare and of a long conflict with enormous casualties. American and British forces had problems in acclimatising to conditions in the desert as they made their preparations in a climate that varied from hot and humid to cold and damp. Troops were exposed to respiratory and diarrhoeal disease, but good health was maintained by active policies of disease prevention and surveillance. Environmental health officers advised on sanitation, food and water supplies and immunisation. The bodies of dead animals, such as sheep, goats and camels left to rot in the desert, were sprayed with strong insecticides. Health specialists were aware of the dangers of corneal abrasions from blowing and drifting sand, shigellosis, haemorrhagic fever, dengue and sand fly fever and advised on their prevention. It could have been a textbook approach to the maintenance of military hygiene.[80]

However, the greatest danger was believed to come from the biological and chemical weapons of mass destruction that might be used by Iraq. Saddam had used mustard gas during the Iran-Iraq War a decade earlier and was expected to resort to such weapons against his latest enemies. American and British troops were issued with 'chemical warfare warning kits', containing pyridostigmine bromide tablets to be taken every eight hours to prevent the lethal effects of nerve gases. These tablets were supposed to be safe, but many soldiers went down with gastrointestinal and urinary problems after taking them. Anthrax was also believed to be a major threat and troops were vaccinated against it and botulinum. Automatic anthrax detectors were set up around military camps. There were also frequent false alarms, some of them triggered by vehicle exhaust fumes setting off the automatic detectors, which compelled the troops to don their uncomfortable protective gear and take their protective tablets.[81] Chris Craig, serving with the Royal Navy, believed that 'the emotional preoccupation with chemical weapons was out of proportion with their real threat ... we increased our already regular drills and were often unsettled by spurious alarms from the upper-deck chemical alarms'.[82]

In the aftermath of the war, many ex-servicemen were to complain of chronic fatigue, lack of appetite, skin rashes, headaches, arthralgia, myalgia, difficulty in concentrating, irritability, forgetfulness and even of 'burning semen' during sexual intercourse. This was initially put down to them having been exposed to the dust, sand and smoke of warfare in the desert, made worse by the burning of Kuwait's oil wells. Some of the sufferers had also been exposed to leaking chemical weapons stored at Khamisiyah. Others had handled enriched uranium shells or been exposed to organophosphates used as insecticide sprays. Some people ascribed the symptoms to the cocktail of vaccines they had received in preparation for the health hazards of the campaign; the combination of botulinum, polio, typhoid, cholera, tetanus, pertussis and anthrax vaccines in particular were blamed for damaging the immune system. Psychiatrists suggested that it had a psychological origin. Yet the cause of the condition, soon to be known as 'Gulf War Syndrome', remained a mystery; British servicemen had to fight long and hard for any official recognition that their illness might be linked to their service in the Gulf.[83]

Iraqi civilians fared little better. The smart bombing of the early days of the conflict destroyed Iraq's power grid and damaged facilities guarding against water pollution. The result was severe food shortages, outbreaks of cholera and typhoid and a severely disrupted medical care system that had scarcely recovered by the outbreak of the Second Gulf War and the fall of Saddam.[84] Once one of the best health systems in the Middle East, the Iraqi health services had been neglected since the early 1980s when Iraq's oil revenues were earmarked for buying military equipment. The damage caused by the First Gulf War to hospitals was simply patched up. The only way into one of the children's hospitals in Baghdad was by wading through a pool of raw sewage. When medical equipment broke down it was not replaced. Doctors and nurses were poorly paid and the system was on the verge of collapse by 2003, only for it to continue to disintegrate even further in the aftermath of the invasion during the Second Gulf War.[85]

The call-up of medical reservists for service in the First Gulf War raised fears that militarily and medically Britain might now be overstretched, concerns that seemed all too reminiscent of the First World War. There had been massive cuts in the armed forces following the 'peace dividend' that came with the end of the Cold War. There no longer seemed to be a need for massive defence expenditure. In order to provide adequate medical cover in the Gulf, doctors and nurses in the reserve forces were mobilised and it was feared that if the war turned out to be a prolonged one there might be a danger of civilian health services at home collapsing through a lack of National Health Service staff at a time when many hospitals back in Britain were preparing wards for the receipt of military casualties which happily were never needed. The short duration of the war meant that the anticipated problem never materialised, but a lack of investment in defence spending was to again raise problems during the war in Afghanistan of 2001 and in Iraq in 2003 and the subsequent troubled occupation of both countries. Military hospitals had been closed down and the wounded when returned to Britain now found themselves treated in the general wards of National Health Service hospitals alongside civilians who would have little idea of what they had endured and could not offer the emotional support of a fellow soldier. Many found themselves on hospital waiting lists and felt bitter that the armed forces had failed to support them when incapacitated in service of Queen and country.[86] Psychiatric patients with post-traumatic stress disorder especially felt abandoned.[87] It was as if, in the face of economy cuts, the long-standing, unspoken pact between state and citizen to compensate the war injured in return for their sacrifices was apparently falling apart.

Soldiers, though, were not the only victims of modern warfare, Civilians have always suffered too. In response to this, the years since the Second World War have seen the growth of international humanitarian organizations dedicated to the relief of the innocent victims of warfare and of natural and manmade disasters. The United Nations Relief and Rehabilitation Administration was formed by the Allies in 1944 to give aid to the people of newly liberated Italy, who faced starvation and epidemics. For a time it provided Italy with seventy per cent of the food its people required.[88] It was wound up when the World Health Organization was founded in 1948 with the idealistic vision of creating 'a state of complete physical, mental and social well-being and not merely the absence of disease or infirmity'. In pursuit of this goal, it has had a role in coordinating responses to the medical crises brought on by war as well as launching campaigns for the eradication of disease and the provision of better public health services in the developing world, areas where warfare often reduces already low standards of medical care. The World Health Organization was the more effective successor to the interwar Health Organization of the League of Nations, which had collapsed along with its parent body on the outbreak of war in 1939 and had been set up as a body completely separate from the United Nations in order to ensure its survival in the event of another world war. That did not stop it from collaborating with the United Nations International Children's Emergency Fund (UNICEF) in organizing relief programmes in the war zones of the world.[89]

The World Health Organization also coordinated the work of other governments in providing bilateral medical aid in emergencies. Much of this had become necessary when the armed forces of a developed country had had a role to play as peace-keeping forces under the aegis of the United Nations in countries wracked by war. However, there was much criticism of the failure of the World Health Organization and the United Nations to deal with the health crisis resulting from the disintegration of the former Yugoslavia in the early 1990s and the subsequent wars between the former republics. Medical care disintegrated in many of the warring states. Hospitals were destroyed, health workers fled from Bosnia and Croatia and the displacement of refugees created enormous problems associated with poor sanitation and infectious disease. Simple sanitary items such as soap, disinfectants, toilet paper and tampons were urgently needed. War victims with physical and psychological injuries were in need of treatment and later of rehabilitation. In Bosnia, Muslim patients were afraid to go into predominantly Serbian hospitals. The State Hospital in Sarajevo was in such a dangerous location that potential patients only went to it when absolutely necessary after seventeen of the staff were killed by snipers or bombs while on duty. Nevertheless, despite the personal danger, the lack of medical supplies and the bitterly cold conditions in a hospital without electricity or heating, one doctor, shivering beneath the overcoat and layers of clothing he habitually wore on night duty, declared that they 'would fight each other like animals if necessary to survive but they would never leave' their posts at the hospital.[90] Yet the international agencies were seen as doing little to improve the situation. At Vukovar Hospital 'the Yugoslav Federal Army perfidiously killed 200 patients, medical staff and civilians' in November 1991 and, according to the memorial stone later erected to the victims, this atrocity was committed 'in the midst of the International Red Cross Committee's attention and in the presence of the European Community Observer Mission'.[91] The Croatian public health specialist Slobodan Lang blamed this on the failure of the World Health Organization to speak out against what was happening in first Bosnia and then Croatia.[92]

Other agencies such as the International Red Cross continued to spearhead famine relief, epidemic interventions and programmes of medical relief in war zones, although they were as heavily criticised as the World Health Organization for not being ineffective enough at times. The Red Cross had been involved in humanitarian aid to the civilian victims of war, as well as combatants, since the Russo-Ottoman War of 1875. In the inter-war years, between the First and Second World Wars, it had extended its remit from aiding the victims of war to the noble aim of improving, health, preventing disease and giving relief to the victims of natural disasters. Such activities are always going to be linked in the modern world where many wars are fought in developing countries with primitive healthcare systems that are further destroyed by conflict. In recent years the Red Cross has been active in the fight to have landmines banned, a cause also taken up, and given great publicity, by Diana, Princess of Wales. In 1997 the Ottawa Treaty banned anti-personnel landmines as weapons likely to cause 'superfluous injury or unnecessary suffering'. However, the International Red Cross has had to deal with the plight of victims of these barbarous weapons. Limb fitting workshops have been opened in Afghanistan, Cambodia, Iraq and Angola where lightweight prostheses are manufactured locally from polypropylene. Local self-sufficiency is promoted in such activities as much as the medical aid offered by them.[93] Relief work has not only attracted idealistic health workers wishing to do something practical to work overseas, but has also inspired other doctors to try to improve healthcare provision for disadvantaged groups at home. Paul Ambrose, a public health campaigner working with immigrants from El Salvador while acting as a clinical adviser to the Surgeon General of the United States before his untimely death at thirty-two aboard the aeroplane that crashed into the Pentagon on 11 September 2001, was keen to 'figure out how he could use these lessons from the old days to make a better world of today – particularly for the underserved population and health professionals in training.'[94]

The International Red Cross has always adopted a policy of strict neutrality and is dependent on its host government for permission to operate in a country. It was this failure to speak out against injustice, incompetence and inhumanity that drove aid workers to form Médecins Sans Frontières in 1971. Its founder Bernard Kouchner was a recently qualified doctor working with the Red Cross in Biafra during the 1967–70 Nigerian Civil War, who found it hard to keep quiet about the corruption he witnessed that was compromising the care of the refugees he was tending. Instead of following the official Red Cross diplomatic tactic of silence, he was unable to stand by and stay silent about the basic questions of human justice and 'had to bear witness to what was happening, and this meant denouncing political corruption, the plight of children'. He got together with a like-minded group of doctors to set up a relief agency that would speak out and exercise 'the moral right to interfere inside someone else's country'.[95] They were concerned that medical relief was being impeded by the excessive bureaucracy and diplomatic manoeuvrings of government agencies and big international agencies like the Red Cross. A nongovernmental agency seemed to be the answer, one able to respond much more quickly to a crisis and act independently of the government of the country in which they were working. Soon, there were branches of Médecins Sans Frontières all over the world with idealistic doctors and nurses ready to go where they were needed.[96] Kouchner was himself expelled in 1979 from the organization he had founded when he hired a hospital ship to save Vietnamese boat people amidst accusations from his erstwhile colleagues that he was putting self-promotion before humanitarian concerns.[97]

Kouchner may have been the victim of the greater scope offered by Médecins Sans Frontières for individual action when he took it too far, but the flexibility of the agency allowed it to rapidly deploy teams of volunteers where needed, such as Kosovo in 1999 when the expulsion of ethnic

Albanians from their country caused a humanitarian crisis. The Kosovan refugees, many of whom had been forced to leave their homes or jobs at gun point, included young professional people, whose business suits and mobile telephones seemed incongruous in the refugee camps and offered a reminder that not all victims of modern conflict are from the third world. Unlike more usual refugees elsewhere in the world, the Kosovans had been beneficiaries of a decent health system and were not malnourished, so only needed simple primary acute care and treatment for chronic conditions that the older and feebler of the refugees were already suffering from before their expulsion.[98] Médecins Sans Frontières, having given primary medical care to the exhausted refugees, believed that the Kosovan refugees should be encouraged to help themselves to avoid conditioning them with a sense of helplessness, something that was especially viable when already they had built up an effective social and medical network as an ethnic minority in their homeland. It seemed important that Kosovan doctors and nurses should be involved in treating their own people where possible. Once they had coped with the immediate practical problems of hygiene, feeding and pressing medical care, Médecins Sans Frontières, unlike many of the other relief agencies, urged immediate psychiatric support for any one traumatised by their experiences rather than waiting until later.[99] The United Nations response to the crisis was predictably more bureaucratic and slower.[100]

Relief work in war zones is one way in which military and civilian medicine converge, but for most people in the Western world this all seemed to be something that went on in less civilised parts of the world. The events of Tuesday 11 September 2001 were to bring the message home that everyone was equally vulnerable and shock the world. When the passenger planes hijacked by Al-Qaeda crashed into the twin towers of the World Trade and the Pentagon, the emergency medicine procedures for handling casualties that had been developed in the military context of the Korean and Vietnam Wars and then introduced into civilian accident and emergency medicine came into effect. The emergency rooms of New York and Washington DC were put on standby, blood donation stations were set up and teams of paramedics and doctors went out to see what they could do. The expected mass casualties never came. All that remained recognizable of the passengers and crew aboard United Airlines Flight 93, which crashed into a field in Pennsylvania, was a still knotted necktie lying on the ground, scattered teeth and bone fragments.[101] There and at the Pentagon and World Trade Center, it was the work of the forensic pathologists in identifying the victims from random body parts and

DNA samples that was to reflect medical advances and build upon experience gained in investigating war crimes in the former Yugoslav republics where Andrew Thomson, a doctor working with the United Nations, had sighed that 'I set out to save lives and have ended up collecting the dead'.[102] Only 289 whole bodies were recovered in New York; it was easy to identify 'a man in a suit and tie who had fallen from Cantor Fitzgerald in the North Tower and was sitting upright, now somewhat shrivelled but whole, with his wallet in his pocket' although he was not found until almost three months after the disaster, but it was not so easy to identify most of the fatalities.[103] It was a painstaking job to match bone fragments of the 2,819 victims, sifted by hand from the rubble and debris, with DNA taken from their toothbrushes and hairbrushes.[104] The London bombings of 7 July 2005, when underground and bus passengers were targeted, were to be a better test of the value of emergency medicine in dealing with the victims of terrorism than the events of 9/11. Meanwhile, military advances in the treatment of post-traumatic stress disorder were to be used in treating the survivors, eyewitnesses, rescuers and families of the victims of 9/11 and 7/7.[105]

Since 2001, the world has been as dangerous a place as it ever was, but has been perceived as being even more perilous than ever before in the aftermath of 9/11. In the United States, for so long physically removed from the field of war, the effects of international terrorism were especially traumatic on a people not accustomed to being vulnerable. In the months after the Al-Qaeda attacks, bioterrorism became an urgent issue in medical defence preparations as there were scares of anthrax and smallpox attacks.[106] A national programme of smallpox immunization was begun in the United States in December 2002 to counter the threat of the malicious release of the variola virus. However, it was anthrax that was seen as the major threat from bioterrorism since the spores could easily be dispersed by such innocent means as the United States postal service as happened in autumn 2001 and once released they could persist for many years.[107] Both service personnel and civilians today are at risk from the weapons of terror, including biological warfare.[108] Cold War dread of atomic annihilation has been superseded by fears of dirty bombs and mass terrorism. In the twenty first century warfare will continue to devise ever-nastier ways of killing people using all the tools of modern technology. Equally, modern medicine will continue to meet the challenge of repairing the damage of war just as it has done over the last hundred years.

Notes

Preface

1 W. Osler, 'The War and Typhoid Fever', *British Medical Journal*, 2 (1914), 909–13.

2 See R. Cooter, M. Harrison and S. Sturdy (ed.), *War, Medicine and Modernity* (1998), pp. 1–17.

3 W. Osler, 'Science and War', *The Lancet*, 2 (1915), 795–801.

4 R. Cooter, 'War and Modern Medicine' in W.F. Bynum and R. Porter (ed), *Companion Encyclopaedia of the History of Medicine* (1993), pp. 1536–73.

5 Political Warfare Executive, *Instructions for British Servicemen in France, 1944* (2005), p.6.

6 Virgilio Retrosi, *Guerra* (1914–15), exhibited at Estorick Collection of Modern Italian Art, London, 'Barbed Wit: Italian Satire of the Great War' exhibition, January–March 2007.

7 Gaetano Donizetti, *La Fille du Régiment*, (DVD, Decca Music Group 074 3146, 2006).

8 T. Cassidy, *Birth: A History* (2007), pp. 175–7. I wish to thank Elise Younger for this reference.

9 *Independent on Sunday*, 11 March 2007.

10 R. Holmes, *Dusty Warriors* (2007), p. 35.

Chapter 1: National Inefficiency

1 'Government Service', *St Mary's Hospital Gazette*, 5/8 (October 1899), 115–6.

2 Thomas Hardy, 'The Darkling Thrush', in H. Gardner (ed.), *New Oxford Book of English Verse* (1972), p. 757.

3 A.W. Sanders, 'Civilian Surgery in South Africa', *St Mary's Hospital Gazette*, 6/3 (March 1900), 45.

4 G.R. Searle, *A New England?* (2004), p. 274.

5 A. Conan Doyle, *The Great Boer War* (1901), p. 1.

6 V. Warren Low, 'Some Modern Bullet Wounds', *St Mary's Hospital Gazette*, 8/4 (April 1902), 54.

7 *Ibid.*

8 J. Laffin, *Combat Surgeons* (1999), p. 142.

9 V. Warren Low, 'Some Modern Bullet Wounds' (1902), 54.

10 TNA, WO 108/252, 'Report on the Organisation and Equipment of Medical Units', Pretoria, 1900, p. 8.

11   Lt. Wingate, letter, *St Mary's Hospital Gazette*, 6/4 (May 1900), 47.

12 F. Treves, *The Tale of a Field Hospital* (1900), pp. 14–15.

13 *Ibid.*, pp. 15–23.

14 Unattributed letter on 'Army Medical Reform', *St Mary's Hospital Gazette*, 6/7 (September 1900), 96–7.

15 TNA, WO 108/252, 'Report on the Organisation and Equipment of Medical Units', Pretoria, 1900, p. 2.

16 *The Times*, 14 April 1900.

17 TNA, WO 108/252, 'Report on the Organisation and Equipment of Medical Units', Pretoria, 1900, p. 3.

18 F. Treves, *The Tale of a Field Hospital* (1900), pp. 74–6.

19 M.K. Gandhi, *An Autobiography* (1930), pp. 142–8.

20 G.R. Searle, *A New England?* (2004), p. 283; D. Low-Beer, M. Smallman-Raynor and A. Cliff, 'Disease and Death in the South African War: Changing Disease Patterns from Soldiers to Refugees', *Social History of Medicine*, 17/2 (2004), 223–45.

21 V.J. Cirillo, *Bullets and Bacilli: the Spanish-American War and Military Medicine* (2004), p. 139.

22 E.W. Herrington, 'Further News from South Africa', *St Mary's Hospital Gazette*, 6/10 (December 1900), 149. See also V.J. Cirillo, 'Winged Sponges: Houseflies as Carriers of Typhoid Fever in Nineteenth- and Early-Twentieth-Century Military Camps, *Perspectives in Biology and Medicine*, 49/1 (2006), 52–63.

23 W. Osler, *The Principles and Practice of Medicine* (1914), pp. 2–3; W.G. Macpherson, W.P. Herringham, T.R. Elliot and A. Balfour (ed.), *History of the Great War: Medical Services* (1922), vol. 1, p. 11.

24 K.F. Kiple (ed)., *Cambridge Historical Dictionary of Disease* (2003), pp. 345–9.

25 W. Osler, *The Principles and Practice of Medicine* (1914), p.2.

26 'Recollections of the Siege of Ladysmith from the Diary of Miss Charleson', *St Mary's Hospital Gazette*, 7/6 (June 1901), 91.

27 *Ibid.*, 92.

28 *Ibid.*, 91.

29 *Ibid.*, 92–3.

30 *Ibid.*, 7/7 (July 1901), 104.

31 H.W. Nevinson, *Ladysmith: the Diary of a Siege* (1900), pp. 285–90.

32 G.W. Steevens, *From Cape Town to Ladysmith* (1900), pp. 122–5.

33 T. Packenham, *The Boer War* (1992), pp. 353–4.

34 Quoted in *ibid.* p. 355.

35 Letter from J.A.H. Brinker, *St Mary's Hospital Gazette*, 6/4 (May 1900), 56–7.

36 Letter to *British Medical Journal*, 7 July 1900.

37 *The Times*, 27 June 1900.

38 *Ibid.*, 11 April 1900.

39 A.A. Bowlby, *A Civilian War Hospital: Being an Account of the Work of the Portland Hospital and Experience of Wounds and Sickness in South Africa* (1900).

40 TNA, WO 33/195, Recommendations of the Committee Directed to Consider Sir Thomas Gallwey's Medical Report on the Campaign in Natal, 1899–1900, p. 2.

41 P. Hoare, *Spike Island* (2001), pp. 164–70.

42 L. Colebrook, *Almroth Wright* (1954), p. 123.

43 *Ibid.*, p. 46.

44 A.E. Wright and F. Smith, 'On the Application of the Serum Test to the Differential Diagnosis of Typhoid and Malta Fever', *The Lancet*, 1 (1897), 656.

45 A.E. Wright, 'On Vaccination against Typhoid Fever', *British Medical Journal*, 1 (1897), 256.

46 'Notes from India', *The Lancet*, 1 (1899), 929–34; *ibid.*, 2, 182; A.E. Wright and W.B. Leishman, 'Results Which Have Been Obtained by Anti-Typhoid Inoculations', *British Medical Journal*, 1 (1900), 122–4; A.E. Wright, 'On the Results Which Have Been Obtained by Anti-Typhoid Inoculation, *The Lancet*, 2 (1902), 652–3.

47 See N. Durbach, *The Anti-Vaccination Movement in England, 1853–1907* (2005).

48 L. Colebrook, *Almroth Wright* (1954), p. 38.

49 L. Colebrook, 'Obituary of Almroth Edward Wright', *The Lancet*, 1(1947), 654.

50 'Letter from a Civilian Surgeon', *St Mary's Hospital Gazette*, 6/4 (May 1900), 54–5.

51 Letter from E.W. Herrington, No. 9 General Hospital, Bloemfontein, *St Mary's Hospital Gazette*, 6/5 (July 1900), 82.

52 'Report of Advisory Board for Army Medical Services, 25 September 1902', *Journal of Royal Army Medical Corps*, 5 (1905), 242.

53 Interim report of the Anti-Typhoid Inoculation Committee, Cd. 26989 July 1904.

54 K. Pearson, Letters to the Editor, *British Medical Journal*, 1 (1904), 1243, 1259, 1614, 1667.

55 See further L. Colebrook, *Almroth Wright, Provocative Doctor* (1954); V.Z. Cope, *Almroth Wright, Founder of Modern Vaccine Therapy* (1966); M. Dunnill, *The Plato of Praed Street: the Life and Times of Almroth Wright* (2000).

56 M. Worboys, 'Almroth Wright at Netley: Modern Medicine and the Military in Britain, 1892–1902' in R. Cooter, M. Harrison and S. Sturdy (ed.) *Medicine and Modern Warfare* (1999), pp. 77–97.

57 An outbreak of bubonic plague in Cape Town in 1901 also revealed a lack of collaboration between military and civilian authorities on account of the desire of army doctors to remain aloof from, and unimpeded by, their civilian counterparts, M. Sutphen, 'Striving to be Separate? Civilian and Military Doctors in Cape Town During the Anglo-Boer War' in R. Cooter, M. Harrison and S. Sturdy (ed.), *War, Medicine and Modernity* (1998), 48–64.

58 E. Lynn Jenkins, 'Life in a Flying Column', *St Mary's Hospital Gazette*, 8/6 (June 1902), 86.

59 Report on the Concentration Camps in South Africa by the Committee of Ladies, Cd. 893, 1902 pp. 170, 174–9.

60 *Ibid.*, 179.

61 R.J.S. Simpson, *Medical History of the War in South Africa* (1911), pp. 229–36.

62 Report on the Concentration Camps in South Africa by the Committee of Ladies, Cd. 893, 1902, p. 89.

63 *Ibid*, p. 93.

64 E. Hobhouse, *Report of a Visit to the Camps of Women and Children in the Cape and Orange Rivers* (1902), p. 135.

65 M. Hasian, 'The Hysterical Emily Hobhouse and Boer War Concentration Camp Controversy', *Western Journal of Communication*, 67/2 (2003), 138–63.

66 E. Hobhouse, *Report of a Visit to the Camps of Women and Children in the Cape and Orange Rivers* (1902), pp.9–13.

67 *The Times*, 27 June 1900.

68 Care and Treatment of the Sick and Wounded During the South African Campaign, Cd. 453, 1901.

69 TNA, WO 108/252, Report on the Organisation and Equipment of Medical Units, Pretoria, July 1900.

70 E.W. Herrington, 'Further News from South Africa', *St Mary's Hospital Gazette*, 6/9 (November 1900), 126.

71 R. McLaughlin, *The Royal Army Medical Corps* (1972), p. 16.

72 Letter on Army Medical Reform, *St Mary's Hospital Gazette*, 6/76 (September 1900), 96–7.

73 Report to Consider the Re-organization of the Army Medical Services, Cd. 791, 1901; TNA, WO 30/114, Discussion of War Office Committee on Reorganisation of the Army Medical and Army Nursing Services, 5 July 1901.

74 *Ibid.*, p. 11.

75 TNA, WO 163/581, Minutes of Permanent Executive Committee of the War Office, 6 April 1902.

76 TNA, WO 30/114, Summary of reorganisation of various branches of the Army, including the RAMC, *c.* 1902.

77 *Ibid.*, Extracts from the Report of the Royal Commission on the Care and Treatment of the Wounded in South Africa, 1901.

78 *Ibid.*, Proposed scheme for the reorganisation of the Army and Indian Nursing Services, 19 July 1901.

79 TNA, WO 32/9338, comments of Queen Alexandra on reorganisation of Army and Indian Nursing Services, 1901–2. The motto of QAIMNS *Sub Cruce Candida* ('Under the White Cross') was adopted as a tribute to the Queen's Danish birth and referred to the white cross on the flag of Denmark.

80 Quoted in F. Prochaska, *Royal Bounty* (1995), p. 126.

81 A. Summers, *Angels into Citizens*, (1988), p. 241.

82 B.S. Rowntree, *Poverty: A Study of Town Life* (1901), pp. 216–220.

83 J.F. Maurice, 'Where to Get Men', *Contemporary Review*, 81 (1902), 78–86; 'National Health: A Soldiers' Study', *Contemporary Review*, 83 (1903), 41–56.

84 See G.R. Searle, *Quest for National Efficiency* (1971).

85 Report of the Inter-Departmental Committee on Physical Deterioration, Cd. 2175, 1904, p. 8, quoting Professor Cunningham.

86 *Ibid.*, p. 8.

87 K. Pearson, *The Groundwork of Eugenics* (1912), pp. 27–30; Huxley Lecture, 1903, quoted in Report of the Inter-Departmental Committee on Physical Deterioration, Cd. 2175, 1904, p. 38.

88 Quoted in D. Dwork, *War is Good for Babies and Other Young Children: A History of the Infant and Child Welfare Movement in England 1898–1918* (1987), p. 30.

89 J. Lewis, *The Politics of Motherhood: Child and Maternal Welfare in England 1900–1939* (1980), p. 65.

90 *Ibid.*, p.90.

91 H.D. Harben, *The Endowment of Motherhood* (1910).

92 B. Harris, *The Health of the School Child: A History of the School Medical Service in England and Wales* (1995), p. 64; J.D. Hirst, 'The Growth of Treatment Through the School Medical Service, 1908–18', *Medical History*, 33 (1989), 318–42.

93 P. Horn, *The Victorian and Edwardian Schoolchild* (1989), p. 90.

94 Report of the Inter-Departmental Committee on Physical Deterioration, Cd. 2175, 1904, pp. 5–6.

95 Report of the Royal Commission on the Poor Laws and Relief of Distress, Cd. 4499, 1909, p. 659.

96 E. Noble-Smith, *Growing Children: Their Clothes and Deformity* (1899), p. 7.

97 TNA, ED 24/37, Report of Physical Training Committee, 1901.

98 M. Girourad, *The Return to Camelot: Chivalry and the English Gentleman* (1981), pp. 250–8; see also K. Townsend, *Manhood at Harvard* (1996), pp. 102–4, for a consideration of the role of sport in promoting military qualities among American students at Harvard University.

99 Obituary, A.E. Bullock, *St Mary's Hospital Gazette*, 21/8 (October 1915), 126.

100 W. Osler, *The Principles and Practice of Medicine* (1914), p. 3.

101 TNA, WO 106/6359, 'Medical notes on the Japanese Army' by Captain B. Vincent, 17 May 1905, p. 133.

102 *Ibid.*, 'Medical and Sanitary Reports from Officers Attached to the Japanese Force in the Field', 1906, p. 2.

103 *Ibid.*, pp. 3–4.

104 *Ibid.*, p. 7.

105 *Ibid.*, 'Medical Service of the Second Japanese Army During and After the Battle of the Sha Ho (10–16 October 1904)', report by W.G. Macpherson, Manchuria, February 1905.

106 *Ibid.*, pp. 176, 179.

107 *Ibid*, p. 190.

108 *Ibid.*, 'The Battle of Mukden', report by W.G. Macpherson, July 1905, p. 219.

109 TNA, WO 106/6360, 'Report on the Russian Medical Service' by Colonel W.H.H. Waters, 1905, p. 539.

110 *Ibid.*, 'Report on Russian Medical Administration in the Field' by Major J.M. Horne, 1905.

111 TNA, WO 106/6359, 'Report on Condition of the Hospitals in Port Arthur After the Capitulation' by W.G. Macpherson, April 1905, p. 268.

112 *Ibid.*, p. 270.

113 TNA, WO 106/6360, 'Report on the Health of the Russian Troops' by Colonel W.H.H. Waters, 1905, p. 558.

114 C. Herrick, 'The Conquest of the Silent Foe: British and American Military Medical Reform Rhetoric and the Russo Japanese War' in R. Cooter, M. Harrison and S. Sturdy (ed.) *Medicine and Modern Warfare* (1999), pp. 99–129.

Chapter 2: Medicine in Khaki

1 Dr Slavka Mihaljlovic, cited in H. Strachan, *The First World War* (2003), pp. 20–1.

2 A.A. Martin, *A Surgeon in Khaki* (1915), pp. 9–10. The reason for doctors being advised to equip themselves with revolver and sword was that they might need to defend the wounded.

3 H.S. Souttar, *A Surgeon in Belgium* (1915), p. 59.

4 'Extracts from a Letter from a Late Houseman at the Front', *St Mary's Hospital Gazette*, 20/8 (October 1914), 120–1. For a collection of similar letters from doctors from the Front, see O. Craig and A. Fraser, *Doctors at War* (2007).

5 B. Ziegler, 14 September 1914, in P. Witkop (ed.), *German Students' War Letters* (2002), p. 5.

6 Report upon the Physical Examination of Men of Military Age by National Service Boards from November 1st 1917 – October 31st 1918, Cmd. 504 (1919), 6.

7 A.A. Martin, *A Surgeon in Khaki* (1915), pp. 11–13. See also, D. Silbey, 'Bodies and Cultures Collide: Enlistment, the Medical Exam and the British Working Class, 1914–1916', *Social History of Medicine*, 17/1 (2004), 61–76.

8 Report upon the Physical Examination of Men of Military Age by National Service Boards from November 1st 1917 – October 31st 1918, Cmd. 504 (1919), 308.

9 D.H. Lawrence, *Kangaroo* (1950), p. 238.

10 J. Bourke, *Dismembering the Male* (1999), p. 172; I.R. Bet-El, *Conscripts* 2003, 33–7.

11 Letter from Aubrey W. Venables, 4 February 1915, *St Mary's Hospital Gazette*, 21/2 (February 1915), 25–6.

12 L.B. Clarke, 'Active Service and the Unfit', *St Mary's Hospital Gazette*, 23/6 (June 1917), 66.

13 D.J. Kevles, 'Testing the Nation's Intelligence: Psychologists in World War I', *Journal of American History*, 55 (1968), 565–81.

14 Letter from A.A. Bowlby, *The Lancet*, 2 (1914), 1427.

15 B. Ziegler, 14 September 1914 in P. Witkop (ed.), *German Students' War Letters* (2002), p. 6. The wounded man had his leg amputated at the knee. Ziegler himself was killed less than a month later aged 22.

16 'Extract from a Letter from a Late Houseman', *St Mary's Hospital Gazette*, 20/9 (November 1914), 143.

17 C.H. Sorley, *Collected Letters* (1990), p. 245.

18 *Ibid.*, p. 254.

19 Obituary of Harold Ackroyd, *Guy's Hospital Reports (War Memorial Number)*, 70 (1922), 17–18.

20 R. McLaughlin, *The Royal Army Medical Corps* (1972), pp. 57–9.

21 Obituary of Arthur Ernest Bullock, *St Mary's Hospital Gazette*, 21/8 (October 1915), 125–6.

22 Obituary of Reginald Joseph Wooster, *St Mary's Hospital Gazette*, 22/8 (October 1916), 107.

23 G. Dyer, *The Missing of the Somme* (1994), p. 73. The Boer War memorial at Hull shows two wounded soldiers defending a wounded comrade, an earlier depiction of an iconic scenario.

24 Letter from J. Errol M. Boyd, 18 January 1915, *St Mary's Hospital Gazette*, 21/1 (January 1915), 11–12.

25 TNA, WO 159/16, Letter from Arthur Lee to Lord Kitchener, 12 October 1914.

26 S. Maynard Smith, 'With the Armies in France', *St Mary's Hospital Gazette*, 24/3 (March 1919), 28–33.

27 Private information, Harry Lazenby.

28 S. Maynard Smith, 'With the Armies in France', *St Mary's Hospital Gazette*, 24/3 (March 1919), 28–33.

29 Postcard of German wounded in the church at Neufmoutiers showing the injured lying on straw before the altar in F. Pairault, *Images de Poilus* (2005), p. 93.

30 I.R. Whitehead, *Doctors in the Great War* (1999), pp. 181–2.

31 A.A. Martin, *Surgeon in Khaki* (1915), 120–3.

32 TNA, WO 159/16, Letter from Arthur Lee to Lord Kitchener, 21 October 1914.

33 *Ibid.*, 12 October 1914.

34 A.J.P. Taylor, *English History 1914–1945* (1965), p. 5.

35 TNA, WO 159/16, Letter from Arthur Lee to Lord Kitchener, 6 November 1914.

36 M. Lloyd, *The London Scottish in the Great War* (2001), p. 31.

37 TNA, WO 32/4751, Report on Medical Services in France by the Commission on Medical Establishments, 1917.

38 Private Donald Bliss cited in M. Lloyd, *The London Scottish in the Great War* (2001), p. 91.

39 H.S. Souttar, *A Surgeon in Belgium*, (1915) pp. 124–5.

40 A. Carrel and G. Debelly, *The Treatment of Infected Wounds* (1917), pp. 215–17.

41 W.H. Schneider, 'Blood Transfusion in Peace and War, 1900–1918', *Social History of Medicine*, 10/1 (1997), 105–26.

42 X-ray equipment had first been used on the battlefield during the 1897 Tirah campaign when British forces quelled an uprising on the Khyber Pass; its value was proven in 1898 during the Spanish-American War when seventeen X-ray units were deployed to hospitals and three hospital ships. W.C. Borden, *The Use of the Röntgen Ray by the Medical Department of the United States Army in the War with Spain* (1900).

43 H. Cushing, *From a Surgeon's Journal* (1936), p. 404–6.

44 *Ibid.*, pp. 49–51.

45 M. Bliss, *Harvey Cushing* (2005), p. 314.

46 *Ibid.*, p. 325.

47 S. Westman, *Surgeon with the Kaiser's Army* (1968), p. 75.

48 Otto Heinebach, 22 September 1915, in P. Witkop (ed.), *German Students' War Letters* (2002), p. 239.

49 A.S. Daly, 'Anaesthetics' in S. Barling and J.T. Morrison (ed), *A Manual of War Surgery* (1919), pp. 397–412.

50 C.T. Edmunds, 'Experiences in a German Field Hospital', *St Mary's Hospital Gazette* 23/3 (March 1917), 33.

51 S. Westman, *Surgeon with the Kaiser's Army* (1968), p. 69–70.

52 E.M. Remarque, *All Quiet on the Western Front* (1980), p. 27.

53 *Ibid.*, p. 25.

54 R. Graves, *Goodbye to All That* (1979), p. 198.

55 M. Lloyd, *The London Scottish in the Great War* (2001), p. 31.

56 TNA, FO 383/43, Report by Captain Middleton, 24 August 1915.

57 W. Ellison, *Escaped!* (1918), p. 117.

58 S. Westman, *Surgeon with the Kaiser's Army* (1968), pp. 159–60.

59 TNA, FO 383/43, Report by Captain Middleton, 24 August 1915.

60 A.A. Martin, *A Surgeon in Khaki* (1915), p. 177.

61 I.R. Whitehead, *Doctors in the Great War* (1999), p. 157.

62 L. Colebrook, *Almroth Wright* (1954), p. 70.

63 K. Brown, 'The Inoculation Department at Boulogne', *St Mary's Gazette*, 103/1 (1997), 32–5. The facilities offered to Wright for his laboratory were perhaps as bad as those being endured in the trenches: a basement with a pipe leaking sewage from the gaming rooms, now wards, above. He was then offered the former fencing school in the attic with no running water, gas or drainage. Alexander Fleming improvised laboratory equipment using pumps, petrol cans, a paraffin stove and fire bellows, and claimed it was the best lab he had ever worked in. BL Add. MS 56214, W. Claydon.

64 TNA, FD 5/97, 'Memorandum on the Necessity of Creating at the War Office, a Medical Intelligence and Investigation Department to Get the Best Possible Treatment for the Wounded, Diminish Invaliding; and Return the Men to the Ranks in the Shortest Possible Time', 1916.

65 *Ibid.*

66 *Ibid.*, Letter from Wright to Major Astor, January 1917; Letter from Wright to C.M. Fletcher, 30 January 1917. Wright disingenuously claimed to Fletcher that 'the fact that a man thinks me wrong or my actions ill-judged and tells me so will never make bad blood between him and me' yet throughout his acrimonious career he made many enemies and was merciless in his attacks on them.

67 TNA, WO 32/4751, Report on Medical Services in France by the Commission on Medical Establishments, 1917.

68 *The Times*, 28 September 1914.

69 A.A. Martin, *A Surgeon in Khaki* (1915), pp. 10–11.

70 A.P. Long, 'Immunizations in the United States Army', *American Journal of Public Health*, 34 (1944), 27–33; G.R. Callendar and G.F. Luippold, 'The Effectiveness of Typhoid Vaccine Prepared by the U.S. Army', *Journal of American Medical Association*, 123 (1943), 319–21.

71 *Journal of Royal Army Medical Corps*, 18 (1912), 600.

72 St Mary's Hospital Archives, SM/MX4/16, brochure *Who Won the Great War?*, *c.* 1931; WF/AD, Inoculation Department, House Committee for Therapeutic Inoculation Minutes, 15 October 1914; *ibid.*, 26 March 1915. After 10 months of war, 3 million doses of typhoid vaccine had been given to the British army, 500,000 to the Belgians, 300,000 to the Serbian army; 130,000 doses of cholera vaccine were issued to the British and 450,000 doses to the Serbian army; both the French and Russian armies each got

100,000 doses of an antisepsis vaccine, *St Mary's Hospital Gazette* 21/6 (June 1915), 87.

73   L. Colebrook, *Almroth Wright* (1954), p. 42.

74   W.G. Macpherson, W.P. Herringham, T.R. Elliot, and A. Balfour, *Official History* (1922), p. 153.

75   *The Lancet*, 1 (1905), 1453.

76   TNA, WO 32/9797, 'Note on Typhoid', 1941.

77   TNA WO32/4752, 'Report on Medical Services in France', 1917.

78   *Ibid.*

79   TNA, WO 159/16, Letter from Lee to Kitchener, 16 February 1915.

80   TNA, WO 162/67, Medical Arrangements at Gallipoli, 1915.

81   Letter from 'Old Student', Anzac Cove, Gallipoli, 15 May 1915, *St Mary's Hospital Gazette*, 21/6 (June 1915), 92–3.

82   TNA, CAB 19/27, Appendices to Report of Commission on the Medical Arrangements in Mesopotamia, July 1916; St Mary's Hospital Archives, DP 42/7/14, 'Third Interim Report: the Prospects of Epidemic Plague in Mesopotamia in 1917' by J.C.G. Kunhardt, 1 March 1917.

83   W.H. Willcox, 'Mesopotamia 1916–1919', *St Mary's Hospital Gazette*, 25/5 (May 1919), 67.

84   *Ibid.*, 25/7 (July 1919), 98.

85   T.E. Lawrence, *Seven Pillars of Wisdom* (1983), p. 677.

86   *Ibid.*, 682.

87   P. Gosse, *Memoirs of a Camp Follower* (1950), 109–10.

88   *Ibid.*, pp. 144–7.

89   'Interim Report of the War Office Committee for the Study of Trench Fever', *Journal of the Royal Army Medical Corps*, 30 (1918), 352–3.

90   Isaac Rosenberg, 'Louse Hunting' (1917), in T. Cross (ed.), *The Lost Voices of World War I* (1998), p. 73.

91   TNA, WO 159/16, Letter from Arthur Lee to Lord Kitchener, 13 December 1914.

92   Walter Schmidt, 27 September 1915, in P. Witkop (ed.), *German Students' War Letters* (2002), p. 309.

93   TNA, WO 95/47, Director of Medical Services, 12 May 1918.

94   TNA, WO 188/146, 'Treatment of Clothing by Antiseptic Substances in Relation to Wound Infections' by W.H. Horrocks, 23 November 1916.

95   J.S. Haller, 'Trench Foot: A Study in Military Medical Responsiveness in the Great War', *Western Journal of Medicine*, 152 (June 1990), 729–33.

96   A.A. Martin, *Surgeon in Khaki* (1915), p. 72.

97   TNA, WO 159/16, Letter from Lee to Kitchener, 28 November 1914.

98   TNA, WO 32/9797, Note on Typhoid, 1941; I.W. Brown, 'The Amazing Adventures of Wilburt C. Davison, Wilder G. Penfield, and Emile F. Holman While Rhodes Scholars in Medicine at Oxford During World War I, 1913–1917', *Annals of Surgery*, 211/2 (1990), 228.

99 M. St Clair Stobart, *The Flaming Sword* (1917), pp. 50–1.

100 *Ibid.*, p. 242.

101 TNA, FO 383/43, Report on Camp Visit at Wittenberg, 2 July 1915.

102 Cited in K.D. Patterson, 'Typhus and its Control in Russia, 1870–1940', *Medical History*, 37 (1993), 379; see also R. Porter, *The Greatest Benefit to Mankind* (1997), p. 399.

103 Letter from B.W. Armstrong, *St Mary's Hospital Gazette*, 20/9 (November 1914), 141.

104 Ninety per cent of the samples from uncontaminated clothing when cultured grew *Clostridium welchii*, the bacterium that caused gas gangrene, forty per cent produced streptococci, thirty per cent the tetanus bacilli and fifteen per cent staphylococci. A. Fleming, 'Some Notes on the Bacteriology of Gas Gangrene', *The Lancet*, 2 (1915), 376–8; 'On the Bacteriology of Septic Wounds', *The Lancet*, 2 (1915), 638–43; S.R. Douglas, A. Fleming and L. Colebrook, 'On the Question of Bacterial Symbiosis in Wound Infections', *The Lancet*, 1 (1917, 604–7.

105 S. Westman, *Surgeon with the Kaiser's Army* (1968), p. 82.

106 A.E. Wright, *Pathology and Treatment of War Wounds* (1942), p.30.

107 In fresh wounds, the leucocytes, the white blood cells that act as the body's own natural defences, were actively devouring the invading bacteria. Yet when antiseptics were used on the wounds, very few live white blood cells could be seen. This led to the conclusion that the antiseptics were killing off the body's own defences. Moreover, organisms such as those causing gas gangrene and tetanus that are anaerobic and do not grow in the presence of oxygen were multiplying in exposed wounds and affecting tissues which were oxygenated by blood. Further investigation showed that aerobic bacteria such as streptococci, which only grow in the presence of oxygen, were growing in the surrounding fluid of these wounds and consuming the oxygen. This allowed the lethal anaerobic bacteria free range in the oxygen-free dead tissue in the depths of the wound.

108 S.R. Douglas, L. Colebrook and A. Fleming, 'On the Growth of Anaerobic Bacilli in Fluid Media under Apparently Anaerobic Conditions', *The Lancet*, 2 (1917), 530–2.

109 A.E. Wright and A. Fleming, 'Further Observations on Acidaemia in Gas Gangrene and the Conditions which Favour the Growth of its Infective Agent in the Blood Serum', *The Lancet*, 1 (1918), 205–10; 'The Aerobic Infections of War Wounds', *Medical Research Council Special Report Series*, no. 39 (1919), 70–8.

110 He did this by filling a series of test tubes with blood serum and differing concentrations of carbolic acid. He then inoculated them with the bacterium that causes gas gangrene and covered the surface of the liquid with a layer of melted Vaseline. When the test tubes were incubated, any gas produced by the growth of the bacteria forced the Vaseline up the tube;

the further it went, the more bacteria had been produced. A. Fleming and F.J. Clemenger, 'A Simple Method of Recording Automatically the Gas Produced by Bacteria in a Culture and of the Oxygen Absorbed by Aerobic Non-Gas-Forming Bacteria', *British Journal of Experimental Pathology*, 1 (1920–1), 66–9.

111 A.E. Wright, A. Fleming and L. Colebrook, 'The Conditions under which the Sterilisation of Wounds by Physiological Agency can be Obtained', *The Lancet*, 1 (1918), 831–7.

112 A.E. Wright, *British Medical Journal*, 2 (1915), 629, 670, 717; W.W. Cheyne, *British Journal of Surgery*, 3 (1917), 427.

113 A. Fleming, 'The Physiological and Antiseptic Action of Flavine, with Some Observations on the Testing of Antiseptics', *The Lancet*, 2 (1917), 341–5; Letter to *The Lancet*, 2 (1917), 508–9.

114 A. Porritt, *'Treatment of War Wounds'* in *History of the Second World War, United Kingdom Medical Services, Surgery* (1953), p. 927.

115 *The Times*, 1 May 1919.

116 D. Richter, 'The Experience of the British Special Brigade in Gas Warfare' in H. Cecil and P.H. Liddle (ed.), *Facing Armageddon* (1996), pp. 353–64.

117 TNA, WO 32/5169, Report on Gas Attack, 23–24 May 1915.

118 S. Westman, *Surgeon with the Kaiser's Army* (1968), pp. 122–4.

119 TNA, WO 32/5176, Report on German Mustard Gas attacks on Ypres, 12–13 June 1917.

120 TNA, WO 32/5951, Report on Casualties Caused by Gas Warfare, 17 December 1918.

121 IWM, ART 1460. The painting was commissioned by the British War Memorials Committee in April 1918 for a projected Hall of Remembrance to be built on Richmond Hill. Sargent was originally asked to depict British-American co-operation but instead chose to depict the aftermath of a gas attack. The Hall of Remembrance was never built and the painting was purchased by the Imperial War Museum for £600 in March 1919.

122 M. Brown, *The Imperial War Museum Book of the First World War* (1991), pp. 76–7.

123 IWM, Q 11586, Photograph of Men suffering from Gas at Advanced Dressing Station, Bethune, by Tom Aitken, April 1918.

124 Wilfred Owen, 'Dulce et Decorum Est' in T. Cross (ed.), *The Lost Voices of World War I* (1998), p. 78.

125 See *moulages* made by Fritz Kolbow showing facial war wounds in the Deutsche Hygiene Museum, Dresden, 1914, DHM 1991/233, 1991/257.

126 Royal College of Ophthalmologists, London, papers of William Wallace, case 2380, Private A. Wheatcroft, aged 25, wounded in France 10 October 1917.

127 *Ibid.*, case 8267, Bombardier Thomas, aged 26, wounded at Arras, 25 January 1918.

128 *Ibid.* I am grateful to Richard Keeler, Honorary Curator at the Royal College of Ophthalmologists for drawing my attention to the work of William Wallace and giving me access to his records.

129 Medical records of Gillies' patients, including clinical notes, photographs, watercolours, *moulages* and model of surgical techniques at Queen Mary's Hospital, Sidcup; H.D. Gillies, *Plastic Surgery of the Face* (1920); A. Bamji, 'Facial Surgery: the Patient's Experience' in H. Cecil and P.H. Liddle (ed.), *Facing Armageddon* (1996), pp. 490–501.

130 Gillies Archive, Queen Mary's Hospital, Sidcup, Macalister collection of watercolours of plastic surgery patients; Tonks's watercolours at the Royal College of Surgeons; see also, S. Callister, '"Broken Gargoyles": the Photographic Representation of Severely Wounded New Zealand Soldiers', *Social History of Medicine*, 20/1 (2007), 111–30.

131 *Ibid.*, file 28118, Private Frank Whipp, Border Regiment, 28 March 1919 – 9 November 1920.

132 Burns were the major injuries on many ships at the Battle of Jutland, TNA, ADM 101/399, surgeon's log of Fleet Surgeon W.W. Keir, HMS *Warspite*, 31 May 1916.

133 Gillies Archive, file 2324, Able Seaman W. Vicarage, Royal Navy, 2 August 1917–8 September 1920. This patient was the first one to be treated with a 'tube pedicle' when Gillies sutured two flaps from his chest together into a tube and found that this enhanced the blood supply.

134 *Ibid.*, file 90667, Private S. Beldam, 28 November 1917–25 January 1921.

135 *Ibid.*, file 13745, Private W. Fairweather, Second London Regiment, 7 July 1916–11 October 1921.

136 C. S. Myers, 'A Contribution to the Study of Shell-shock', *The Lancet*, 1 (1915), 316–20.

137 F.S. Fitzgerald, *Tender is the Night* (1993), pp. 102–3.

138 C.S. Myers, *Shell-shock in France 1914–1918* (1940), p. 90.

139 *Ibid.*, pp. 96–7.

140 T. Salmon, 'The Care and Treatment of Mental Diseases and War Neuroses ("Shell-shock") in the British Army', *Mental Hygiene*, 1 (1917), 509–547.

141 TNA, CSC 5/93, Letter from Seymour Taylor to L.C.H. Weekes, July 1917.

142 R.C. Sherriff, *Journey's End* (1929).

143 W.H.R. Rivers, 'An Address on the Repression of War Experience', *The Lancet*, 1 (1918), 173–7.

144 C.M. Wilson, *Anatomy of Courage* (1945), p. 75.

145 J. Buchan, *Greenmantle* (1999), p. 235.

146 See P. Barham, *Forgotten Lunatics of the Great War* (2004) for the treatment of rank and file servicemen in lunatic asylums.

147 G. Oram, *Worthless Men* (1998), 89–101.

148 S. Sassoon, *Sherston's Progress* (1988), pp. 50–1.

149 *Ibid.*, p. 51.

150 IWM, P444, WH. Rivers's medical case notes for Siegfried Sassoon, 1917.

151 W. Owen, 'Mental Cases', T. Cross (ed.), *The Lost Voices of World War I* (1998), p. 79.

152 L.R. Yealland, *Hysterical Disorders of Warfare* (1918), p. 7.

153 B. Shephard, *A War of Nerves* (2002), pp. 98–101.

154 T.C. Allbutt, *Greek Medicine in Rome With Other Historical Essays* (1921), p. 542.

155 F. Garrison, *Introduction to the History of Medicine* (1929), p. 790.

156 P. Mitchell, *Memoranda on Army General Hospital Administration* (1917), p.1.

157 See N. Bosanquet, 'Health Systems in Khaki: the British and American Medical Experience' in H. Cecil and P.H. Liddle (ed.), *Facing Armageddon* (1996), pp. 451–65; I. Whitehead, 'Not a Doctor's War? The Role of the British Regimental Medical Officer in the Field' in *ibid.*, pp. 466–74.

158 G. Duhamel, *Souvenirs de la Grande Guerre* (1985), p. 139.

159 W. Osler, 'The War and Typhoid Fever', *British Medical Journal*, 2 (1914), 909–13.

Chapter 3: Business not as Usual

1 IWM, ART 2759, J. Hodgson Lobley, 'Outside Charing Cross Station, July 1916', 1918. See also W. Muir, *Observations of an Orderly at an English War Hospital 1915–1917* (2006), pp. 99–107 for more details on the unloading of patients from such trains.

2 *Reports by the Joint War Committee and Joint War Finance Committee of the British Red Cross Society and the Order of St John of Jerusalem in England on Voluntary Aid Rendered to the Sick and Wounded at Home and Abroad, and to British Prisoners of War 1914–19* (1921), p. 211.

3 K. Brown, 'History of the Newcastle upon Tyne Church High School 1885–1985' in H.G. Scott and E.A. Wise (ed.), *Centenary Book of the Newcastle upon Tyne Church High School 1885–1985* (1985), pp. 13, 30.

4 K. Rose, *King George V* (2000), p. 189.

5 B. Abel Smith, *The Hospitals, 1800–1948* (1964), p. 255.

6 Lord Rothschild, Chairman, British Red Cross Society, Letter to *The Times*, 15 August 1915.

7 *Brighton Herald* and *Hove Chronicle*, 28 November 1914.

8 *Ibid.*, 5 December 1914.

9 B. Abel Smith, *The Hospitals, 1800–1948* (1964), pp. 263–4.

10 A. Powell, *The Metropolitan Asylums Board and its Work, 1867–1930* (1930), pp. 84–92.

11 'Editorial', *St Mary's Hospital Gazette*, 20/10 (December 1914), p. 151.

12 K. Lees, 'Wounded Soldiers at St Mary's', *St Mary's Hospital Gazette*, 20/10 (December 1914), p.163.

13 K, Brown, 'Another Day, Another War', *St Mary's Gazette,* 97/2 (April 1991), 35–7; 'Tested Under Pressure: St Mary's During the Great War', *St Mary's Hospital Past and Present Nurses' League Journal,* 43 (2006), 14–20.

14 TNA, MH 10/80, Local Government Circular, 18 February 1916.

15 Letter signed 'Scarified', *British Medical Journal,* 1 (1917), 245.

16 *The Times,* 15 July 1918.

17 TNA, NATS 1/833, Report on Further Withdrawal of Doctors from Civil Medical Practice, March 1918.

18 'Editorial', *St Mary's Hospital Gazette,* 20/9 (November 1914), 131.

19 TNA, WO 293/3, Military Training for Medical Students, 10 December 1915.

20 TNA, NATS 1/711, Memorandum on the Shortage of Medical Students, August 1917.

21 St Mary's Hospital Archives, MS/AD 28/725, T.S. North, October 1915– October 1922. North died in 1924, his health undermined by his brief but bloody war service.

22 I.R. Whitehead, *Doctors in the Great War* (1999), pp. 92–3.

23 St Mary's Hospital Archives, MS/AD 28/942, D. Dimitrejevich, October 1920. Dimitrejevitch returned to Serbia and service as a doctor in the Yugoslav navy.

24 Robert Otto Marcus, 15 April 1915 in P. Witkop (ed.), *German Students' War Letters* (2002), p. 80.

25 I. Mann, *Ida and the Eye* (1996), p. 62. The typescript of Mann's autobiography gives a fuller account of her experiences as a woman medical student in a male world than the published version, St Mary's Hospital Archives, DP 21.

26 C. Dyhouse, 'Women Students and the London Medical Schools, 1914–39: the Anatomy of a Masculine Culture', *Gender and History* 10/1 (1998), 110–132.

27 St Mary's Hospital Archives, MS/AD 1/5, Medical School Committee, 2 February 1915.

28 'Notes', *St Mary's Hospital Gazette,* 22/7 (July 1916), 88.

29 St Mary's Hospital Archives, DP 21, typescript autobiography of Ida Mann, p. 126.

30 J.S. Garner, 'The Great Experiment: the Admission of Women Students to St Mary's Hospital Medical School, 1916–1925', *Medical History,* 42 (1998), 77–8.

31 I. Mann, *Ida and the Eye* (1996), p, 40.

32 St George's Hospital admitted 5 women only in 1915, Charing Cross Hospital Medical School followed in 1916, Westminster in 1917 and the London, King's College and University College Hospitals all had women students by 1918. Only the older and more socially exclusive medical schools at St Bartholomew's, St Thomas's, Guy's and the Middlesex Hospitals remained free of women medical students. See University of London, *Report*

of the Special Committee to Consider the Medical Education of Women in London (1944).

33 University of London, *Conference on Medical Education of Women in London* (1917), p. 3

34 *Ibid.*, p. 2.

35 St Mary's Hospital Archives, MS/AD 46/1–4, petition requesting exclusion of women, 1 April 1924.

36 H. Bourdillon, *Women as Healers* (1988), p. 40.

37 E.S. McLaren, *A History of the Scottish Women's Hospitals* (1919); SKIA, 'A Hospital in France', *Blackwood's Magazine*, 204 (1918), 613–40. The lower death rate was ascribed to copious use of hot water and scrupulous cleanliness. In the early twenty-first century, such an approach to hospital infection has aroused renewed interest in the work at Royaumont as a result of concern about the rise of antibiotic resistant bacteria; HRH The Princess Royal is a great admirer of the achievement of Elsie Inglis and considers her methods of infection control might offer lessons to modern hospitals: conversation with author, April 2004. There is something in this argument. When soap and water are used to clean hospital wards, the same bacteria that were there return within 24 hours, but when antiseptics are used it is the more resilient and harmful bacteria that quickly return and fill the space vacated by the weaker germs that have succumbed to the antibiotics (conversation of author with Dr John Wain, June 2007).

38 *Ibid.*, 633.

39 F. Murray, *Women as Army Surgeons* (1920), pp. 53–4; B. McLaren, *Women of the War* (1920), p. 2.

40 F. Thébaud, *La Femme au Temps de la Guerre de 14* (1994), p. 92.

41 L. Leneman, 'Medical Women at War, 1914–1918', *Medical History, 38* (1994), 160–77; *In the Service of Life: the Story of Elsie Inglis and the Scottish Women's Hospitals,* (1994).

42 *The Daily Telegraph*, 8 October 1916.

43 O. Wilberforce, *Octavia Wilberforce: the Autobiography of a Pioneer Woman Doctor* (1989), p. 77.

44 Musée International de la Croix Rouge et du Croissant Rouge, Geneva, Inv. BBT-1997-16-64, French postcard 'Le Brassard'; Inv. BBT-1997-16-69, German postcard 'und ein nuer Frühling folgt dem Winter nad'; Inv. BBT-199-16-60, 'The Real Angel of Mons'.

45 F. Thébaud, *La Femme au Temps de la Guerre de 14* (1994), p. 82.

46 I. Hay, *One Hundred Years of Army Nursing* (1953), pp. 89–90.

47 G. Duhamel, *Souvenirs de la Grande Guerre* (1985), pp. 135–6.

48 TNA, WO 32/9342, Report of Committee on Supply of Nurses, 14 November 1916.

49 A. Christie, *The Mysterious Affair at Styles* (2001), p. 96.

50 Alexandra, *A Nurse's Story (1954)*; K. Brown, '"Contact with the Seamy Side of Life": a Nurse's Story', *St Mary's Gazette*, 96/3 (October1990), 38–9.

51 TNA, DT 13/65, General Nursing Council record for Princess Arthur of Connaught, 1922.

52 TNA, WO 32/9342, Report of Committee on Supply of Nurses, 14 November 1916.

53 V. Brittain, *Testament of Youth* (1979), p. 206.

54 *Ibid.*, p. 209.

55 *Ibid.*, p. 279.

56 H. Speake, 'From a St Mary's Nurse in Brussels', *St Mary's Hospital Gazette*, 21/5 (May 1915), 76–7.

57 Letter from Edward Brittain to Vera Brittain, 14 September 1917, A. Bishop and M. Bostridge (ed.), *Letters from a Lost Generation* (1999), p.374.

58 Letter from Vera Brittain to W.H.K. Bervon, 9 August 1917, A. Bishop and M. Bostridge (ed.), *Letters from a Lost Generation* (1999), p. 370.

59 TNA, FO 383/15, arrest and execution of Edith Cavell, 1915; M. de Croy, *Le Martyre des Pays Envahis* (1933); R. Ryder, *Edith Cavell* (1975), p. 228–9, 238.

60 Inter-Allied Conference on the Aftercare of Disabled Men, *Reports* (1918), pp. 14–15.

61 *Reports by the Joint War Committee and Joint War Finance Committee of the British Red Cross Society and the Order of St John of Jerusalem in England on Voluntary Aid Rendered to the Sick and Wounded at Home and Abroad, and to British Prisoners of War 1914–19* (1921), pp. 733–4; Manoel II, 'Scheme and Organization of Curative Workshops' in R. Jones (ed.), Orthopaedic Surgery of Injuries (1921), 629–44; TNA, WO 32/5334, *Orthopaedic work of King Manoel, 1920*; A.H. Bizarro, *El-Rei Dom Manoel II na Grande Guerra* (1952).

62 S. Koven, 'Remembering and Dismemberment: Crippled Wounded Soldiers and the Great War in Great Britain', *American Historical Review*, 99/4 (1994), 1167–1202.

63 R. Jones, 'The Problem of the Disabled', *American Journal of Orthopaedic Surgery*, 16/5 (1918), 273.

64 R. Cooter, *Surgery and Society in Peace and War* (1993), pp. 113–21; J.S. Reznick, 'Work Therapy and the Disabled British Soldier in the First World War: the Case of Shepherd's Bush Military Hospital, London' in D.A. Gerber (ed.), *Disabled Veterans in History* (2000), pp. 185–203.

65 St Dunstan's Association for Blind Ex-Servicemen and Women, *The Spirit of St Dunstan's* (2006), pp. 1–2.

66 N. Venus and P. Willis, *The Home on the Hill* (2006).

67 D. Cohen, 'Will to Work: Disabled Veterans in Britain and Germany after the First World War' in D.A. Gerber (ed.), *Disabled Veterans in History* (2000), pp. 295–321.

68 C. Rollet, 'The Other War: Setbacks in Public Health', in J. Winter and J.L. Robert (ed.), *Capital Cities at War* (1999), pp. 456–86.

69 I. MacDougall (ed.), *Mid and East Lothian Miners' Association Minutes, 1894–1918* (2003), pp.334–5. See also K. Brown, 'The Lodges of the Durham Miners' Association, 1869–1926, *Northern History*, 23 (1987), 138–52.

70 F.B. Smith, *The Retreat of Tuberculosis, 1850–1950* (1988), p. 222.

71 P.J. Bishop, B.D.P. Lucas and B.G.B. Lucas, *The Seven Ages of the Brompton* (1991), p. 113.

72 H. Sellier, *La Lutte Contre la Tuberculose dans la Région Parisienne* (1928), p. 638.

73 G. Vitoux, 'L'Oeuvre des Comités Départementaux d'Assistance aux Soldats Réformés', *Revue d'Hygiène* 1 (1918), 561–70.

74 *The Lancet*, 1 (1918), 646–7.

75 A. Marwick, *The Deluge* (1973), p. 199.

76 S. Westman, *Surgeon with the Kaiser's Army* (1968), p. 139–40.

77 J.D.C. Bennett, 'Medical Advances Consequent to the Great War, 1914–1918', *Journal of the Royal Society of Medicine*, 83 (1990), 738–42; I. Loudon, 'On Maternal and Infant Mortality 1900–1960', *Social History of Medicine*, 4 (1991), 43–4.

78 J.M. Winter, *The Great War and the British People* (1985), pp. 105, 132–3, 138, 157; L. Bryder, 'The First World War: Healthy or Hungry?', *History Workshop*, 24 (1987), 141–55; B. Harris, 'The Demographic Impact of the First World War: An Anthropometric Perspective', *Journal of the Society for the Social History of Medicine*, 6 (1993), 343–66.

79 *The Times*, 1 March 1915.

80 *Ibid.*, 30 March 1915.

81 Report of Central Control Board, Cd. 8243, 1916.

82 K. Rose, *King George V* (2000), p. 179. Lloyd George had suggested the King's vow of abstinence, prompting Queen Mary to comment that 'We have been carted'. The Prince of Wales was later to cast aspersions on the contents of his mother's fruit cup and the nature of the business his father regularly retired to attend to after dinner.

83 'I don't want to be a Soldier' in M. Stephen (ed.), *Never Such Innocence* (1991), p. 97.

84 TNA, MH 55/530, deputation from Association of Municipal Councils to Lord Rhondda, statement of Sir Hamar Greenwood, 24 January 1917.

85 K. Brown, *The Pox* (2006), pp. 123–5.

86 National Archives, College Park, Maryland, Record Group 165, War Department and General Staff, box 433, syllabus accredited for use in official supplementary lectures on sex hygiene and venereal diseases, February 1918.

87 *Ibid.*, box 426, letter from Hilton Railey to Raymond B. Fosdick, 17 September 1917.

88 *Ibid.*, Record Group 120, American Expeditionary Forces, 1917–23, box 5259, 'Something to Think about for Men Going on Leave', 12 April 1919.

89 *Ibid.*, Record Group 165, War Department and General Staff, box 433, syllabus accredited for use in official supplementary lectures on sex hygiene and venereal diseases, February 1918.

90 D.M. Kennedy, *Over Here* (1982), p. 187.

91 G. Walker, *Venereal Disease in the American Expeditionary Forces* (1922), pp. 10–19.

92 National Archives, College Park, Maryland, Record Group 165, War Department General and Special Staff, box 586, letter from J. Frank Chase to Raymond B. Fosdick, 13 October 1917.

93 TNA, MEPO 2/3434, Metropolitan Police figures obtained from a study of 2,312 social case sheets at Canadian hospital, Etchinghill, Lyminge, 25 August 1918.

94 TNA, HO 45/10893/359931, Order in Council, 22 March 1918.

95 *Ibid.*, letter from Womens' Cooperative Guild, 28 October 1918.

96 TNA, WO 32'4745, War Cabinet memorandum, 28 August 1918.

97 Final Report of the Commissioners, Royal Commission on Venereal Diseases, Cd. 8189, 1916.

98 *The Lancet* (1917), 236–7.

99 TNA, FO 383/524, Report by Eric Higgins on Ruheleben, 10 March 1919.

100 O. Lindsay and J.R. Harris, *The Battle for Hong Kong* (2005), pp. 218–9.

101 Trinitrotoluene.

102 TNA, WO 142/274, report on Ministry of Munitions National Filling Factory No. 23, 1918.

103 I.W.F. Beckett, *Home Front 1914–1918* (2006), p. 124.

104 *The Daily Telegraph*, 1 July 1917.

105 *Ibid.*, 7 May 1916.

106 Solicitors' Journal and Weekly Reporter, 7 July 1917.

107 St Mary's Hospital Archives, PG/AD 7/17, annual report of Paddington Green Children's Hospital, 1917.

108 *Westminster Gazette*, 2 July 1917.

109 Letter from A.H.D. Acland, *The Times*, 7 April 1916.

110 Medical Correspondent, *The Times*, 5 April 1916.

111 Letter from W.A. Brend, *The Times*, 8 April 1916.

112 S. Westman, *Surgeon with the Kaiser's Army* (1968), p. 139.

113 G.R. Searle, *A New England?* (2004), p. 817.

114 D. Jeffreys, *Aspirin: The Story of a Wonder Drug* (2004), pp. 97–122.

115 J. Slinn, 'The Development of the Pharmaceutical Industry' in S. Anderson (ed.), *Making Medicines* (2005), pp. 165–6.

116 P.A. Willcox, *The Detective Physician* (1970), pp. 83–4.

117 Paul Ehrlich Institut, PEI/S59, laboratory book testing toxicity of salvarsan, 1909–10, Hoechst tests, pp. 72–4.

118 K. Brown, *The Pox* (2006), p. 107.

119 S.M. Tomkins, 'The failure of Expertise: Public Health Policy in Britain During the 1918–1919 Influenza Epidemic', *Social History of Medicine*, 5 (1992), 435–54; E. Tognotti, 'Scientific Triumphalism and Learning from the Facts: Bacteriology and the Spanish Flu Challenge of 1918', *Journal of the Society for the Social History of Medicine*, 16 (2003), 97–110.

120 V.C. Vaughan and G.T. Palmer, 'Communicable Disease in the United States Army During the Summer and Autumn of 1918', *Journal of Laboratory Clinical Medicine*, 3 (1918), 587–623, 647–86.

121 T. Cross (ed.), *The Lost Voices of World War* I (1998), p. 204.

Chapter 4: Spanish Rehearsal

1 L. Portillo, 'Unamuno's Last Lecture' in C. Connolly (ed.), *The Golden Horizon* (1953), pp. 397–409.

2 Cervantes wrote *Don Quixote*, his great satire on chivalry, after he was wounded at the Battle of Lepanto in 1571.

3 H. Thomas, *The Spanish Civil War* (1977), p. 501.

4 Editorial, 'The War in Spain' *British Medical Journal*, 1 (1939), 68.

5 E. Bosch i Monegal, *L'Hospital del Mar en la historia de Barcelona* (1992), p. 67.

6 *Ibid.*, p. 121.

7 'Foreign letters: Madrid', *Journal of the American Medical Association*, 113 (1939), 159–60.

8 H. Thomas, *The Spanish Civil War* (1977), p. 269.

9 L. Stainton, *Lorca: A Dream of Life* (1998), pp. 465, 472.

10 N. Coni, *Medicine and Warfare* (2007), pp. 19– 20.

11 E. Martinez Alonso, *The Adventures of a Doctor* (1962), pp. 50–63.

12 Hospital of Our Lady of the Sea.

13 E. Bosch i Monegal, *L'Hospital del Mar en la historia de Barcelona* (1992), pp. 67–8.

14 T. Buchanan, *The Impact of the Spanish Civil War on Britain: War, Loss and Memory* (2007), pp. 53–4.

15 St Mary's Hospital Archives, MS/AD28/1358, Randall Sollenberger; see also N. Coni, *Medicine and Warfare* (2007), p. 137.

16 TNA, FO 889/2, report on Norman King, 18 May 1937.

17 P. Fyvel, *English Penny* (1992), pp. 32–44.

18 W.H. Auden, 'Spain, 1937' in *Selected Poems* (1979), p. 54.

19 TNA, FO 371/22681, extract from Sir George Maunsey's conversation with the Duke of Alba, 10 May 1938.

20 H. Thomas, *The Spanish Civil War* (1977), p. 979.

21 R.R. Macintosh and F.B. Pratt, 'Anaesthesia in Wartime', *British Medical Journal*, 2 (1939), 1077–9.

22 P. Scott-Ellis, *The Chances of Death* (1995); P. Preston, *Doves of War* (2002), pp. 11–118.

23 M. Junod, *Le Troisième Combattant.* (1947), p. 53.

24 *Ibid.*, p. 98.

25 *Ibid.*, pp. 97–8.

26 *Ibid.*, p. 107.

27 *Ibid.*, pp, 174–83.

28 During the Second World War there were suggestions in the USA and Britain that Red Cross aid relief should be 'made in return for an assurance by Spain that she will not enter into the war, and that in any case this kind of assistance might assist a policy of independence from Germany', TNA, FO 371/24527, 'Special Distribution and War Cabinet', cipher, 10 September 1940.

29 D.W. Jolly, *Field Surgery in Total War* (1941), p. 25.

30 K. Sinclair-Loutit, 'An Ambulance in Spain', *The Lancet*, 2 (1939), 1295–6.

31 'Medicine in Republican Spain', *St Mary's Hospital Gazette*, 45/1 (January 1939), 2–4.

32 D.W. Jolly, *Field Surgery in Total War* (1941), pp. 11–14, 33; N. Coni, *Medicine and Warfare* (2007), pp. 66–7.

33 A. Beevor, *The Battle for Spain: The Spanish Civil War 1936–1939* (2006), p. 215.

34 F. Borkenau, *The Spanish Cockpit: An Eyewitness Account of the Spanish Civil War* (2000), pp. 161–2.

35 *Ibid.*, p.159.

36 G. Orwell, *Homage to Catalonia* (2000), p. 53.

37 *Ibid.*, p. 147.

38 *Ibid.*, p. 140.

39 *Ibid.*, p. 143.

40 C. Moorehead, *Martha Gellhorn* (2003), p. 143.

41 P. Fyvel, *English Penny* (1992), p. 33.

42 *Ibid.*, p. 28.

43 A. Beevor, *The Battle for Spain* (2006), pp. 215–7.

44 J. Bescós Torres, 'Las enfermeras en la guerra de España 1936–1939', *Revista de la Historia Militar*, 26 (1982), 97–143; 'La sanidad military en la Guerra d'España 1936–1939', *Medicina Militar*, 43 (1987), 88–99, 434–47.

45 P. Kemp, *Mine Were of Trouble* (1957), p. 197.

46 J. Villarroya and E. Juliana, 'El bombardeo de Barcelona en 1938: Y Mussolini decidió experimentar', *La Vanguardia* (12 March 2003), 3–5.

47 *The Times*, 28 April 1937.

48 R. Titmuss, *History of the Second World War: Problems of Social Policy* (1950), pp. 13–14.

49 G. Leval, *L'Espagne libertaire, 1936–1939: L'oeuvre constructive de la revolution espagnole* (1971), p. 296.

50 H. Thomas, *The Spanish Civil War* (1977), pp. 536–7.

51 'Medicine in Republican Spain', *St Mary's Hospital Gazette*, 45/1 (January 1939), 3.

52 H. Thomas, *The Spanish Civil War* (1977), pp. 297–8.

53 J. Trueta, 'Closed Treatment of War Fractures', *The Lancet, 1* (1939), 1452–5; *The Treatment of War Wounds and Fractures* (1939); *The Principles and Practice of War Surgery* (1943).

54 J. Trueta, *The Treatment of War Wounds and Fractures* (1939), p. 135.

55 A.M. Low, *Benefits of War* (1945), pp. 137–40.

56 J. Trueta, *The Treatment of War Wounds and Fractures* (1939), p. xi.

57 M. Broggi, *Memories d'un Cirugia* (2001), p. 62.

58 'Sulphanilamide and War Wounds', *The Lancet*, 1 (1939), 740.

59 E. Grundmann, *Gerhard Domagk: The First Man to Triumph over Infectious Diseases* (2004), pp. 14–15.

60 G. Domagk, 'Ein Beitrag zur Chemotherapie der bacteriellen Infektionen', *Deutsche Medizinische Wochenshrift*, 61 (1935), 250–3; *Chemotherapie bakterieller Infektionen* (1944); 'Further Progress in Chemotherapy of Bacterial Infections: Nobel Lecture 12 December 1947' in *Nobel Lectures: Physiology or Medicine* (1965), pp. 490–529.

61 Army Directorate of Pathology, 'Memorandum Concerning the Use of Sulfonamide Derivatives for Prophylaxis and Treatment of Wound Infections, Journal of the Royal Army Medical Corps, 73 (1939), 298–300.

62 L. Colebrook, 'Gerhard Domagk, 1895–1964', *Biographical Memoirs of Fellows of the Royal Society* (1964), vol. 10, p.39.

63 'The Barcelona Blood Transfusion Services', *The Lancet, 1* (1939), 768.

64 F. Duran i Jordà, 'The Barcelona Blood Transfusion Service', *The Lancet*, 1 (1939), 773–5.

65 W.H. Schneider, 'Blood Transfusion Between the Wars', *Journal of the History of Medicine and the Allied Sciences*, 58 (2003), 187–224.

66 'Visita a un Hospital: Cómo se efectúa la transfusión de sangre en el frente', *La Vanguardia* (25 November 1936), 10–11.

67 F. Duran i Jordà, 'El Servei de Tranfusio de sang al front: Organització i utillatge', *La Medicina Catalana* 7 (1936), 45–46; J. Grífols i Espés, *Frederic Duran i Jordà: Un métido, una época* (1997), 51–2.

68 L. Martinez, 'Perque la sang és vida', *Avui* (22 May 2005), 28–33; J.E. Baños and E. Guardiolo, 'Eponímia mèdica catalana: El mètode de Duran', *Annals de Medicina*, 89 (2006), 41–5; M. Lozano and J. Cid, 'Frederic Duran-Jorda: A Transfusion Medicine Pioneer', *Transfusion Medicine Reviews*, 21/1 (2007), 75–81. I am grateful to Miguel Lozano for allowing me to see this article before its publication.

69 A. Franco, J. Cortes and J. Alvarez, 'The Development of Blood Transfusion: The Contribution of Norman Bethune in the Spanish Civil War', *Canadian Journal of Anaesthesia*, 10 (1996), 1076–8; I.B. Rosen, 'Dr Norman Bethune as a Surgeon', *Canadian Journal of Surgery*, 39 (1996), 72–7.

70 R.S. Saxton, 'The Madrid Blood Transfusion Institute' *The Lancet*, 2 (1937), 606–7.

71 F. Duran i Jordà quoted in 'Medicine in Republican Spain', *St Mary's Hospital Gazette*, 45/1 (January 1939), 3.

72 F. Borkenau, *The Spanish Cockpit* (2000), p. 135.

73 E. Mira i López, *Psychiatry in War* (1943), p. 1.

74 *Ibid.*, pp. 63–81.

75 E. Mira i López, 'Psychiatric Experience in the Spanish War, *British Medical Journal*, 1 (1939), 1217–20.

76 'Medicine in Republican Spain', *St Mary's Hospital Gazette*, 45/1 (January 1939), 3.

77 TNA, MH 55/707, letter from A. Marignac, Office Internalional d'Hygiene Publique, Paris, to Dr Goodwin, 4 September 1939.

78 TNA, MH 55/707, medical conditions of refugees from Spain, 1936.

79 H.C. Maurice Williams, 'Four Thousand Basque Children', *The Lancet*, 1 (1937), 383.

80 H. Thomas, *The Spanish Civil War* (1977), p.863.

81 TNA, FO 371/24527, situation report, 1 May 1940.

82 *Ibid.*, p. 485.

83 N. Coni, 'Medicine and the Spanish Civil War', *Journal of the Royal Society of Medicine*, 95/3 (2002), 148–9.

84 TNA, FO 371/24142, letter from R.C. Skrine Stevenson to Walter Roberts, 22 December 1938.

85 'Medicine in Republican Spain', *St Mary's Hospital Gazette*, 45/1 (January 1939), 3–4.

86 TNA, KV 5/46, Secret Service, report on camp at Gurs, June 1939.

87 J. Trueta, *Trueta: Surgeon in War and Peace* (1980).

88 M. Lozano and J. Cid, 'Frederic Duran-Jorda: A Transfusion Medicine Pioneer', *Transfusion Medicine Reviews*, 21/1 (2007), 75.

89 Private information, Montserrat Mira; Lluis Martinez.

90 H. Thomas, *The Spanish Civil War* (1977), p. 945.

91 G.B. Shirlaw and C. Troke, *Medicine versus Invasion: The Home Guard Medical Service in Action* (1941), p. x.

Chapter 5: Healing for Victory

1 J.C. Watts, *Surgeon at War* (1955), pp. 88–9.

2 *Ibid.*, p. 90.

3 Obituary, *The Daily Telegraph*, 16 August 2006.

4 TNA, WO 177/3, H. Walker, account of events, May–June 1940.

5 TNA, WO 222/9, survey of work of War Wounds Committee, 1940–45.

6 TNA, WO 222/89, reorganisation of medical services in the field, 3 November 1942.
7 R. McLaughlin, *The Royal Army Medical Corps* (1972), p. 76.
8 M. Harrison, *Medicine and Victory* (2004), pp. 280–1.
9 TNA, WO 373/39, citation for H.D. Cockburn, 15 September 1944.
10 Private information.
11 M.H. Kater, *Doctors Under Hitler* (1989), p. 52.
12 B. Carruthers, *Servants of Evil* (2001), pp. 52–3.
13 Wellcome Library, RAMC 651/3, Eighth Army Medical Report, 1943.
14 C. Merridale, *Ivan's War* (2005), pp. 90–1.
15 N. Davies, *Europe at War* (2006), p. 262.
16 H.N. Cole, *On Wings of Healing* (1963), pp. 34–50.
17 TNA, WO 222/23, A.A. Eagger, 'Development of Airborne Medical Services', 1945.
18 TNA, AIR 2/11/87/9528, Report of Air Board Research Committee (Medical), 25 April 1917.
19 TNA, AIR 2/11/87, J.G. Priestley, report on 'Flight at High Altitudes', 30 April 1917.
20 *Ibid.*, J.S. Haldane, report to Air Board Research Committee (Medical), 1917.
21 TNA, AIR 2/5016, extract from War Cabinet Scientific Advisory Committee, 7 July 1944.
22 *Ibid.*, creation of RAF Institute of Aviation Medicine, 1943–4.
23 T.M. Gibson and M.H. Marshall, *Into Thin Air* (1984), pp. 109–12.
24 *Ibid.*, p. 81.
25 *Ibid.*, p. 125.
26 *Ibid.*, p. 198.
27 TNA, FD1/6300, memorandum by A.H. McIndoe on treatment of burns in the RAF, 1942.
28 R. Hillary, *The Last Enemy* (1997), p. 3.
29 TNA, FD 1/6300, letter from L. Colebrook to Dr Drury, 17 April 1942.
30 W.C. Noble, *Coli: Great Healer of Men* (1974), p. 89.
31 TNA, FD 1/6300., memorandum by A.H. McIndoe on treatment of burns in the RAF, 1942.
32 TNA, WO 222/65, report on casualties in AVFs, 20 July 1942.
33 S.M. Cohen, 'Experience in the Treatment of War Burns', *British Medical Journal* (1940), 251–4.
34 TNA, FD1/6300, memorandum by A.H. McIndoe on treatment of burns in the RAF, 1942.
35 TNA, AIR 20/10269, George H. Morley, 'Plastic Surgery in the Royal Air Force', May 1948.
36 Emergency Medical Service, 'The Local Treatment of War Burns', *British Medical Journal* (1940), 489.

37 TNA, AIR 49/354, talk by Flight-Lieutenant D.C. Bodenham, 19 August 1943.

38 TNA, FD 1/6300, letter to Professor R.A. Peters, 27 April 1942.

39 *Ibid.*, memorandum by A.H. McIndoe on treatment of burns in the RAF, 1942.

40 TNA, FD1/5892, blood transfusion research, 1940.

41 L. Whitby, 'Blood Transfusion in the Field: Organisation of Supplies' in H. Letherby Tidy (ed.), *Inter-Allied Conferences on War Medicine 1942–1945* (1947), pp. 123–6.

42 TNA, WO 222/1480, Campaign in Norway, April–June 1940.

43 TNA, WO 222/1479, Army Transfusion Service, 1940; FD 1/5290, Progress Report of Blood Transfusion Emergency Depots Committee covering the period from the outbreak of war to 30 September 1940.

44 J.C. Watts, *Surgeon at War* (1955), p. 42.

45 A.E. Cowdrey, *Fighting for Life* (1994), pp. 165–73.

46 L. Whitby, 'Blood Transfusion in the Field: Organisation of Supplies' in H. Letherby Tidy (ed.), *Inter-Allied Conferences on War Medicine 1942–1945* (1947), pp. 123–6.

47 A. Hood, 'Army Medical Services in Action,', *Journal of the Royal Army Medical Corps*, 38 (1943), 287–90.

48 TNA, FD1/6300, memorandum by A.H. McIndoe on treatment of burns in the RAF, 1942.

49 Report to the Army Council of the Army Advisory Committee on Maxillo-Facial Injuries (1940), p. 3.

50 L. Miller, *Lee Miller's War* (2005), p. 17.

51 TNA, FD1/6300, memorandum by A.H. McIndoe on treatment of burns in the RAF, 1942.

52 J.P. Bennett, 'A History of the Queen Victoria Hospital, East Grinstead', *British Journal of Plastic Surgery*, 41 (1988), 422–40.

53 Bob Marchant, who worked as McIndoe's operating theatre attendant in the 1950s has commented that McIndoe was definitely 'the boss' but was not as difficult as he has often been made out and always thanked everyone if they met his demanding standards (conversation with author, July 2007); E.R. Mayhew, *The Reconstruction of Warriors* (2004), pp. 62–4.

54 *Ibid.*, p. 138.

55 TNA, AIR 49/354, report on maxillo-facial and plastic injuries in the RAF, 1942.

56 R. Hillary, *The Last Enemy* (1997), pp. 146–7.

57 *Ibid.*, p. 159–60.

58 S. Faulks, *The Fatal Englishman* (1996), pp. 111–208.

59 TNA, AIR 20/10269, press cutting from *The Daily Sketch*, 20 October 1942.

60 *Ibid.*, 'The Guinea Pig', Christmas number, December 1947, p. 5.

61 TNA, INF 6/519, 'Plastic Surgery in Wartime', Realist Film Unit, 23 October 1941.

62 TNA, WO 222/1513, scheme for medical arrangements, March 1940.

63 TNA, ADM 116/5559, minute by S.F. Dudley, 10 July 1943.

64 TNA, ADM 116/5559, 'Psychology for the Fighting Man', 1943.

65 B. Shephard, *War of Nerves* (2002), pp. 187–9.

66 Letter from H.J Starling, *Proceedings of the Royal Society of Medicine*, 34 (1941), 542.

67 TNA, ADM 116/5559, Ministerial Committee on the Work of Psychologists and Psychiatrists in the Services, 31 January 1945.

68 L. Kennett, *GI: the American Soldier in World War II* (1987), pp. 34–5.

69 *Ibid.*, p. 96.

70 War Department, Washington DC, Instructions for American Servicemen in Britain, 1942 (1994).

71 TNA, WO 222/158, divisional psychiatry report by P.J.R. Davies, March 1946.

72 TNA, 222/8, notes on administration of army psychiatry, September 1939–May 1943.

73 TNA, ADM 116/5559, Ministerial Committee on the Work of Psychologists and Psychiatrists in the Services, 31 January 1945.

74 J.R. Rees, 'Three Years of Military Psychiatry in the United Kingdom', *British Medical Journal*, 1 (1943), 6.

75 TNA, WO 222/158, divisional psychiatry report by P.J.R. Davies, March 1946.

76 J. Heller, *Catch-22* (1994), p. 52.

77 H.S. Gear, 'Hygiene Aspects of the El Alamein Victory', *British Medical Journal*, 1 (1944), 383.

78 R.B. Frank, *Guadalcanal* (1990), p. 588.

79 M. Harrison, *Medicine and Victory* (2004), pp.201–13.

80 P.W. Sewell (ed.), *Healers in World War II* (2001), pp. 21–2.

81 TNA, WO 222/159, malaria control in mobile warfare, Italian campaign, by A.W.S. Thompson, 15 November 1945.

82 TNA, WO 204/4945, malaria control dusting by aircraft, 23 March 1944.

83 TNA, WO 222/159, malaria control in mobile warfare, Italian campaign, by A.W.S. Thompson, 15 November 1945.

84 TNA, WO 222/150, report on malaria in 6th Infantry Brigade Arakan Operations by Major R. Bevan, 1943.

85 C.M. Wilson (Lord Moran), *Winston Churchill: The Struggle for Survival, 1940–1965* (1966), pp. 163–4.

86 TNA, WO 222/1479, conference on VD held at GCHQ, 9 December 1939.

87 C. Paul, *Zwangs Prostitution: Staatlich Erricht Bordelle im Nationalsozialismus* (1994).

88 Political Warfare Executive, Germany 1944: The British Soldier's Pocketbook (2006), p. 30.

89 TNA, WO 204/6725, leaflet issued to soldiers, 1944.

90 M. Harrison, 'Sex and the Citizen Soldier: Health, Morals and Discipline in the British Army during the Second World War' in R. Cooter, M. Harrison and S. Sturdy (eds), *Medicine and Modern Warfare* (1999), p. 235.

91 TNA, MH 55/2317, notes of meeting at Home Office, 29 October 1942.

92 *Ibid.*, letter from Richard Law to Osbert Peake, 7 April 1943.

93 TNA, MH 55/1341, Ministry of Health circular, 8 January 1943.

94 TNA, WO 204/3015, report on VD in the 15th Army by Gordon Cheyne, director of Public Health, 5 December 1943.

95 TNA, WO 204/6725, notes on prophylactic treatment, 1944.

96 M.H. Salaman, A.J. King, D.I. Williams and C.S. Nichol, 'Prevention of Jaundice Resulting from Antisyphilitic Treatment', *The Lancet*, 1 (1944), 7–10. See further P.P. Mortimer, 'Arsphenamine Jaundice and the Recognition of Instrument-Borne Virus Infection', *Genitourinary Medicine*, 71 (1995), 109–119.

97 S. Longden, *To the Victor the Spoils* (2004), p. 119.

98 TNA, WO 222/1300, report of Robert Lees, 13 April 1945; W.F. Mellor (ed.), *Casualties and Medical Statistics* (1972), pp. 119, 192, 240, 242, 246, 264, 282, 334.

99 J. Howie, 'Gonorrhoea: A Question of Tactics', *British Medical Journal*, 2 (1979), 1631.

100 K. Brown, 'A Night with Venus, A Lifetime with Mercury: the Treatment of Syphilis', *Pharmaceutical Historian*, 37/3 (2007), 37.

101 National Academy of Sciences, National Research Council Archives, Institute of Medicine, Committees on Military Medicine, VD folder, *Venereal Diseases Bulletin*, minutes of conference of the sub-committee on venereal diseases, 29 June 1944.

102 E. Martinez Alonso, *The Adventures of a Doctor* (1962), p. 164.

103 K. Brown, *The Pox* (2006), p. 194.

104 TNA, FO 938/90, note by John Simpson, 14 January 1947.

105 A. Fleming, 'On the Antibacterial Action of Cultures of a Penicillium with Special Reference to their Use in the Isolation of *B. Influenzae*', *British Journal of Experimental Pathology*, 10 (1929, 226–36.

106 K. Brown, *Penicillin Man* (2004); 'The History of Penicillin from Discovery to the Drive to Production', *Pharmaceutical Historian*, 34/3 (2004), 37–43.

107 Rockefeller Archive Center, North Tarrytown, NY, RF RG 1-1, Project Series 40D, England, Box 36, F 458, Grant-in-aid to the Department of Pathology, University of Oxford, under Professor H.W. Florey, 21 February 1940; Grant-in-aid, 30 December 1941; Trustees Bulletin, October 1943.

108 E.B. Chain, 'Thirty Years of Penicillin Therapy', *Proceedings of the Royal Society of London*, B, 179 (1971), 293.

109 Wellcome Library, PP/EBC/B41, E. Chain, 'What is Penicillin?'

110 Personal information, Norman Heatley (1999).
111 Wellcome Library, GC/48/B5, Norman Heatley's Diary, 30 May 1940, 3 June 1940, 4 June 1940, 18 October 1940, 31 October 1940, 18 November 1940, 23 December 1940.
112 Wellcome Library, PP/EBC/B104, Ernst Chain.
113 Wellcome Library, GC 48,/A1, Heatley's notebook, 20 July 1939–29 March 1940; E. Chain, H.W. Florey, A.D. Gardner, N.G. Heatley, M.A. Jennings, J. Orr-Ewing and A.G. Sanders, 'Penicillin as a Chemotherapeutic Agent', *The Lancet*, 2 (1940), 226–8; E.P. Abraham, E. Chain, C.M. Fletcher, H.W. Florey, A.D. Gardner, N.G. Heatley and M.A. Jennings, 'Further Observations on Penicillin', *The Lancet*, 2 (1941), 177–88.
114 TNA, FD 1/3331, Medical Research Council, file on grants to Professor H.W. Florey.
115 Wellcome Library, CG/48/B5, Heatley's diary, 15 July 1940.
116 S. Mines, *Pfizer: an Informal History* (1978), p. 73.
117 Pfizer Records Centre, Sandwich, Kent, Kemball Bishop records, Box 96B-2E, file 1, letter from J.E. Whitehall, Managing Director, to H.W. Florey, 20 August 1942.
118 *Ibid.*, Box 96B-2E, file 7, J.G. Barnes, 'Early Work on Penicillin in England with Special Reference to Bromley', May 1971.
119 National Archives, College Park, Maryland, Record Group 227, series 41, Northern Regional Research Office of Scientific Research and Development, series E-165, CMR, minutes of penicillin conference, 8 October 1941.
120 National Archives, College Park, Maryland, Record Group 97, Bureau of Agricultural and Industrial Chemistry, series 41, Northern Regional Research Laboratory, file 1, conference minutes, 15 July 1941.
121 National Archives, College Park, Maryland, Record Group 97, Bureau of Agricultural and Industrial Chemistry, series 41, Northern Regional Research Laboratory, file 2, memorandum by R.D. Coghill on penicillin conference and visit to various companies in New York, 16–23 December 1941.
122 National Center for Agricultural Utilization Research, Peoria, Illinois, mycology registers.
123 National Archives, College Park, Maryland, Record Group 227, Office of Scientific Research and Development, series E-165, Committee for Medical Research, general records, letter from J.T. Connor to Oscar Cox, Solicitor General, requesting assistance of anti-trust expert to work out contractual relationships of commercial firms to avoid 'monopolistic control ... contrary to the public interest', 5 October 1943.
124 *Ibid.*, penicillin file, sample letter from A.N. Richards to W.J. McManus endorsing requests for priority in allocation of materials, 18 March 1943.

125 R.D. Coghill, 'The Development of Penicillin Strains' in A. Elder (ed.), *The History of Penicillin Production*, American Institute of Engineers, Chemical Engineering Progress Symposium, 66/100 (1970), 14–15; P. Neushul, 'Science, Government and the Mass Production of Penicillin', *Journal of the History of Medicine and the Allied Sciences*, 48 (1993), 371–95.

126 National Archives, College Park, Maryland, Record Group 227, Office of Scientific Research and Development, series E-162, Committee on Medical Research, minutes of 65th meeting, 27 May 1943.

127 Pfizer, New York City, Pfizer Penicillin papers, Gladys Hobby records, series 5, box 38, report by Jasper Kane to J.L. Smith on expansion of penicillin submerged fermentation, 27 August 19423.

128 R. Hare, *Birth of Penicillin and the Disarming of Microbes,* (1970), p. 177.

129 A. Elder, 'The Role of the Government in the Wartime Penicillin Program', in A. Elder (ed.), *The History of Penicillin Production*, American Institute of Engineers, Chemical Engineering Progress Symposium, 66/100 (1970) 3–11.

130 BL, Add. MS 56112, minutes of first meeting of General Penicillin Committee, 25 September 1942.

131 Ibid.

132 *Ibid.*, 22 February 1944.

133 Pfizer Records Centre, Sandwich, Kent, Kemball Bishop records, Box 96B-2E, file 1, correspondence between J.E. Whitehall, Arthur Mortimer and H.W. Florey, 23 September 1942–24 September 1943.

134 BL, Add. MS 56112, minutes of General Penicillin Committee, 5 April 1944.

135 *Ibid.*, 5 April 1944, 11 May 1944.

136 H.W. Florey and H. Cairns, *A Preliminary Report to the War Office and Medical Research Council on Investigations Concerning the Use of Penicillin in War Wounds* (1943); L.P. Garrod, 'The Treatment of War Wounds with Penicillin', *British Medical Journal, 2* (11 December 1943), 755–6; H.W. Florey and H. Cairns, 'Penicillin in Warfare', *British Journal of Surgery, 32* (1944), 110–224.

137 L. Miller, *Lee Miller's War* (2005), p. 17.

138 *The Daily Herald*, 15 June 1944.

139 *Sunday Express*, 9 July 1944.

140 A.E. Porritt and G.A.G. Mitchell, 'Wounds and Gas Gangrene' in A. Fleming (ed.), *Penicillin: Its Practical Application* (1946), p. 163.

141 J. Hofmeyr, *The Testament of a Doctor: A Life of Contrasts* (2003), pp. 159–60. Fuyschott did not recover from the osteomyelitis infecting his leg and died many years later from amyloid as a result of chronic sepsis from the osteomyelitis.

142 R.D. Coghill, 'The development of penicillin strains', in *The history of penicillin production*, American Institute of Chemical Engineers, Chemical Engineering Progress Symposium, 66/100 (1970), 15.

143 BL, Add. MS 56221, R.J. Pulvertaft.

144 J. Vonkennel, J. Kimmig and A. Lembke, 'Die Mycoine, eine Neue Gruppe Therapeutisch Wirksamer Substanzen aus Pilzen', *Klinische Wochenschrift*, 22 (1943), 321; T. Wagner-Jauregg, 'Die Neueren Biochemischen Erkentnisse und Probleme der Chemotherapie', *Die Naturwissenschaften*, 31 (1943), 335–44; M. Kiese, 'Chemotherapie mit Antibakteriellen Stoffen aus Niederen Pilzen und Bakterien', *Klinische Wochenschrift* , 22 (1943), 505–11.

145 Royal Society, HF/1/3/2/12/2, letter from H.W. Florey to A. Fleming, 24 February 1941.

146 I. Pieroth, 'Penicillin: A Survey from Discovery to Industrial Production', in H. Kleinkauf and H. van Dohren (ed.), *Fifty Years of Penicillin Application* (1980), pp. 33–6; G. Shama and J. Reinarz, 'Allied Intelligence Reports on Wartime German Penicillin Research and Production', *Historical Studies in the Physical and Biological Sciences*, 32/2 (2002), 347–68.

147 TNA, FO 1031/9, Combined Intelligence Objectives report, file xxiv–16, 'Pharmaceutical Targets Visited in Southern Germany, 19–26 May 1945, pp. 4–5.

148 *Ibid.*,' Pharmaceuticals : Research and Manufacture at I.G., Farbenindustrie', 1946.

149 J.-P. Gaudillière, *Inventer la biomedicine: la France, l'Amérique et la production des savoirs de vivant* (2002), pp. 36–68.

150 M. Burns and P.W.M. van Dijk, 'The Development of the Penicillin Production Process in Delft, the Netherlands, during World War II, under Nazi Occupation', *Advances in Applied Microbiology*, 51 (2002), 185–99; M. Burns, J.W. Bennett and P.W.M. van Dijk, 'Code Name Bacinol', *American Society of Microbiology News*, 69/1 (2003), 25–31.

151 R. Bud, *Penicillin: Triumph and Tragedy* (2007), pp. 78–9.

152 Y. Yagisawa, 'Early History of Antibiotics in Japan' in J. Parascandola (ed.), *The History of Antibiotics* (1980), pp. 69–81.

153 A. Cotterell, *R.A.M.C.* (1943), pp. 7–8.

Chapter 6: The Road to Utopia

1 C.L. Dunn, *The Emergency Medical Services* (1952), vol. 1, pp. 42–3.

2 TNA, MH 77/2, description of Emergency Hospital Service, 21 February 1942.

3 TNA, MH 80/24, letter from A.S. McNalty to E.R. Forber, 8 January 1940.

4 TNA, HO 186/92, scheme for an organized Emergency Medical Service, 30 June 1939.

5 TNA, MH 76/99, Emergency Medical Service survey of London voluntary hospitals, May 1938.

6 TNA, MH 76/284, letter to Miss E.A. Sharpe, 16 June 1938.

7 TNA, MH 76/128, interim report of Wilson Committee, July 1938.

8 TNA, MH 76/284, letter to Miss E.A. Sharpe, 16 June 1938.

9 TNA, MH 76/242, review of requirements for hutted hospitals, July 1939.

10 M.P. Shepherd, *Heart of Harefield* (1990), p. 54.

11 'Hospitals in Emergency', *The Lancet*, 1 (1939) 723. Sectors I and II were led
by the London Hospital, III by St Bartholomew's and the Royal Free, IV by
University College Hospital and Charing Cross, V by Middlesex Hospital,
VI by St Mary's, VII by St George's and Westminster Hospital, VIII by
St Thomas's, IX by King's College Hospital, and X by Guy's.

12 TNA, MH 76/128, comments on interim report of Wilson Committee, July
1939.

13 'The Emergency Hospital Scheme'. *The Lancet*, 2 (1939), 938.

14 TNA, HO 186/92, minutes of a meeting held at Ministry of Health, 27 June
1939.

15 'The Emergency Hospital Scheme: Political and Economic Planning',
The Lancet, 2 (1941), 413.

16 TNA, MH 76/284, notes on provision of an ambulance service in the event
of a national emergency, 20 June 1938. The reference to 'the great strike' is
to the 1926 General Strike when the government-sponsored Organization
for the Maintenance of Supplies had used a pool of private cars to maintain
communications and essential services.

17 TNA, MH 76/248, evacuation of London Hospitals, September 1939; 'Town
into Country', *The Lancet*, 2 (1939), 605.

18 J. Ellis, *LHMC 1785–1985: the Story of the London Hospital Medical College,
England's First Medical School* (1986), p. 85.

19 A.E. Clarke-Kennedy, *London Pride* (1979), p. 214.

20 J. Ellis, *LHMC 1785–1985* (1986), p. 85.

21 TNA, HO 186/92, minutes of a meeting held at Ministry of Health, 27 June
1939.

22 *The Times*, 24 November 1939.

23 TNA, HO 186/92, memorandum on formation of civilian hospital EMS,
17 May 1939.

24 *Ibid.*, note on EMS, 21 June 1939.

25 Letter from 'Disillusioned', *St Mary's Hospital Gazette*, 46/1 (1940), 20.

26 'Dispatch no 5', *St Mary's Hospital Gazette*, 46/1 (1940), 34.

27 Letter from Sir Charles Wilson, *The Times*, 6 December 1939.

28 M. Kater, *Doctors under Hitler* (1989), p.p. 153–4.

29 F.A.E. Crew, *The Army Medical Services: Administration* (1953), vol. 1, pp. 206–
14.

30 *Ibid.*, pp. 194–5.

31 St Mary's Hospital Archives, DP 5/19, letter from F.M. McRae to A.H. Buck,
18 August 1943.

32 *Ibid.*, DP 5/16, letter from McRae to Buck, 13 February 1943.

33 *The Times*, 19 October 1945. Attempts by his friends after the war to gain McRae an award for gallantry were frustrated by the lack of contemporary first hand accounts of his heroism from survivors of *HMS Mahratta* or their rescuers; see St Mary's Hospital Archives, DP 5/31, letter from PBC Moore to N.M. Simon, 2 August 1950.

34 *In Which We Serve* (Two Cities, 1942), dir. Noel Coward (DVD, Carlton Visual Entertainment 37115 01663, 2003).

35 Letter from 'Nelson Expects', *St Mary's Hospital Gazette*, 49/3 (1943), 53–4.

36 R.P.M. Miles, 'OHMS', *ibid.*, 49/8 (1943), 143.

37 Letter from 'Surgeon-Lieutenant, RNVR', *ibid*, 46/2 (1940), 36.

38 P. Ziegler, *London at War* (1995), p. 61.

39 St Mary's Hospital Archives, SM/AD 46/14, annual report for 1939.

40 *Ibid.*, SM/AD 46/15, annual report for 1944.

41 'Editorial', *St Mary's Hospital Gazette*, 46/8 (1940), 115. One of the old ladies had been Queen Mary's housekeeper (private information, Barbara Gammon).

42 R.M. Titmuss, *History of the Second World War: Problems of Social Policy* (1950), p. 103.

43 J. Sheldrake, 'The L.C.C. Hospital Service', in A. Saint (ed.), *Politics and the People of London: the London County Council, 1889–1965* (1989), pp. 187–98.

44 Mass Observation, *War Begins at Home* (1940), p. 305.

45 J. Macnichol, 'The Effects of the Evacuation of Schoolchildren on Official Attitudes to State Evacuation' in H.L. Smith (ed.), *War and Social Change in British Society in the Second World War* (1996), p. 3.

46 V. Brittain, *England's Hour* (1981), p. 21.

47 J. Gardiner, *Wartime Britain, 1939–1945* (2005), pp. 36–7.

48 Women's Group on *Social* Welfare, *Our Towns: A Close Up* (1943), pp. 1–6.

49 V. Brittain, *England's Hour* (1981), p. 170.

50 R.M. Titmuss, *History of the Second World War: Problems of Social Policy* (1950), p. 113.

51 Private information, Ellen Reace.

52 J. Gardiner, *Wartime Britain, 1939–1945* (2005), p. 61.

53 TNA, MH 96/165, 'A Fixed First Aid Post under Civil Defence' by L.W. Heffermann, Swansea, July 1941.

54 T.H. O'Brien, *History of the Second World War: Civil Defence* (1955) pp. 321–4.

55 TNA, MH 55/2317, notes of conference at Home Office, 16 April 1943.

56 T.H. O'Brien, *History of the Second World War: Civil Defence* (1955) p. 330.

57 M. Allingham, *The Oaken Heart* (1941), p. 35.

58 S. Garfield (ed.), *We Are at War* (2006), p. 324.

59 V. Woolf, *Diary of Virginia Woolf* (1984), vol. 5, p. 289.

60 J. Gardiner, *Wartime Britain, 1939–1945* (2005), pp. 207–8.

61 W. Sargant, *The Unquiet Mind* (1967), p.p. 86–7.

62 'Editorial', *St Mary's Hospital Gazette*, 46/8 (1940), 115.

63 D. Maurice, *From Cradle to War* (1998), p. 24.

64 'St Mary's Home Guard Company', *St Mary's Hospital Gazette*, 46/10 (1940), 129.

65 *The Daily Express*, 30 December 1940.

66 A.E. Clarke-Kennedy, *London Pride* (1979), pp. 218–9.

67 *Ibid.*, p. 223.

68 C. Graves, *The Story of St Thomas's, 1106–1947* (1947), pp. 61–6.

69 J. Gardiner, *Wartime Britain, 1939–1945* (2005), p. 351.

70 F. Taylor, *Dresden* (2004), pp. 265, 299.

71 M. Kater, *Doctors under Hitler* (1989), pp. 45–6.

72 *Ibid.*, p. 49.

73 J. Ostry, 'St George's Hospital 1940', *George's Magazine*, 7 (2004), 16–17.

74 M. F. Gamble, 'Mary Milne: A Personal Tribute', *St Mary's Hospital Past and Present Nurses' League Journal*, 12 (1975), 32–3.

75 *Johannesburg Star*, 22 May 1947.

76 W. Parkes, 'Miss Mary G. Milne', *St Mary's Hospital Gazette*, 50 (1949), 118–20.

77 *The Lamp Still Burns*, dir. Maurice Elvey (Two Cities, 1943).

78 IWM 536/172/K9540, recruitment poster.

79 TNA, MH 51/602, Nurses Act 1943.

80 P. Starns, *March of the Matrons* (2000), p. 35.

81 TNA, LAB 8/796, nursing cadets, 1943.

82 TNA, CAB 75/10, Cabinet minutes, 1 August 1941.

83 S.M. Sacharski, *To Be a Nurse* (1990), p. 51.

84 V.K. Brown, *Cathedral of Healing* (1981), pp. 123–5.

85 V.K. Brown, *The Story of Passavant Memorial Hospital 1865–1972* (1976), p. 104.

86 TNA, FD 1/5290, progress report on Blood Transfusion Emergency Depots from the outbreak of the War to 30 September 1940.

87 *Ibid.*, minutes of the Blood Transfusion Emergency Depots Committee, 1 May 1940.

88 *Ibid.*, progress report on Blood Transfusion Emergency Depots from the outbreak of the War to 30 September 1940.

89 TNA, FD 1/5892, report on research at Sutton Depot, 1940.

90 TNA, HLG 7/693, note by A.H. King on casualty records, 14 October 1943.

91 Crepitus is a cracking sound caused by friction between the bone and cartilage or between the fractured parts of a bone.

92 TNA, MH 96/165, minutes of meeting at Guildhall, Swansea on treatment of air raid casualties, 9 July 1941.

93 *Ibid.*, 'A Fixed First Aid Post under Civil Defence' by L.W. Heffermann, Swansea, July 1941.

94 *Ibid.*, minutes of meeting at Guildhall, Swansea on treatment of air-raid casualties, 9 July 1941.

95 C. Perry, *Boy in the Blitz* (2000), p. 212.

96 *Ibid.*, p. 213.

97 TNA, MH 96/165, 'A Fixed First Aid Post under Civil Defence' by L.W. Heffermann, Swansea, July 1941.

98 R. Calder, *Carry on London* (1941), p. 39.

99 J. Gregg, *The Shelter of the Tubes* (2001), p. 28.

100 TNA, HLG 7/641, minutes of meeting to discuss incorporation of nursing staff of Shelter Medical Aid Posts into the First Aid Post Service, 29 September 1942.

101 TNA, HO 207/488, London Civil Defence Region circular 327, 8 March 1941.

102 TNA, HO 207/445, report on deep tunnel shelters by Dr Stock, 28 October 1941.

103 C. Perry, *Boy in the Blitz* (2000), p. 160.

104 F. Brown, 'Civilian Psychiatric Air-Raid Casualties', *The Lancet*, 1 (1941), 686–91.

105 H. Wilson, 'Mental Reactions to Air-Raids', *The Lancet*, 1 (1942), 284–7.

106 A. Lewis, 'Incidence of Neurosis', *The Lancet*, 2 (1942), 175–83.

107 B. Banham, *Snapshots in Time* (1991), p. 32.

108 St Mary's Hospital Archives, SM/AD 46/14, annual report for 1940.

109 B. Shephard, *A War of Nerves* (2002), p. 179.

110 *North London Press*, 3 November 1944.

111 Ministry of Information, *How to Keep Well in Wartime* (2007), p. 44.

112 Ministry of Information, *Make Do and Mend* (2007), p. 45.

113 J. Gardiner, *Wartime Britain, 1939–1945* (2005), pp. 186–7.

114 P. Ziegler, *London at War* (1995), p. 248.

115 J. Gardiner, *Wartime Britain, 1939–1945* (2005), p. 178.

116 TNA, MAF 75/68, supplementary ration book, 1942.

117 M. Kater, *Doctors under Hitler* (1989), p. 47.

118 BL Add MS 56112, minutes of General Penicillin Committee, 22 December 1943.

119 *The Daily Telegraph*, 14 February 1944.

120 *Sun Chicago*, 18 August 1943; *Tribune Chicago*, 18 August 1943.

121 Personal information, Barbara Gammon, née Parry; Betty Ashton.

122 Mary Verrier in R. Miller (ed.), *Nothing Less than Victory* (1993), p. 446.

123 BL Add MS 56220, Arthur Mortimer.

124 *The Best Years of Our Lives* (Metro Goldwyn Mayer, 1946), dir. William Wyler (DVD, Metro Goldwyn Mayer Home Entertainment 10001141 MZ1, 2004).

125 Lord Dawson, 'Medicine and the State', *The Medical Officer*, 23 (1920), 223–4.

126 *The Lancet*, 2 (1939), 947.

127 *The Times*, 19 November 1943.

128 'Editorial', *St Mary's Hospital Gazette*, 47/3 (1941), 44.

129 TNA, PREM 4/89/2, evidence of TUC to Beveridge Report, p. 14, 1941.

130 'Draft Interim Report of Medical Planning Commission', *British Medical Journal*, 1 (1942), 743–53.

131 *The Times*, 15 January 1941.

132 J. Harris, *William Beveridge: A Biography* (1977), pp. 378–418.

133 Report of the Interdepartmental Committee on Social Insurance and Allied Services, Cmd. 6404, 1942.

134 TNA, CAB 66/30, Cabinet papers, 24 November 1942.

135 National Health Service, Cmd. 6502, 1944.

136 British Medical Journal, 1 (1944), 293–5.

Chapter 7: Behind the Wire

1 J. Hankinson, 'Belsen', *St Mary's Hospital Gazette*, 51/5 (1945), 74–8.

2 A.M. Brandt, *No Magic Bullet* (1987), illustration between pp. 164 and 165.

3 K. Binding and A. Hoche, *Die Freigabe zur Vernichtung lebensunwerten Lebens. Ihr Maß und ihr Form* (1920).

4 F. Lommel, 'Volkische Aufartung und Arzt', 63 (1933), 221–4; M. Schwartz, 'Euthanasie: Debatten in Deutschland 1895–1945', *Vierteljahreshefte fur Zeitgeschichte*, 46 (1998), 629.

5 Cited in M. Burleigh and W. Wippermann, *The Racial State: Germany 1933–1945* (1991), p. 69.

6 H.M. Hanauske-Abel, 'Not a Slippery Slope or Sudden Subversion: German Medicine and National Socialism in 1933', *British Medical Journal*, 313 (1996), 1453–63; See also M. Kater, *Doctors under Hitler* (1989), pp. 54–74.

7 *Deutsches Arzteblatt*, 1 July 1933.

8 M. Kater, 'Hitler's Early Doctors: Nazi Physicians in Pre-Depression Germany', *Journal of Modern History*, 59 (1987), 25–52; D.M. Pressel, 'Nuremberg and Tuskegee: Lessons for Contemporary American Medicine, *Journal of the National Medical Association*, 95/12 (2003), 1218. For an account of the exclusion of Jewish doctors during the occupation of France, see B. Halioua, *Blouses Blanches, Étoiles Jaunes* (2000).

9 A. Hitler, *Mein Kampf* (1971), pp. 403–4.

10 G. Bock, 'Nazi Sterilization and Reproductive Policies' in S.D. Bachrach (ed.), *Deadly Medicine* (2004), pp. 70–3, 85.

11 G. Bock, *Zwangsterilisation im Nationalsozialismus* (1986), pp. 152,156.

12 Cited in M. Burleigh, *The Third Reich: a New History* (2001), p. 356.

13 R.J.B. Bosworth, *Mussolini's Italy* (2005), p. 221–2, 289–90.

14 *Ibid.*, p. 450.

15 M. Fulbrook, *Germany 1918–1990* (1991), p.80.

16 K.D. Bracher, *The German Dictatorship* (1973), pp. 330–334.

17 R.J.B. Bosworth, *Mussolini's Italy* (2005), p. 290.

18 R. Proctor, *The Nazi War on Cancer* (1999), pp. 183, 195, 213–14.

19 G. Bock, 'Nazi Sterilization and Reproductive Policies' in S.D. Bachrach (ed.), *Deadly Medicine* (2004), pp. 67–9.

20 G. Broberg and N. Rolls-Hansen, *Eugenics and the Welfare State* (1996), pp. 104–5.

21 National Archives, College Park, Maryland, Record Group 238, interrogation of Karl Brandt, 1 October 1945.

22 M. Burleigh, 'Nazi Euthanasia Programs', in S.D. Bachrach (ed.), *Deadly Medicine* (2004), pp. 131–4.

23 Operation T-4 was named after the headquarters of this secret programme at Tiergartenstaße 4 in Berlin.

24 These centres were at Brandenburg, Bernburg, Grafeneck, Hadamar, Sonnenstein (Pirna) and Hartheim.

25 H. Friedlander, *Origins of Nazi Genocide*, (1995) pp. 86–110. See also E. Klee, *Euthanasie im NS-Staat* (2004).

26 H. Steppe, 'Nursing under Totalitarian Regimes: The Case of National Socialism' in A.M. Rafferty, J. Robinson and R. Elkan (ed.), *Nursing History and the Politics of Welfare* (1997), p. 21.

27 M. Burleigh, *Death and Deliverance* (1994), pp. 113–19.

28 P. Löffler (ed.), *Clemens August Graf von Galen: Akten, Briefe und Predigten 1933–1946* (1988), vol. 2, p. 543.

29 M. Burleigh, 'Nazi Euthanasia Programs', in S.D. Bachrach (ed.), *Deadly Medicine* (2004), pp. 149–153.

30 N. Davies, *Rising '44: The Battle for Warsaw* (2003), p.95.

31 M. Burleigh, *The Third Reich: a New History* (2001), p. 589.

32 H. Friedlander, 'From Euthanasia to the Final Solution' in S.D. Bachrach (ed.), *Deadly Medicine* (2004), pp.155–183.

33 R. Hilberg, *Destruction of the European Jews* (2003), p. 1320.

34 Quoted in R.J. Aldrich, *Witness to War* (2005), p.466.

35 N. Davies, *God's Playground* (1981), vol 2, pp. 459–60.

36 L. Rees, *Auschwitz* (2005), p. 184.

37 E. Kogon, H. Langbein and A.Ruckerl, *Nazi Mass Murder* (1993), p. 73.

38 M. Nyiszli, *Auschwitz: A Doctor's Eyewitness Account* (1973), p. 53.

39 L. Alexander, 'Medical Science Under Dictatorship', *New England Journal of Medicine*, 241 (1949), 39–47.

40 TNA, WO 309/468, Military Tribunal no. 1. case no, 1, USA v. Karl Brandt, Siegfried Handler, Paul Rostock et al., 1947.

41 *Ibid.*

42 J.M. Le Minor, 'Des Dérives de la Craniologie aux Crimes Contre l'Humanité: August Hirt (1898–1945) à Strasbourg de 1941 à 1945', in B. Schnitzler (ed.), *Histoire(s) de Squelettes* (2006), pp. 291–3; J. Heran, 'Les Sinistres Expériences Médicales du Struthof,', *Saisons d'Alsace*, 121 (1993), 64–73.

43 A. Faramus, *Journey into Darkness* (1990), p. 369.

44 P. Levi, *If This is a Man* (1987), p. 61.

45 *Ibid.*, pp. 160–1.

46 N. Davies, *God's Playground* (1981), vol 2, p. 451.

47 G. Herling, *A World Apart* (2005), p. 97.

48 *Ibid.*, p. 101.

49 Personal information, Michael Wolach, a Polish prisoner of the Russians 1939–41.

50 TNA, WO 222/20A, War Diary of Lt. Col. L.W. Shackleton, Hong Kong, 1940–2, appendix D, report of Corporal N.J. Leath.

51 *Ibid.*, appendix F, report of Sergeant J.H. Anderson.

52 TNA, WO 141/101, atrocities committed by the Japanese in Hong Kong, 1942.

53 TNA, WO 222/20A, War Diary of Lt. Col. L.W. Shackleton, Hong Kong, 1940–2, appendix F, report of Sergeant J.H. Anderson.

54 TNA, CO 980/52, Report on atrocities by J.R.P. Ridgeway, 18 August 1942.

55 *Ibid.*

56 TNA, WO 106/2579B, notes on the campaign in Malaya by Lieutenant Colonel Robinson, July 1942.

57 CMAC, RAMC 840/2, report by Private Ray.

58 D.M. Kennedy, *Freedom from Fear* (1999), pp. 529–31.

59 TNA, WO 222/22, Report by Captain A.J.N Warrack on conditions experienced as a prisoner of war from a medical point of view, 1945.

60 TNA, CO 980/52, Telegram from Foreign Office to International Red Cross Committee, Geneva, 7 February 1942.

61 Personal information, Bill Frankland.

62 CMAC, RAMC 1016/2, annual medical report for Changi Camp, 1942–3.

63 TNA, WO 222/22, Report by Captain A.J.N Warrack on conditions experienced as a prisoner of war from a medical point of view, 1945.

64 *Ibid.*

65 IWM, EPH, artificial leg made by Prisoners of War in Siam for Sergeant W. Berber, Royal Artillery.

66 IWM, EPH, spectacles made by Prisoner of War on Burma-Siam Railway.

67 Private information, Bill Frankland.

68 CMAC, RAMC 1016/2, Annual medical report for Changi Camp, 1942–3.

69 TNA, WO 222/22, Report by Captain A.J.N Warrack on conditions experienced as a prisoner of war from a medical point of view, 1945.

70 R.J. Aldrich (ed.), *The Faraway War* (2005), pp. 303–4.

71 Private information, Bill Frankland.

72 B. MacArthur, *Surviving the Sword* (2006), p. 38.

73 D.A. Smith, 'Barbed Wire and Beri-beri', *St Mary's Hospital Gazette*, 52/3 (April 1946), 32–34.

74 TNA, WO 222/22, Report by Captain A.J.N Warrack on conditions experienced as a prisoner of war from a medical point of view, 1945.

75 TNA, WO 106/2550B, 'The last days of Singapore' by Val Kobouky, 1942.

76 D.A. Smith, 'Barbed Wire and Beri-beri', *St Mary's Hospital Gazette*, 52/3 (April 1946), 32.

77 TNA, CO 537/1220, report on the internment of civilians in Changi, compiled from camp records by C.E. Courtney, August 1945.

78 D.A. Smith, 'Barbed Wire and Beri-beri', *St Mary's Hospital Gazette*, 52/3 (April 1946), 33–4.

79 O. Lindsay and J.R. Harris, *The Battle for Hong Kong, 1941–1945* (2005), pp. 176, 219.

80 A. Keith, *Three Came Home* (1985), p. 78.

81 TNA, CO 980/52, Telegram from Foreign Office to International Red Cross Committee, Geneva, 7 February 1942.

82 TNA, CO 537/1220, report on the internment of civilians in Changi, compiled from camp records by C.E. Courtney, August 1945.

83 IWM 01/24/1, death certificate of Alexander Edmond Macgregor Mitchell, assistant with the firm of Harrisons, Barker & Co. of Singapore, 28 December 1944.

84 R.J. Aldrich (ed.), *The Faraway War* (2005), pp. 308–10.

85 E.E. Dunlop, *The War Diaries of Weary Dunlop*, (1987), pp. 172–3.

86 Letter from E.E. Dunlop, *St Mary's Hospital Gazette*, 52/1 (1946), 11.

87 B. MacArthur, *Surviving the Sword* (2006), pp. 228–32.

88 R. Porter, *The Greatest Benefit to Mankind* (1997), p. 650.

89 G. Carter and B. Balmer, 'Chemical and Biological Warfare and Defence' in R. Bud and P. Gummett (ed.), *Cold War, Hot Science* (1999), pp. 309–11.

90 R. Mayou (ed.)., International Red Cross and Red Crescent Museum (2000).

91 TNA, CO 980/52, Telegram from Foreign Office to International Red Cross Committee, Geneva, 7 February 1942.

92 TNA, WO 222/22, Report by Captain A.J.N Warrack on conditions experienced as a prisoner of war from a medical point of view, 1945.

93 TNA, CO 537/1220, report on the internment of civilians in Changi, compiled from camp records by C.E. Courtney, August 1945.

94 TNA, WO 32/11678, note on discussions with IRCC at Geneva on matters affecting prisoners of war and civilian internees in the Far East, 7–10 June 1945.

95 M. Junod, *Le Troisième Combattant* (1947), pp. 219–20.

96 TNA, FO 9/6/761, report of Red Cross on prisoner of war camps in Hong Kong, 3 July 1942.

97 TNA, CO 980/155, supplementary report on the work of the ICRC in Hong Kong under Japanese occupation by Rudolph Zindel, 15 July 1946.

98 *Ibid.*, report on conditions in Stanley camp by a recent repatriate, R.D. Gillespie, 1946.

99 *Ibid.*, supplementary report on the work of the ICRC in Hong Kong under Japanese occupation by Rudolph Zindel, 15 July 1946.

100 International Committee of the Red Cross, Report of the International Committee of the Red Cross on its activities during the Second World War (1947).

101 M. Gilbert, *The Righteous* (2002), p. 235.

102 R. Wallenberg, *Letters and Dispatches, 1924–1944* (1995), p. 261, 266.

103 J. Bierman, *Righteous Gentile* (1982), p. 95. Belgian resistance worker Anne Brusselsmans similarly played on German fears of typhoid when she hid a young member of the Secret Army in her house and stopped the Gestapo from searching it by saying her son had the disease, R.J. Aldrich, *Witness to War* (2005), pp. 739–40.

104 W.E. Seidelman, 'Nuremberg: Lamentation for the Forgotten Victims of Medical Science', *British Medical Journal*, 313 (1996), 1463–7.

Chapter 8: Trauma & Terror

1 W.S. Churchill, *History of the Second World War: Triumph and Tragedy*, vol. 6 (1954), p. 553.

2 'Nagasaki', *St Mary's Hospital Gazette*, 51/10 (1945), 137.

3 R.J. Lifton, *Death in Life* (1967), p. 27.

4 M. Hachiya, *Hiroshima Diary* (1955), p. 101.

5 *Ibid.*, p. 15.

6 R.J. Lifton, *Death in Life* (1967), p. 57.

7 *Ibid.*, p. 66.

8 *Ibid.*, p. 61.

9 TNA, WO 32/13461, pamphlet on 'Defence Against the Atom Bomb', July 1951.

10 TNA, FO 371/87185, notes on export of Podbielniak extractors to Eastern Europe, 30 December 1949, 8 January 1950, 25 January 1950; TNA, MH 79/416, report of Joint Intelligence Committee on sale of penicillin plant, 6 March 1948.

11 St Mary's Hospital Archives, SM/AD Civil Defence files, minutes of meeting of Civil Defence Hospital and First Aid Services, 25 June 1953.

12 *Ibid.*, 19 September 1951.

13 TNA, WO 32/16000, note by Director General of Army Medical Services on deployment of units, 27 February 1956.

14 St Mary's Hospital Archives, SM/AD Civil Defence files, minutes of meeting of Civil Defence Hospital and First Aid Services, 23 May 1951.

15 A. Winkler, *Life Under a Cloud* (1993), pp. 94–6.

16 J.T. Patterson, *Grand Expectations* (1996), p. 277.

17 A. Winkler, *Life Under a Cloud* (1993), pp. 91–3.

18 G. Carter and B. Balmer, 'Chemical and Biological Warfare and Defence' in R. Bud and P. Gummett (ed.), *Cold War, Hot Science* (1999), pp. 297–8

19 T. Hickman, *The Call-up* (2005), pp. 257–64.

20 J.T. Patterson, *Grand Expectations* (1996), p. 223.

21 J.T. Greenwood and F.C.Berry, *Medics at War* (2005), p. 123.

22 S.H. Neel, 'Medical Considerations in Helicopter Evacuation', *United States Armed Forces Medical Journal*, 1 (1954), 224–5.

23 R.S. Driscoll, 'US Army Medical Helicopters in the Korean War', *Military Medicine*, 166/4 (2001), 292–3.

24 O.F. Apel, *MASH* (1998), p. 80.

25 W.I. White, *Back Down the Ridge* (1953), pp. 45–6.

26 J.T. Greenwood and F.C. Berry, *Medics at War* (2005), p. 126.

27 TNA, WO 32/13525, report by K. Fry on American helicopters in Korea, 12 September 1951.

28 *Ibid.*, letter from J.C. Barnetson to J.M. Matheson, 14 November 1948.

29 *Ibid.*, letter from J.M. Matheson to J.C. Barnetson, 2 December 1948.

30 *Ibid.*, report on casualty evacuations from Sungei Segamat, 13 October 1950.

31 *Ibid.*, letter from J.C. Barnetson, Nairobi, 13 May 1955.

32 S.C. Woodward, 'The Story of the Mobile Army Surgical Hospital', *Military Medicine*, 168/7 (2003), 507.

33 National Archives, College Park, Maryland, Record Group 112, Office of the Surgeon General (Army), Historical Division, US AMEDD records 1946–61, Box 196, Eighth Army annual reports, Army Medical Service activities, 1950, 1951.

34 O.F. Apel, *MASH* (1998), p. 57.

35 D.G. Horwitz (ed.), *We Will Not Be Strangers* (1997), pp. 99, 212.

36 O.F. Apel, *MASH* (1998), pp. 15, 35.

37 D.G. Horwitz (ed.), *We Will Not Be Strangers* (1997), p. 7.

38 O.F. Apel, *MASH* (1998), p. 49.

39 *Battle Circus*, dir. Richard Brooks (Metro Goldwyn Mayer, 1952).

40 O.F. Apel, *MASH* (1998), p. 136.

41 *Ibid.*, p. 126.

42 J.T. Greenwood and F.C. Berry, *Medics at War* (2005), p. 129.

43 B. King and I. Jatoi, ''The Mobile Army Surgical Hospital: A Military and Surgical Legacy, *Journal of the National Medical Association*, 97/5 (2005), 651–2.

44 F.C. Spencer and R.V. Grewe, 'The Management of Arterial Injuries in Battle Casualties', *Annals of Surgery*, 141 (1953), 304–12.

45 TNA, WO 32/14285, report of Committee on Physical Training in the Army, 1950.

46 A.J. Glass, 'Preventive Psychiatry in the Combat Zone', *United States Armed Forces Medical Journal*, 4 (1953), 683–92.

47 National Archives, College Park, Maryland, Record Group 112, Office of the Surgeon General (Army), Historical Division, US AMEDD records 1946–61, Box 196, Eighth Army annual reports, Army Medical Service activities, 1950.

48 A.J. Glass, 'Psychiatry in the Korean Campaign', *United States Armed Forces Medical Journal*, 4 (1953), 1387–1583.

49 C.L. Anderson, A.M. Boysen, S. Estensen, G.N. Lam and W.R. Shadish, 'Medical Experiences in Communist POW Camps in Korea', *Journal of American Medical Association*, 156 (1954), 120–2.

50 S.C. Woodward, 'The Story of the Mobile Army Surgical Hospital', *Military Medicine*, 168/7 (2003), 511.

51 B. King and I. Jatoi, ''The Mobile Army Surgical Hospital: A Military and Surgical Legacy, *Journal of the National Medical Association*, 97/5 (2005), 655.

52 R. Hooker, *MASH: A Novel About Three Army Doctors* (1968).

53 *M*A*S*H* (Twentieth Century Fox, 1969), dir. Robert Altman (DVD, Twentieth Century Fox Home Entertainment F1-0GB 01038, 2002). The subsequent television series based on the book and film ran from 1972–1983, lasting far longer than the war itself, and returned to the Korean War origins of the characters and their MASH.

54 B. King and I. Jatoi, 'The Mobile Army Surgical Hospital: A Military and Surgical Legacy', Journal of the National Medical Association, 97/5 (2005), 653.

55 R.J. Glasser, *365 Days* (1980), p. 8.

56 P. Dorland and J. Nanney, Dust Off: Aeromedical Evacuation in Vietnam (1982).

57 R.J. Glasser, *365 Days* (1980), p. 9.

58 J.T. Greenwood and F.C.Berry, *Medics at War* (2005), p. 141.

59 S. Levitsky, P.M. James and R.W. Anderson, 'Vascular Trauma in Vietnam Battle Casualties: An Analysis of 55 Consecutive Cases', *Annals of Surgery*, 168 (1968), 831–6.

60 Rodney Hardin in M.R. Littleton and C. Wright (ed.), *Doc* (2005), p, 219.

61 E.L. Jones, A.F. Peters and R.M. Gasior, 'Early Management of Battle Casualties in Vietnam: An Analysis of 1011 Consecutive Cases Treated at a Mobile Army Surgical Hospital', *Archives of Surgery*, 97 (1968), 1–15.

62 J.A. Moncrief, 'The Use of a Topical Sulphonamide in the Control of Burn Wound Sepsis', *Journal of Trauma*, 6 (1966), 407–19; R.M. Hardaway, 'Surgical Research in Vietnam', *Military Medicine*, 132 (1967), 873–87.

63 J.T. Greenwood and F.C.Berry, *Medics at War* (2005), p. 140.

64 B. King and I. Jatoi, 'The Mobile Army Surgical Hospital: A Military and Surgical Legacy', *Journal of the National Medical Association*, 97/5 (2005), 654.

65 James Chaffee in M.R. Littleton and C. Wright (ed.), *Doc* (2005), p. 245.

66 J.T. Greenwood and F.C.Berry, *Medics at War* (2005), p. 145.

67 R.J. Wilensky, 'The Medical Civic Action Program in Vietnam: Success or Failure', *Military Medicine*, 166/9 (2001), 815–9.

68 R.J. Glasser, *365 Days* (1980), p. 5.

69 T. A. Verdon and E. T. Thomas, 'Current problems with Neisseria Gonorrhoea in Vietnam', *United States Army in Vietnam Medical Bulletin*, 40/22 (1970), 9–10.

70 S. Sun, 'Where the Girls Are: the Management of Venereal Disease by United States Military Forces in Vietnam', *Literature and Medicine*, 23/1 (2004), 69.

71 Ibid., 70.

72 S. Mirin and G. McKenna, 'Combat Zone Adjustment: Role of Marijuana Use', *Military Medicine*, 140 (1975), 482–6.

73 R. A. Ratner, 'Drugs and Despair in Vietnam', *University of Chicago Magazine*, 64 (1972), 15–23.

74 H. C. Holloway, 'Epidemiology of Heroin Dependency among Soldiers in Vietnam', *Military Medicine*, 139 (1974), 108–13.

75 Jim Tolomay in M.R. Littleton and C. Wright (ed.), Doc (2005), p. 233.

76 J. T. Patterson, *Grand Expectations* (1996), p. 619.

77 P. Bourne, 'Military Psychiatry and the Vietnam Experience', *American Journal of Psychiatry*, 127 (1970), 481–8.

78 J. Kaylor, D. King and L. King, 'Psychological Effects of Military Service in Vietnam: A Meta Analysis', *Psychological Bulletin*, 102 (1987), 257–71.

79 A. R. Marsh, 'A Short but Distant War: the Falklands Campaign', *Journal of the Royal Society of Medicine*, 76 (1983), 972–82; D.S. Jackson, C.G. Batty, J.M. Ryan and W.S.P. McGregor, 'The Falklands War: Army Field Surgical Experience', *Annals of the Royal College of Surgeons*, 65 (1983), 281–5.

80 H. M. Souka, 'Management of Gulf War Casualties', *British Journal of Surgery*, 79 (1992), 1307–8.

81 J. R. Riddle, M. Brown, T. Smith, E.C. Ritchie, K.A. Brix and J. Romano, 'Chemical Warfare and the Gulf War: A Review of the Impact on Gulf Veterans' Health', *Military Medicine*, 168/8 (2003), 606–13.

82 J. Laffin, *Combat Surgeons* (1999), p. 232.

83 C. Unwin, N. Blatchley, W. Coker, S. Ferry, M. Hotopf, L. Hull, K. Ismail, I. Palmer, A. David and S. Wessely, 'Health of UK Servicemen who Served in the Persian Gulf War', *The Lancet*, 1 (1999), 169–78.

84 J. T. Patterson, *Restless Giant* (2005), p. 234.

85 *Independent*, 20 October 2006.

86 Tonight with Trevor McDonald, television programme on 'War Wounds', ITV 1, 30 October 2006; *Independent*, 8 October 2006.

87 *Independent*, 16 May 2006, 13 January 2007.

88 United Nations Relief and Rehabilitation Administration, Report of the Director General to the Council for the Period 1 January 1946 to 31 March 1946 (1946).

89 M. I. Roemer, 'Internationalism in Medicine' in W.F. Bynum and R. Porter (ed.), *Companion Encyclopaedia of the History of Medicine* (1993), pp. 1408–26; P. Weindling, *The Rise of Medical Internationalism* (1996).

90 D. Acheson, 'Conflict in Bosnia, 1992–3', *British Medical Journal*, 319 (1993), 1639–42.

91 R. Horton, 'Croatia and Bosnia: the Imprints of War', *The Lancet*, 353 (1999), 2223–8.

92 S. Lang, 'The Third Balkan War: Red Cross Bleeding', *Croatian Medical Journal*, 34 (1993), 5–20.

93 R. Mayou (ed.), *International Red Cross and Red Crescent Museum* (2000), pp. 154–5.

94 *Journal of American Board of Family Medicine*, 15/1 (2002), 80–3.

95 *Financial Times*, 17 January 2004.

96 'Médecins Sans Frontières: Bearing Witness', *Canadian Medical Association Journal*, 161/10 (1999), 1221.

97 *Financial Times*, 17 January 2004.

98 *British Medical Journal*, 318 (1999), 1616.

99 K. de Jong, N. Ford and R. Kleber, 'Mental Health Care for Refugees from Kosovo: the Experience of Médecins Sans Frontières ', *The Lancet*, 353 (1999), 1616–7.

100 *British Medical Journal*, 318 (1999), 961.

101 J. Longman, *Among the Heroes* (2002), p. 216.

102 K. Cain, H. Postlewait and A. Thomson, *Emergency Sex* (2005), p. 255.

103 *Atlantic Monthly*, September 2002.

104 *The Week Magazine*, 13 September 2002.

105 R. Bally in M.R. Littleton and C. Wright (ed.), *Doc* (2005), pp. 274–5.

106 T.V. Inglesby, T. O'Toole, and D.A. Henderson, 'Anthrax as a Biological Weapon, 2002: Updated Recommendations for Management', *Journal of American Medical Association*, 287 (2002), 2236–52.

107 J.D. Grabenstein, P.R. Pittman, J.T. Greenwood and R.J.M. Engler, 'Immunization to Protect the U.S. Armed Forces: Heritage, Current Practice and Prospects', *Epidemiology Review*, 28 (2006), 3–26.

108 C. Catlett, and J.E. Farley, 'Infection Control Challenges for the New Century: Lessons Learned from Past Epidemics are Valuable in Healthcare System Bioterrorism Disaster Planning', *Seminars in Infection Control*, 2/1 (2002), 2–9.

Bibliography

Primary Archival Sources

British Library, London
Alexander Fleming papers, BL Add. MSS 56106-225

Gillies Archive, Queen Mary's Hospital, Sidcup
Case notes of Harold Gillies, 1917–25

Imperial War Museum, London, IWM

Musée International de la Croix Rouge et du Croissant Rouge, Geneva

National Academy of Sciences, National Research Council Archives, Institute of Medicine, Washington DC (USA)
Committee on Chemotherapeutic and Other Agents records
Committees on Military Medicine records
Venereal Diseases Bulletin

National Archives (Public Records Office), London
Admiralty records, TNA, ADM
Air Ministry records, TNA, AIR
Cabinet papers, TNA, CAB
Colonial Office records, TNA, CO
Civil Service Commission, TNA, CSC
Education Board records, TNA, ED
General Nursing Council, TNA, DT
Home Office records, TNA, HO

Medical Research Council Archives, TNA, FD
Metropolitan Police records, TNA, MEPO
Ministry of Food, TNA, MAF
Ministry of Health records, TNA, MH
Ministry of Health and Local Government, TNA, HLG
Ministry of Information records, TNA, INF
Ministry of Labour records, TNA, LAB
Ministry of National Service records, TNA, NATS
Prime Minister's Office, TNA, PREM
Secret Service, TNA, KV
War Office records, TNA, WO

National Archives, Washington DC (USA)
Public Health Service records, RG 90
Office of the Surgeon General (Army) records, RG 112
Bureau of Agricultural and Industrial Chemistry records, RG 97
American Expeditionary Forces, 1917–23, records, RG 120,
War Department General and Special Staff records, RG 165
Office of Scientific Research and Development, RG 227

National Center for Agricultural Utilization Research, Peoria, Illinois (USA)
Mycology registersi

Paul Ehrlich Institut, Langen, Frankfurt-am-Main (Germany)
Paul Ehrlich papers

Pfizer Information Center, Corporate Affairs Division, New York (USA)
Pfizer penicillin papers, Gladys Hobby records, series 5, Pfizer history

Pfizer Records Centre, Sandwich, Kent
Kemball Bishop and Co. records, Box 96B-2E

Rockefeller Archive Center, North Tarrytown, NY (USA)
Rockefeller Foundation archives, records of projects funded, RF, RG 1.1, projects
    series 401, boxes 36–7, folders 457–70, 481–4

Royal College of Ophthalmologists
William Wallace papers.

Royal Society, London
Howard Walter Florey papers, HF

St Mary's Hospital. Archives, London
St Mary's Hospital records, SM/AD
St Mary's Hospital Medical School records, MS/AD
Paddington Green Children's Hospital records, PG/AD
Papers of F.M. McRae, DP 5
Papers of Ida Mann, DP 21
Papers of Sir William Willcox, DP 46
Inoculation Department records, WF/AD

Wellcome Library, Contemporary Medical Archives Centre, London
Ernst Boris Chain papers, PP/EBC
Norman George Heatley papers, GC48
Royal Army Medical Corps collection, RAMC

Official Papers

Care and Treatment of the Sick and Wounded During the South African
    Campaign, Cd. 453, 1901
Report to Consider the Re-organization of the Army Medical Services, Cd.
    791, 1901
Report on the Concentration Camps in South Africa by the Committee of
    Ladies, Cd. 893, 1902
Report of the Inter-Departmental Committee on Physical Deterioration, Cd.
    2175, 1904
Interim Report of the Anti-Typhoid Inoculation Committee, Cd. 26989
    July 1904
Report of the Royal Commission on the Poor Laws and Relief of Distress, Cd.
    4499, 1909
Final Report of the Commissioners, Royal Commission on Venereal Diseases,
    Cd. 8189, 1916
Report of Central Control Board, Cd. 8243, 1916
Report upon the Physical Examination of Men of Military Age by National
    Service Boards from November 1st 1917 – October 31st 1918, Cmd.
    504, 1919
Report of the Interdepartmental Committee on Social Insurance and Allied
    Services, Cmd. 6404, 1942
White Paper on A National Health Service, Cmd. 6502, 1944

Primary Published Sources

Abraham, E.P., Chain, E., Fletcher, C.M., Florey, H.W., Gardner, A.D., Heatley, N.G. and Jennings, M.A., 'Further Observations on Penicillin', *The Lancet*, 2 (1941), 177–88

Acheson, Donald, 'Conflict in Bosnia, 1992–3', *British Medical Journal*, 319 (1993), 1639–42

Aldrich, Richard J., *Witness to War: Diaries of the Second World War in Europe and the Middle East*, London, Corgi, 2005

_____, *The Faraway War: Personal Diaries of the Second World War in Asia and the Pacific*, London, Doubleday, 2006

Alexander, L., 'Medical Science Under Dictatorship', *New England Journal of Medicine*, 241 (1949), 39–47

Alexandra, Duchess of Fife (Princess Arthur of Connaught), *A Nurse's Story*, London, privately published, 1954

Allingham, Marjorie, *The Oaken Heart*, London, Michael Joseph, 1941

Anderson, C.L., Boysen, A.M., Estensen, S., Lam, G.N., and Shadish, W.R., 'Medical Experiences in Communist POW Camps in Korea', *Journal of American Medical Association*, 156 (1954), 120–2

Apel, Otto F., *MASH: An Army Surgeon in Korea*, Lexington, University Press of Kentucky, 1998

Army Advisory Committee on Maxillo-Facial Injuries, *Report to the Army Council of the Army Advisory Committee on Maxillo-Facial Injuries*, London, HMSO, 1940

Army Directorate of Pathology, 'Memorandum Concerning the Use of Sulphonamide Derivatives for Prophylaxis and Treatment of Wound Infections, *Journal of the Royal Army Medical Corps*, 73 (1939), 298–300

Auden, W.H., *Selected Poems*, London, Faber and Faber, 1979

Banham, Belinda, *Snapshots in Time: Some Experiences in Health Care 1936–1991*, Newmill, Patten Press, 1991

Barling, S. and Morrison, J.T. (ed.), *A Manual of War Surgery*, London, Hodder and Stoughton, 1919

Binding, Karl and Hoche, Alfred, *Die Freigabe zur Vernichtung lebensunwerten Lebens. Ihr Maß und ihr Form*, Leipzig, privately published, 1920

Bishop, Alan and Bostridge, Mark (ed.), *Letters from a Lost Generation: First World War Letters of Vera Brittain and Four Friends*, London, Abacus, 1999

Borden, William Cline, *The Use of the Röntgen Ray by the Medical Department of the United States Army in the War with Spain*, Washington DC, Government Printing Office, 1900

Borkenau, Franz, *The Spanish Cockpit: An Eyewitness Account of the Spanish Civil War*, London, Phoenix Press, 2000

Bourne, P., 'Military Psychiatry and the Vietnam Experience', *American Journal of Psychiatry*, 127 (1970), 481–8

Bowlby, A.A., *A Civilian War Hospital: Being an Account of the Work of the Portland Hospital and Experience of Wounds and Sickness in South Africa,* London, John Murray, 1900

British Red Cross and Order of St John, *Reports by the Joint War Committee and Joint War Finance Committee of the British Red Cross Society and the Order of St John of Jerusalem in England on Voluntary Aid Rendered to the Sick and Wounded at Home and Abroad, and to British Prisoners of War 1914–19,* London, HMSO, 1921

Brittain, Vera, *Testament of Youth: An Autobiographical Study of the Years 1900–1925,* London, Fontana, 1979

_____, *England's Hour: An Autobiography, 1939–1941,* London, Futura, 1981

Broggi, Moises, *Memories d'un Cirugia,* Barcelona, Edicions, 2001

Brown, F., 'Civilian Psychiatric Air-Raid Casualties', *The Lancet,* 1 (1941), 686–91

Buchan, John, *Greenmantle,* Oxford, Oxford University Press, 1999

Cain, Kenneth, Postlewait, Heidi and Thomson, Andrew, *Emergency Sex (and Other Desperate Measures): True Stories from a War Zone,* London, Ebury Press, 2005

Calder, Ritchie, *Carry on London,* London, English Universities Press, 1941

Callendar, G.R. and Luippold, G.F., 'The Effectiveness of Typhoid Vaccine Prepared by the U.S. Army', *Journal of American Medical Association,* 123 (1943), 319–21

Carrel, A. and Debelly, G., *The Treatment of Infected Wounds,* London, University of London Press, 1917

Catlett, C. and Farley, J.E., 'Infection Control Challenges for the New Century: Lessons Learned from Past Epidemics are Valuable in Healthcare System Bioterrorism Disaster Planning', *Seminars in Infection Control,* 2/1 (2002), 2–9

Chain, Ernst Boris, 'Thirty Years of Penicillin Therapy', *Proceedings of the Royal Society of London,* B, 179 (1971), 293

_____, Florey, H.W., Gardner, A.D., Heatley, N.G., Jennings, M.A., Orr-Ewing, J.and Sanders, A.G., 'Penicillin as a Chemotherapeutic Agent', *The Lancet,* 2 (1940), 226–8

Charleson, Miss, 'Recollections of the Siege of Ladysmith from the Diary of Miss Charleson', *St Mary's Hospital Gazette,* 7/6 (June 1901), 91–3

_____, 'Recollections of the Siege of Ladysmith from the Diary of Miss Charleson', *St Mary's Hospital Gazette,* 7/7 (July 1901), 103–5

Christie, Agatha, *The Mysterious Affair at Styles,* London, Harper Collins, 2001

Churchill, Winston S., *History of the Second World War: Triumph and Tragedy,* vol. 6, London, Cassell, 1954

Clarke, L.B., 'Active Service and the Unfit', *St Mary's Hospital Gazette,* 23/6 (June 1917), 66–8

Cohen, S.M., 'Experience in the Treatment of War Burns', *British Medical Journal* (1940), 251–4

Connolly, Cyril (ed.), *The Golden Horizon*, London, Weidenfeld and Nicolson, 1953

Cotterell, Anthony, *R.A.M.C.*, London, Hutchinson, 1943

Craig, Oscar and Fraser, Alasdair (ed.), *Doctors at War*, Stanhope, The Memoir Club, 2007

Cross, Tim (ed.), *The Lost Voices of World War I: An International Anthology of Writers, Poets and Playwrights*, London, Bloomsbury, 1998

Croy, Marie de, *Le Martyr des Pays Envahis*, Paris, Hachette, 1933

Cushing, Harvey, *From a Surgeon's Journal, 1915–1918*, London, Constable, 1936

Daly, A.S., 'Anaesthetics' in S. Barling and J.T. Morrison (ed.), *A Manual of War Surgery* (1919), pp. 397–412

Dawson, Lord, 'Medicine and the State', *The Medical Officer*, 23 (1920), 223–4

Domagk, Gerhard 'Ein Beitrag zur Chemotherapie der bacteriellen Infektionen', *Deutsche Medizinische Wochenshrift*, 61 (1935), 250–3

———, *Chemotherapie bakterieller Infektionen*, Leipzig, Hirzel, 1944

Douglas, S.R., Fleming, Alexander and Colebrook, Leonard, 'On the Question of Bacterial Symbiosis in Wound Infections', *The Lancet*, 1 (1917), 604–7

———, Colebrook Leonard and Fleming, Alexander, 'On the Growth of Anaerobic Bacilli in Fluid Media under Apparently Anaerobic Conditions', *The Lancet*, 2 (1917), 530–2

Doyle, Arthur Conan, *The Great Boer War*, London, Smith and Elder, 1901

Duhamel, Georges, *Souvenirs de la Grande Guerre*, London, Methuen, 1985

Dunlop, E.E., *The War Diaries of Weary Dunlop*, London, Leonard Publishing, 1987

Duran i Jordà, Frederic, 'El Servei de Tranfusió de sang al front: Organització i utillatge', *La Medicina Catalana* 7 (1936), 45–46

———, 'The Barcelona Blood Transfusion Service', *The Lancet*, 1 (1939), 773–5

Edmunds, C.T., 'Experiences in a German Field Hospital', *St Mary's Hospital Gazette*, 23/3 (March 1917), 32–3

Ellison, Wallace, *Escaped! Adventures in German Captivity*, Edinburgh, William Blackwood and Sons, 1918

Emergency Medical Service, 'The Local Treatment of War Burns', *British Medical Journal* (1940), 489

Faramus, Anthony, *Journey into Darkness*, London, Grafton, 1990

Fitzgerald, F. Scott, *Tender is the Night*, Ware, Wordsworth Editions, 1993

Fleming Alexander, 'Some Notes on the Bacteriology of Gas Gangrene', *The Lancet*, 2 (1915), 376–8

———, 'On the Bacteriology of Septic Wounds', *The Lancet*, 2 (1915), 638–43

———, 'The Physiological and Antiseptic Action of Flavine, with Some Observations on the Testing of Antiseptics', *The Lancet*, 2 (1917), 341–5; Letter to *The Lancet*, 2 (1917), 508–9

_____, 'On the Antibacterial Action of Cultures of a Penicillium with Special Reference to their Use in the Isolation of *B. Influenzae*', *British Journal of Experimental Pathology*, 10 (1929), 226–36

_____, 'Penicillin: Its Practical Application', London, Butterworth, 1946

_____, and Clemenger, F.J., 'A Simple Method of recording Automatically the Gas Produced by Bacteria in a Culture and of the Oxygen Absorbed by Aerobic Non-Gas-Forming Bacteria', *British Journal of Experimental Pathology*, 1 (1920–1), 66–9

Florey, Howard Walter and Cairns, Hugh, *A Preliminary Report to the War Office and Medical Research Council on Investigations Concerning the Use of Penicillin in War Wounds,* London, HMSO, 1943

_____, _____, 'Penicillin in Warfare', *British Journal of Surgery*, 32 (1944), 110–224

Fyvel, Penelope, *English Penny*, Ilfracombe, Arthur H. Stockwell, 1992

Gamble, M. F., 'Mary Milne: A Personal Tribute', *St Mary's Hospital Past and Present Nurses' League Journal*, 12 (1975), 32–3

Gandhi, Mohandras K., *An Autobiography*, London, Phoenix Press, 1930

Garfield, Simon, *We Are at War: The Diaries of Five Ordinary People in Extraordinary Times,* London, Ebury Press, 2006

Garrod, L.P. 'The Treatment of War Wounds with Penicillin', *British Medical Journal*, 2 (11 December 1943), 755–6

Gear, H.S., 'Hygiene Aspects of the El Alamein Victory', *British Medical Journal*, 1 (1944), 383–7

Gillies, Harold Delf, *Plastic Surgery of the Face*, London, Hodder and Stoughton, 1920

Glass, A.J., 'Preventive Psychiatry in the Combat Zone', *United States Armed Forces Medical Journal*, 4 (1953), 683–92

_____, 'Psychiatry in the Korean Campaign', *United States Armed Forces Medical Journal*, 4 (1953), 1387–1583

Glasser, Ronald J., *365 Days*, New York, George Braziller, 1980

Gosse, Philip, *Memoirs of a Camp Follower: a Naturalist Goes to War*, London, Cassell, 1950

Grabenstein, John D., Pittman, Phillip R., Greenwood, John T., and Engler, Renata J.M., 'Immunization to Protect the U.S. Armed Forces: Heritage, Current Practice and Prospects', *Epidemiology Review*, 28 (2006), 3–26

Graves, Robert, *Goodbye to All That*, London, Guild Publishing, 1979

Hachiya, Michihiko, *Hiroshima Diary*, Chapel Hill, University of North Carolina Press, 1955

Hankinson, John, 'Belsen', *St Mary's Hospital Gazette*, 51/5 (1945), 74–8

Harben, Henry D., *The Endowment of Motherhood*, London, Fabian Society Pamphlet no. 149, 1910

Hardaway, R.M., 'Surgical Research in Vietnam', *Military Medicine*, 132 (1967), 873–87

Heller, Joseph, *Catch-22*, London, Vintage, 1994

Herling, Gustav, *A World Apart*, London, Penguin, 2005

Herrington, E.W. 'Further News from South Africa', *St Mary's Hospital Gazette*, 6/9 (November 1900), 125–6

_____, 'Further News from South Africa', *St Mary's Hospital Gazette*, 6/10 (December 1900), 149–50

Hillary, Richard, *The Last Enemy*, London, Pimlico, 1997

Hitler, Adolph, *Mein Kampf*, Boston, Houghton Mifflin, 1971

Hobhouse, Emily, *Report of a Visit to the Camps of Women and Children in the Cape and Orange Rivers*, London, Friars Printing Association, 1901

Hofmeyr, John, *The Testament of a Doctor: A Life of Contrasts*, Cape Town, SAMA Health and Medical Publishing, 2003

Holloway, H.C., 'Epidemiology of Heroin Dependency among Soldiers in Vietnam', *Military Medicine*, 139 (1974), 108–13

Hood, Alexander, 'Army Medical Services in Action', *Journal of the Royal Army Medical Corps*, 38 (1943), 287–90

Hooker, Richard, *MASH: A Novel About Three Army Doctors*, New York, Harper, 1968

Horton, Richard, 'Croatia and Bosnia: the Imprints of War', *The Lancet*, 353 (1999), 2223–8

Horwitz, D.G. (ed.), *We Will Not Be Strangers: Korean War Letters Between a MASH Surgeon and his Wife*, Urbana, University of Illinois Press, 1997

Information, Ministry of, *How to Keep Well in Wartime*, London, Imperial War Museum, 2007

_____, *Make Do and Mend*, London, Imperial War Museum, 2007

Inglesby, T.V., O'Toole, T., and Henderson, D.A., 'Anthrax as a Biological Weapon, 2002: Updated Recommendations for Management', *Journal of American Medical Association*, 287 (2002), 2236–52

Inter-Allied Conference on the Aftercare of Disabled Men, *Reports of Second Annual Meeting of the Inter-Allied Conference on the Aftercare of Disabled Men*, London, HMSO, 1918

International Committee of the Red Cross, *Report of the International Committee of the Red Cross on its Activities during the Second World War*, Geneva, ICRC, 1947

Jackson, D.S., Batty, C.G., Ryan, J.M. and McGregor, W.S.P., 'The Falklands War: Army Field Surgical Experience', *Annals of the Royal College of Surgeons*, 65 (1983), 281–5

Jenkins, E. Lynn, 'Life in a Flying Column', *St Mary's Hospital Gazette*, 8/6 (June 1902), 86–7

Jolly, D.W., *Field Surgery in Total War*, London, Hamish Hamilton, 1941

Jones, E.L., Peters, A.F. and Gasior, R.M., 'Early Management of Battle Casualties in Vietnam: An Analysis of 1011 Consecutive Cases Treated at a Mobile Army Surgical Hospital', *Archives of Surgery*, 97 (1968), 1–15

Jones, Robert, 'The Problem of the Disabled', *American Journal of Orthopaedic Surgery*, 16/5 (1918), 273–90

_____, (ed.), *Orthopaedic Surgery of Injuries*, London, Oxford Medical Publications, 1921

Jong, Kaz de, Ford, Nathan and Kleber, Rolf, 'Mental Health Care for Refugees from Kosovo: the Experience of Médecins Sans Frontières', *The Lancet*, 353 (1999), 1616–7

Junod, Marcel, *Le Troisième Combattant*, Paris, Payot, 1947

Keith, Agnes, *Three Came Home: A Woman's Ordeal in a Japanese Prison Camp*, London, Eland, 1985

Kemp, Peter, *Mine Were of Trouble*, London, Cassell, 1957

Kiese, M., 'Chemotherapie mit Antibakteriellen Stoffen aus Niederen Pilzen und Bakterien', *Klinische Wochenschrift* , 22 (1943), 505–11

Lang, Slobodan, 'The Third Balkan War: Red Cross Bleeding', *Croatian Medical Journal*, 34 (1993), 5–20

Lawrence, D.H., *Kangaroo*, Harmondsworth, Penguin, 1950

Lawrence, T.E., *Seven Pillars of Wisdom: A Triumph*, Harmondsworth, Penguin, 1983

Lees, Kenneth, 'Wounded Soldiers at St Mary's', *St Mary's Hospital Gazette*, 20/10 (December 1914), p.163

Letherby Tidy, H. (ed.), *Inter-Allied Conferences on War Medicine 1942–1945*, London, Staples Press, 1947

Levi, Primo, *If This is A Man*, London, Abacus, 1987

Levitsky, S., James, P.M. and Anderson, R.W., 'Vascular Trauma in Vietnam Battle Casualties: An Analysis of 55 Consecutive Cases', *Annals of Surgery*, 168 (1968), 831–6

Lewis, A., 'Incidence of Neurosis', *The Lancet*, 2 (1942), 175–83

Lifton, Robert Jay, *Death in Life*, New York, Random House, 1967

Littleton, Mark. R. and Wright, Charles (ed.), *Doc: Heroic Stories of Medics, Corpsmen and Surgeons in Combat*, St Paul Minnesota, Zenith, 2005

Löffler, Peter (ed.), *Clemens August Graf von Galen: Akten, Briefe und Predigten 1933–1946*, 2 volumes, Mainz, Matthias Grünewald Verlag, 1988

Lommel, F., 'Volkische Aufartung und Arzt', *Deutsches Arzteblatt*, 63 (1933), 221–4

London, University of, *Conference on Medical Education of Women in London*, London, University of London, 1917

_____, *Report of the Special Committee of the University of London to Consider the Medical Education of Women in London*, London, University of London, 1944

Long, A.P., 'Immunizations in the United States Army', *American Journal of Public Health*, 34 (1944), 27–33

Low, A.M., *Benefits of War*, London, Scientific Book Club, 1945

Low, Vincent Warren, 'Some Modern Bullet Wounds', *St Mary's Hospital Gazette*, 8/4 (April 1902), 52–7

MacDougall, Ian (ed.), *Mid and East Lothian Miners' Association Minutes, 1894–1918*, Edinburgh, Scottish History Society, 2003

Macintosh, R.R. and Pratt, F.B., 'Anaesthesia in Wartime', *British Medical Journal*, 2 (1939), 1077–9

McLaren, Barbara, *Women of the War*, London, Hodder and Stoughton, 1920

McLaren, Eva Shaw, *A History of the Scottish Women's Hospitals*, London, Hodder and Stoughton, 1919

Mann, Ida, *Ida and the Eye: A Woman in British Ophthalmology, Tunbridge Wells*, Parapress, 1996

Manoel II, 'Scheme and Organization of Curative Workshops' in R. Jones (ed.), *Orthopaedic Surgery of Injuries* (1921), 629–44

Marsh, A.R., 'A Short but Distant War: the Falklands Campaign', *Journal of the Royal Society of Medicine*, 76 (1983), 972–82

Martin, Arthur Anderson, *A Surgeon in Khaki*, London, Edward Arnold, 1915

Martinez Alonso, E., *The Adventures of a Doctor*, London, Hale, 1962

Mass Observation, *War Begins at Home*, London, Chatto and Windus, 1940

Maurice, Dick, *From Cradle to War: My First Three Decades, 1915–1945*, Edinburgh, Pentland Press, 1998

Maurice, John Frederick, 'Where to Get Men', *Contemporary Review*, 81 (1902), 78–86

_____, 'National Health: A Soldiers' Study', *Contemporary Review*, 83 (1903), 41–56

Maurice Williams, H.C., 'Four Thousand Basque Children', *The Lancet*, 1 (1937), 383

Maynard Smith, S., 'With the Armies in France', *St Mary's Hospital Gazette*, 24/3 (March 1919), 28–33

Miles, R.P.M., 'OHMS', *St Mary's Hospital Gazette*, 49/8 (1943), 142–4

Miller, Lee, *Lee Miller's War: Photographer and Correspondent with the Allies in Europe 1944–45*, London, Thames and Hudson, 2005

Miller, Russell (ed.), *Nothing Less than Victory: The Oral History of D-Day*, London, Michael Joseph, 1993

Mira i López, Emili, 'Psychiatric Experience in the Spanish War, *British Medical Journal*, 1 (1939), 1217–20

_____, *Psychiatry in War*, New York, Norton, 1943

Mirin, S., and McKenna, G., 'Combat Zone Adjustment: Role of Marijuana Use', *Military Medicine*, 140 (1975), 482–6

Mitchell, P., *Memoranda on Army General Hospital Administration*, London, Bailière, Tindall and Cox, 1917

Moncrief, J.A., 'The Use of a Topical Sulphonamide in the Control of Burn Wound Sepsis', *Journal of Trauma*, 6 (1966), 407–19

Muir, Ward, *Observations of an Orderly at an English War Hospital 1915–1917*, Liskeard, Diggory Press, 2006

Murray, Flora, *Women as Army Surgeons*, London, Hodder and Stoughton, 1920

Myers, C. S., 'A Contribution to the Study of Shell-shock', *The Lancet*, 1 (1915), 316–20

———, *Shell-shock in France 1914–1918*, Cambridge, Cambridge University Press, 1940

Neel, S.H., 'Medical Considerations in Helicopter Evacuation', *United States Armed Forces Medical Journal*, 1 (1954), 224–5

Nevinson, Henry W., *Ladysmith: the Diary of a Siege,* London, Methuen, 1900

Noble-Smith, E., *Growing Children: Their Clothes and Deformity,* London, Smith and Elder, 1899

Nyiszli, Miklos, *Auschwitz: A Doctor's Eyewitness Account*, London, Mayflower Books, 1973

Orwell, George, *Homage to Catalonia*, London, Penguin, 2000

Osler, William, *The Principles and Practice of Medicine*, 8th edition, New York and London, D. Appleton, 1914

———, 'The War and Typhoid Fever', *British Medical Journal*, 2 (1914), 909–13

———, 'Science and War', *The Lancet*, 2 (1915), 795–801

Ostry, Joan, 'St George's Hospital 1940', *George's Magazine*, 7 (2004), 16–17

Parkes, Walter, 'Miss Mary G. Milne', *St Mary's Hospital Gazette*, 50 (1949), 118–20

Pearson, Karl, *The Groundwork of Eugenics*, London, Eugenics Laboratory, 1912

Perry, Colin, *Boy in the Blitz: the 1940 Diary of Colin Perry,* Stroud, Sutton Publishing, 2000

Political Warfare Executive, *Instructions for British Servicemen in France, 1944,* Oxford, Bodleian Library, 2005

———, *Germany 1944: The British Soldier's Pocketbook,* Kew, National Archives, 2006

Porritt, A.E. and Mitchell, G.A.G., 'Wounds and Gas Gangrene' in A. Fleming (ed.), *Penicillin: Its Practical Application* (1946), pp.162–179

Portillo, Luis, 'Unamuno's Last Lecture' in C. Connolly (ed.), *The Golden Horizon* (1953), pp. 397–409

Ratner, Richard A., 'Drugs and Despair in Vietnam', *University of Chicago Magazine*, 64 (1972), 15–23

Rees, J.R., 'Three Years of Military Psychiatry in the United Kingdom', *British Medical Journal*, 1 (1943), 1–6

Remarque, Eric Maria, *All Quiet on the Western Front*, London, Guild Publishing, 1980

Riddle James R., Brown, Mark, Smith, Tyler, Ritchie Elspeth Cameron, Brix, Kelly Ann and Romano, James, 'Chemical Warfare and the Gulf War: A Review of the Impact on Gulf Veterans' Health', *Military Medicine*, 168/8 (2003), 606–13

Rivers, W.H.R., 'An Address on the Repression of War Experience', *The Lancet*, 1 (1918), 173–7

Rowntree, B. Seebohm, *Poverty: A Study of Town Life*, London, Macmillan, 1901

St Clair Stobart, Mabel, *The Flaming Sword in Serbia and Elsewhere*, London, Hodder and Stoughton, 1917

Salaman, M.H., King, A.J., Williams, D.I. and Nichol, C.S., 'Prevention of Jaundice Resulting from Antisyphilitic Treatment', *The Lancet*, 1 (1944), 7–10

Salmon, Thomas, 'The Care and Treatment of Mental Diseases and War Neuroses ("Shell-shock") in the British Army', *Mental Hygiene*, 1 (1917), 509–547

Sassoon, Siegfried, *Sherston's Progress*, London, Faber and Faber, 1988

Sanders, Alfred W., 'Civilian Surgery in South Africa', *St Mary's Hospital Gazette* 6/3 (March 1900), 44–5

Sargant, William, *The Unquiet Mind: The Autobiography of a Physician in Psychological Medicine*, London, Heinemann, 1967

Saxton, Reginald S., 'The Madrid Blood Transfusion Institute' *The Lancet*, 2 (1937), 606–7

Scott-Ellis, Priscilla, *The Chances of Death: a Diary of the Spanish Civil War*, Norwich, Michael Russell, 1995

Sellier, Henri, *La Lutte Contre la Tuberculose dans la Région Parisienne*, Paris, Presses Universitaires de France, 1928

Sewell, Patricia W., *Healers in World War II: Oral Histories of Medical Corps Personnel*, Jefferson, North Carolina, McFarland, 2001

Sherriff, R.C. *Journey's End*, London, Samuel French, 1929

Shirlaw, G.B. and Troke, C., *Medicine versus Invasion: The Home Guard Medical Service in Action*, London, Secker and Warburg, 1941

Simpson, R.J.S., *Medical History of the War in South Africa: an Epidemiological Essay*, London, HMSO, 1911

Sinclair-Loutit, Kenneth, 'An Ambulance in Spain', *The Lancet*, 2 (1939), 1295–6

SKIA, 'A Hospital in France', *Blackwood's Magazine*, 204 (1918), 613–40

Smith, Dean A., 'Barbed Wire and Beri-beri', *St Mary's Hospital Gazette*, 52/3 (April 1946), 32–4

Sorley, Charles Hamilton, *Collected Letters of Charles Hamilton Sorley*, ed. by Jean Moorcroft Wilson, London, Cecil Woolf, 1990

Souka, H.M., 'Management of Gulf War Casualties', *British Journal of Surgery*, 79 (1992), 1307–8

Souttar, Henry Sessions, *A Surgeon in Belgium*, London, Edward Arnold, 1915

Speake, Hilda, 'From a St Mary's Nurse in Brussels', *St Mary's Hospital Gazette*, 21/5 (May 1915), 76–7

Spencer, F.C. and Grewe, R.V., 'The Management of Arterial Injuries in Battle Casualties', *Annals of Surgery*, 141 (1953), 304–12

Steevens, George W., *From Cape Town to Ladysmith*, London, Blackwood, 1900

Stephen, Martin (ed.), *Never Such Innocence: a New Anthology of Great War Verse*, London, J.M. Dent, 1991

Treves, Frederick, *The Tale of a Field Hospital*, London, Cassell, 1900

Trueta, Josep, 'Closed Treatment of War Fractures', *The Lancet*, 1 (1939), 1452–5

———, *The Treatment of War Wounds and Fractures*, London, Heinemann Medical Books, 1939

_____, *The Principles and Practice of War Surgery*, London, Heinemann Medical Books, 1943

_____, *Surgeon in War and Peace*, London, Gollancz, 1980

United Nations Relief and Rehabilitation Administration, *Report of the Director General to the Council for the Period 1 January 1946 to 31 March 1946*, Washington DC, United Nations Relief and Rehabilitation Administration, 1946

Unwin, C., Blatchley, N., Coker, W., Ferry, S., Hotopf, M., Hull, L., Ismail, K., Palmer, I., David, A. and Wessely, S., 'Health of UK Servicemen who Served in the Persian Gulf War', *The Lancet*, 1 (1999), 169–78

Vaughan, V.C. and Palmer, G.T., 'Communicable Disease in the United States Army During the Summer and Autumn of 1918', *Journal of Laboratory Clinical Medicine*, 3 (1918), 587–623, 647–86

Verdon, Thomas A. and Thomas, Evan T., 'Current problems with Neisseria Gonorrhoea in Vietnam', *United States Army in Vietnam Medical Bulletin*, 40/22 (1970), 9–10

Vitoux, Georges, 'L'Oeuvre des Comités Départementaux d'Assistance aux Soldats Réformés', *Revue d'Hygiène* 1 (1918), 561–70

Vonkennel, J., Kimmig, J. and Lembke, A., 'Die Mycoine, eine Neue Gruppe Therapeutisch Wirksamer Substanzen aus Pilzen', *Klinische Wochenschrift*, 22 (1943), 321

Wagner-Jauregg, T., 'Die Neueren Biochemischen Erkentnisse und Probleme der Chemotherapie', *Die Naturwissenschaften*, 31 (1943), 335–44

Walker, George, *Venereal Disease in the American Expeditionary Forces*, Baltimore, Medical Standard Books, 1922

Wallenberg, Raoul, *Letters and Dispatches, 1924–1945*, New York, Arcade, 1995

War Department, Washington DC, *Instructions for American Servicemen in Britain, 1942*, Oxford, Bodleian Library, 1994

Watts, J.C., *Surgeon at War*, London, George Allen and Unwin, 1955

Westman, Stephen, *Surgeon with the Kaiser's Army*, London, William Kimber, 1968

Whitby, Lionel, 'Blood Transfusion in the Field: Organisation of Supplies' in H. Letherby Tidy (ed.), *Inter-Allied Conferences on War Medicine 1942–1945* (1947), pp. 123–6

White, W.I., *Back Down the Ridge*, New York, Harcourt Brace, 1953

Wilberforce, Octavia, *Octavia Wilberforce: the Autobiography of a Pioneer Woman Doctor*, London, Cassell, 1989

Willcox, W.H., 'Mesopotamia 1916–1919', *St Mary's Hospital Gazette*, 25/5 (May 1919), 67–71

_____, 'Mesopotamia 1916–1919', *St Mary's Hospital Gazette*, 25/7 (July 1919), 98–106

Wilson, Charles McMoran (Lord Moran), *Anatomy of Courage*, London, Collins, 1945

_____, *Winston Churchill: The Struggle for Survival, 1940–1965*, London, Constable, 1966

Wilson, H., 'Mental Reactions to Air-Raids', *The Lancet*, 1 (1942), 284–7

Witkop Philipp, (ed.), *German Students' War Letters*, Philadelphia, Pine Street Books, 2002

Women's Group on Social Welfare, *Our Towns: A Close Up*, Oxford, Oxford University Press, 1943

Woolf, Virginia, *Diaries of Virginia Woolf, 1936–1941*, vol. 5, London, Chatto and Windus, 1984

Wright, Almroth E., 'On the Results Which Have Been Obtained by Anti-Typhoid Inoculation, *The Lancet*, 2 (1902), 652–71

_____, *Pathology and Treatment of War Wounds*, London, Heinemann, 1942

_____, and Semple D., 'On Vaccination against Typhoid Fever', *British Medical Journal*, 1 (1897), 256–9

_____, and Smith, F., 'On the Application of the Serum Test to the Differential Diagnosis of Typhoid and Malta Fever', *The Lancet*, 1 (1897), 656–9.

_____, and Leishman, W.B., 'Results Which Have Been Obtained by Anti-Typhoid Inoculations', *British Medical Journal*, 1 (1900), 122–9

_____, and Fleming, Alexander, 'Further Observations on Acidaemia in Gas Gangrene and the Conditions which Favour the Growth of its Infective Agent in the Blood Serum', *The Lancet*, 1 (1918), 205–10; 'The Aerobic Infections of War Wounds', *Medical Research Council Special Report Series*, no. 39 (1919), 70–8

_____, _____, and Colebrook, Leonard, 'The Conditions under which the Sterilisation of Wounds by Physiological Agency can be Obtained', *The Lancet*, 1 (1918), 831–7

Yealland, L.R., *Hysterical Disorders of Warfare*, London, Macmillan, 1918

Secondary Published Sources

Abel Smith, Brian, *The Hospitals, 1800–1948*, London, Heinemann, 1964

Allbutt, Thomas Clifford, *Greek Medicine in Rome With Other Historical Essays*, London, Macmillan, 1921

Anderson, Stuart (ed.), *Making Medicines: A Brief History of Pharmacy and Pharmaceuticals*, London, Pharmaceutical Press, 2005

Bachrach, Susan D., (ed.), *Deadly Medicine: Creating the Master Race*, Washington DC, United States National Holocaust Museum, 2004

Bamji, Andrew, 'Facial Surgery: the Patient's Experience' in H. Cecil and P.H. Liddle (ed.), *Facing Armageddon* (1996), pp. 490–501

Baños, Josep E. and Guardiolo, Elena, 'Eponímia mèdica catalana: El mètode de Duran', *Annals de Medicina*, 89 (2006), 41–5

Barham, Peter, *Forgotten Lunatics of the Great War*, New Haven, Yale University Press, 2004

Beckett, Ian F.W., *Home Front 1914–1918: How Britain Survived the Great War*, London, The National Archives, 2006

Beevor, Antony, *The Battle for Spain: The Spanish Civil War 1936–1939*, London, Phoenix, 2006

Bel-El, Ilana R., *Conscripts: Forgotten Men of the Great War*, Stroud, Sutton Publishing, 2003

Bennett, J.D.C., 'Medical Advances Consequent to the Great War, 1914–1918', *Journal of the Royal Society of Medicine*, 83 (1990), 738–42

Bennett, J.P., 'A History of the Queen Victoria Hospital, East Grinstead', *British Journal of Plastic Surgery*, 41 (1988), 422–40

Bescós Torres, J., 'Las enfermeras en la guerra de España 1936–1939', *Revista de la Historia Militar*, 26 (1982), 97–143

_____, 'La sanidad military en la Guerra d'España 1936–1939', *Medicina Militar*, 43 (1987), 88–99, 434–47

Bierman, John, *Righteous Gentile: the Story of Raoul Wallenberg, Missing Hero of the Holocaust*, London, Penguin, 1982

Bishop, P.J., Lucas, B.D.B. and Lucas, B.G.B., *The Seven Ages of the Brompton: A Saga of a Hospital*, Guildford, Seven Corners Press, 1991

Bizarro, A.H., *El-Rei Dom Manoel II na Grande Guerra: Factos e Testemunhos*, Grimanes, Fundação da Casa de Bragança, 1952

Bliss, Michael, *Harvey Cushing: A Life in Surgery*, Oxford, Oxford University Press, 2005

Bock, Gisela, *Zwangsterilisation im Nationalsozialismus: Studien zur Rassenpolitik und Frauenpolitik,* Opladen, Westdeutscher Verlag, 1986

_____, 'Nazi Sterilization and Reproductive Policies' in S.D. Bachrach (ed.), *Deadly Medicine* (2004), pp. 61–87

Bosanquet, Nick, 'Health Systems in Khaki: the British and American Medical Experience' in H. Cecil and P.H. Liddle (ed.)., *Facing Armageddon* (1996), pp. 451–65

Bosch i Monegal, Enric, *L'Hospital del Mar en la historia de Barcelona*, Barcelona, Ajuntament de Barcelona I.M.A.S., 1992

Bosworth, R.J.B., *Mussolini's Italy: Life under the Dictatorship 1915–1945*, London, Allen Lane, 2005

Bourdillon, Hilary, *Women as Healers: a History of Women and Medicine*, Cambridge, Cambridge University Press, 1988

Bourke, Joanna, *Dismembering the Male: Men's Bodies, Britain and the Great War*, London Reaktion Books, 1999

Brandt, Allen M., *No Magic Bullet: A Social History of Venereal Disease in the United States since 1880*, Oxford, Oxford University Press, 1987

Bracher, Karl Dietrich, *The German Dictatorship: The Origins, Structure and Consequences of National Socialism,* Harmondsworth, Penguin, 1973

Broberg, Gunnar and Rolls-Hansen, Nils, *Eugenics and the Welfare State: Sterilization Policy in Denmark, Sweden, Norway and Finland*, East Lansing, Michigan State University Press, 1996

Brown, Ivan W., 'The Amazing Adventures of Wilburt C. Davison, Wilder G. Penfield, and Emile F. Holman While Rhodes Scholars in Medicine at Oxford During World War I, 1913–1917', *Annals of Surgery*, 211/2 (1990), 224–34

Brown, Kevin, 'History of the Newcastle upon Tyne Church High School 1885–1985' in H.G. Scott and E.A. Wise (ed.)., *Centenary Book of the Newcastle upon Tyne Church High School 1885–1985* (1985), pp. 5–33

_____, 'The Lodges of the Durham Miners' Association, 1869–1926, *Northern History*, 23 (1987), 138–52

_____, ' "Contact with the Seamy Side of Life": a Nurse's Story', *St Mary's Gazette*, 96/3 (October 1990), 38–9

_____, 'Another Day, Another War', *St Mary's Gazette*, 97/2 (April 1991), 35–7

_____, 'The Inoculation Department at Boulogne', *St Mary's Gazette*, 103/1 (January 1997), 32–5

_____, *Penicillin Man: Alexander Fleming and the Antibiotic Revolution,* Stroud, Sutton Publishing, 2004

_____, 'The History of Penicillin from Discovery to the Drive to Production', *Pharmaceutical Historian*, 34/3 (2004), 37–43

_____, *The Pox: the Life and Near Death of a Very Social Disease*, Stroud, Sutton Publishing, 2006

_____, 'Tested Under Pressure: St Mary's During the Great War', *St Mary's Hospital Past and Present Nurses' League Journal*, 43 (2006), 14–20

_____, 'A Night with Venus, A Lifetime with Mercury: the Treatment of Syphilis', *Pharmaceutical Historian*, 37/3 (2007), 34–8

Brown, Malcolm, *The Imperial War Museum Book of the First World War: A Great Conflict Recalled in Previously Unpublished Letters, Diaries and Memoirs*, London, Sidgwick and Jackson, 1991

Brown, Vernon K., *The Story of Passavant Memorial Hospital 1865–1972*, Chicago, Northwestern Memorial Hospital, 1976

_____, *Cathedral of Healing: The Story of Wesley Memorial Hospital 1888–1972*, Chicago, Northwestern Memorial Hospital, 1981

Bryder, Linda, 'The First World War: Healthy or Hungry?', *History Workshop*, 24 (1987), 141–55

Buchanan, Tom, *The Impact of the Spanish Civil War on Britain: War, Loss and Memory*, Brighton, Sussex Academic Press, 2007

Bud, Robert, *Penicillin: Triumph and Tragedy*, Oxford, Oxford University Press, 2007

_____, and Gummett, Philip (ed.), *Cold War, Hot Science: Applied Research in Britain's Defence Laboratories*, London, Science Museum, 1999

Burleigh, Michael, *Death and Deliverance: Euthanasia in Germany, 1900–1945*, Cambridge, Cambridge University Press, 1994

_____, *The Third Reich: a New History*, London, Pan, 2001

_____, 'Nazi Euthanasia Programs', in in S.D. Bachrach (ed.), *Deadly Medicine* (2004), pp. 127–153

_____, and Wippermann, Wolfgang, *The Racial State: Germany 1933–1945*, Cambridge, Cambridge University Press, 1991

Burns, Marlene, and van Dijk, Piet W.M., 'The Development of the Penicillin Production Process in Delft, the Netherlands, during World War II, under Nazi Occupation', *Advances in Applied Microbiology*, 51 (2002), 185–99

_____, Bennett , J.W. and van Dijk, Piet W.M., 'Code Name Bacinol', *American Society of Microbiology News*, 69/1 (2003), 25–31

Bynum, W.F. and Porter, Roy, (ed.), *Companion Encyclopaedia of the History of Medicine*, London, Routledge, 1993

Callister, Sandy, '"Broken Gargoyles": the Photographic Representation of Severely Wounded New Zealand Soldiers', *Social History of Medicine*, 20/1 (2007), 111–30

Carruthers, Bob, *Servants of Evil: New First-Hand Accounts of the Second World War from Survivors of Hitler's Armed Forces*, London, André Deutsch, 2001

Carter, Gradon and Balmer, Brian, 'Chemical and Biological Warfare and Defence' in R. Bud and P. Gummett (ed.), *Cold War, Hot Science* (1999), pp. 295–338

Cassidy, Tina, *Birth: A History*, London, Chatto and Windus, 2007

Cecil, Hugh. and Liddle, Peter H. (ed.), *Facing Armageddon: the First World War Experienced*, Barnsley, Leo Cooper, 1996

Cirillo, Vincent J., *Bullets and Bacilli: the Spanish-American War and Military Medicine*, New Brunswick, Rutgers University Press, 2004

_____, 'Winged Sponges: Houseflies as Carriers of Typhoid Fever in Nineteenth- and Early-Twentieth-Century Military Camps', *Perspectives in Biology and Medicine*, 49/1 (2006), 52–63

Clarke-Kennedy, A.E., *London Pride: the Story of a Voluntary Hospital*, London, Hutchinson Benham, 1979

Coghill, R.D., 'The Development of Penicillin Strains 'in A. Elder (ed.), *The History of Penicillin Production*, American Institute of Engineers, Chemical Engineering Progress Symposium, 66/100 (1970), 14–15

Cohen, Deborah, 'Will to Work: Disabled Veterans in Britain and Germany after the First World War' in D.A. Gerber (ed.), *Disabled Veterans in History* (2000), pp. 295–321

Cole, Howard N., *On Wings of Healing: The Story of the Airborne Medical Services 1940–1960*, Edinburgh, William Blackwood, 1963

Colebrook, Leonard, *Almroth Wright, Provocative Doctor and Thinker*, London, Heinemann, 1954

_____, 'Obituary of Almroth Edward Wright', *The Lancet*, 1(1947), 654

_____, 'Gerhard Domagk, 1895–1964', *Biographical Memoirs of Fellows of the Royal Society* , London, Royal Society, 1964, vol. 10, p.39

Coni, Nicholas, *Medicine and the Spanish Civil War, Journal of the Royal Society of Medicine*, 95/3 (2002), 147–50

_____, *Medicine and Warfare: Spain 1936–1939*, London, Routledge, 2007

Cooter, Roger, *Surgery and Society in Peace and War: Orthopaedics and the Organization of Modern Medicine, 1880–1948*, London, Macmillan, 1993

———, 'War and Modern Medicine' in W.F. Bynum and R. Porter (ed.), *Companion Encyclopaedia of the History of Medicine* (1993), pp. 1536–73

———, Harrison, Mark and Sturdy, Steve (ed.), *War, Medicine and Modernity*, Stroud, Sutton, 1998

———, ———, ———, *Medicine and Modern Warfare*, Amsterdam and Atlanta, Rodopi, 1999

Cope, V. Zachary, *Almroth Wright, Founder of Modern Vaccine Therapy*, London, Nelson, 1966

Cowdrey, A.E., *Fighting for Life: American Military Medicine in World War II*, New York, Free Press, 1994

Crewe, F.A.E., *The Army Medical Services: Administration*, 2 volumes, London, HMSO, 1953

Davies, Norman, *God's Playground: A History of Poland*, 2 volumes, Oxford, Oxford University Press, 1981

———, *Rising '44: The Battle for Warsaw*, London, Macmillan, 2003

———, *Europe at War 1939–1945: No Simple Victory*, London, Macmillan, 2006

Dorland, P. and Nanney, J., *Dust Off: Aeromedical Evacuation in Vietnam*, Washington DC, Center of Military History, 1982

Driscoll, Robert S., 'US Army Medical Helicopters in the Korean War', *Military Medicine*, 166/4 (2001), 290–6

Dunn, C.L., *The Emergency Medical Services*, London, HMSO, 1952

Dunnill, Michael, *The Plato of Praed Street: the Life and Times of Almroth Wright*, London, Royal Society of Medicine, 2000

Durbach, Nadia, *The Anti-Vaccination Movement in England, 1853–1907*, Durham, North Carolina, Duke University Press, 2005

Dwork, Deborah, *War is Good for Babies and Other Young Children: A History of the Infant and Child Welfare Movement in England 1898–1918*, London, Tavistock, 1987

Dyer, Geoff, *The Missing of the Somme*, London, Hamish Hamilton, 1994

Dyhouse, Carol, 'Women Students and the London Medical Schools, 1914–39: the Anatomy of a Masculine Culture', *Gender and History* 10/1 (1998), 110–132

Elder, Albert, 'The Role of the Government in the Wartime Penicillin Program', in *The History of Penicillin Production*, American Institute of Engineers, Chemical Engineering Progress Symposium, 66/100 (1970) 3–11

———, (ed.), *The History of Penicillin Production*, New York, American Institute of Engineers, Chemical Engineering Progress Symposium, 66/100 (1970)

Ellis, John, *LHMC 1785–1985: the Story of the London Hospital Medical College, England's First Medical School*, London, London Hospital Medical Club, 1986

Faulks, Sebastian, *The Fatal Englishman: Three Short Lives*, London, Hutchinson, 1996

Franco, A., Cortes, J. and Alvarez, J., 'The Development of Blood Transfusion: The Contribution of Norman Bethune in the Spanish Civil War', *Canadian Journal of Anaesthesia*, 10 (1996), 1076–8

Frank, Richard B., *Guadalcanal: the Definitive Account of the Landmark Battle*, New York, Random House, 1990

Friedlander, Henry, *Origins of Nazi Genocide: From Euthanasia to the Final Solution*, Chapel Hill, University of North Carolina Press, 1995

_____, 'From Euthanasia to the Final Solution' in S.D. Bachrach (ed.), *Deadly Medicine* (2004), pp. 155–183

Fulbrook, Mary, *Germany 1918–1990: A Divided Society*, London, Fontana, 1991

Gardiner, Juliet, *Wartime Britain, 1939–1945*, London, Review, 2005

Gardner, Helen (ed.), *New Oxford Book of English Verse*, Oxford, Oxford University Press, 1972

Garner, James Stuart, 'The Great Experiment: the Admission of Women Students to St Mary's Hospital Medical School, 1916–1925', *Medical History*, 42 (1998), 68–88

Garrison, Fielding, *Introduction to the History of Medicine*, Philadelphia, W.B. Saunders, 1929

Gaudillière, Jean-Paul, *Inventer la biomedicine: la France, l'Amérique et la production des savoirs de vivant*, Paris, La Découvert, 2002

Gerber, David A. (ed.), *Disabled Veterans in History*, Ann Arbor, University of Michigan Press, 2000

Gibson, T.M. and Marshall, M.H., *Into Thin Air: A History of Aviation Medicine in the RAF*, London, Robert Hale, 1984

Gilbert, Martin, *The Righteous: the Unsung Heroes of the Holocaust*, London, Doubleday, 2002

Girourad, Mark, *The Return to Camelot: Chivalry and the English Gentleman*, New Haven, Yale University Press, 1981

Graves, Charles, *The Story of St Thomas's, 1106–1947*, London, Faber and Faber, 1947

Greenwood, John T. and Berry, F. Clifton, *Medics at War: Military Medicine from Colonial Times to the 21st Century*, Annapolis, Naval Institute Press, 2005

Gregg, John, *The Shelter of the Tubes: Tube Sheltering in Wartime London, Harrow*, Capital Transport Publishing, 2001

Grífols i Espés, Joan, *Frederic Duran i Jordà: Un métido, una época*, Barcelona, Hemo-Institut Grífols, 1997

Grundmann, Ekkehard, *Gerhard Domagk: The First Man to Triumph over Infectious Diseases*, Münster, Lit, 2004

Haller, John S. 'Trench Foot: A Study in Military Medical Responsiveness in the Great War', *Western Journal of Medicine*, 152 (June 1990), 729–33

Halioua, Bruno, *Blouses Blanches, Étoiles Jaunes*, Paris, Liana Levi, 2000

Hanauske-Abel, Hartmut M., 'Not a Slippery Slope or Sudden Subversion: German Medicine and National Socialism in 1933', *British Medical Journal*, 313 (1996), 1453–63

Hare, Ronald, *Birth of Penicillin and the Disarming of Microbes*, London, Allen and Unwin, 1970

Harris, Bernard, *The Health of the School Child: A History of the School Medical Service in England and Wales,* Buckingham, Open University Press, 1995

_____, 'The Demographic Impact of the First World War: An Anthropometric Perspective', *Journal of the Society for the Social History of Medicine*, 6 (1993), 343–66

Harris, José, *William Beveridge: A Biography*, Oxford, Clarendon Press, 1977

Harrison, Mark, 'Sex and the Citizen Soldier: Health, Morals and Discipline in the British Army during the Second World War' in R. Cooter, M. Harrison and S. Sturdy (eds.), *Medicine and Modern Warfare* (1999), pp. 225–50

_____, *Medicine and Victory: British Military Medicine in the Second World War*, Oxford, Oxford University Press, 2004

Hasian, Marouf, 'The Hysterical Emily Hobhouse and Boer War Concentration Camp Controversy', *Western Journal of Communication*, 67/2 (2003), 138–63

Hay, Ian, *One Hundred Years of Army Nursing*, London, Cassell, 1953

Heran, J., 'Les Sinistres Expériences Médicales du Struthof', *Saisons d'Alsace*, 121 (1993), 64–73

Herrick, Claire, 'The Conquest of the Silent Foe: British and American Military Medical Reform Rhetoric and the Russo Japanese War' in R. Cooter, M. Harrison and S. Sturdy (ed.) *Medicine and Modern Warfare* (1999), pp. 99–129

Hilberg, Raul, *Destruction of the European Jews*, New Haven, Yale University Press, 2003

Hickman, Tom, *The Call-up: A History of National Service*, London, Headline, 2005

Hirst, J.D., 'The Growth of Treatment Through the School Medical Service, 1908–18', *Medical History*, 33 (1989), 318–42

Hoare, Philip, *Spike Island: the Memory of a Military Hospital*, London, Fourth Estate, 2001

Holmes, Richard, *Dusty Warriors: Modern Soldiers at War*, London, Harper Perennial, 2007

Horn, Pamela, *The Victorian and Edwardian Schoolchild*, Stroud, Sutton, 1989

Howie, J., 'Gonorrhoea: A Question of Tactics', *British Medical Journal*, 2 (1979), 1631

Jeffreys, Diarmuid, *Aspirin: The Story of a Wonder Drug*, London, Bloomsbury Publishing, 2004

Jones, Edgar and Wessely, Simon, *Shell-shock to PTSD: Military Psychiatry from 1900 to the Gulf War*, Hove, Psychology Press, 2005

Kater, Michael, 'Hitler's Early Doctors: Nazi Physicians in Pre-Depression Germany', *Journal of Modern History*, 59 (1987), 25–52

_____, *Doctors under Hitler*, Chapel Hill, North Carolina, University of North Carolina Press, 1989

Kaylor, J., King, D. and King, L., 'Psychological Effects of Military Service in Vietnam: A Meta Analysis', *Psychological Bulletin*, 102 (1987), 257–71

Kennedy, David M., *Over Here: The First World War and American Society*, Oxford, Oxford University Press, 1982

_____, *Freedom from Fear: the American People in Depression and War, 1929–45*, Oxford, Oxford University Press, 1999

Kennett, Lee, *GI: the American Soldier in World War II*, New York, Charles Scribner, 1987

Kevles, Daniel J., 'Testing the Nation's Intelligence: Psychologists in World War I', *Journal of American History*, 55 (1968), 565–81

King, Booker and Jatoi, Ismail, 'The Mobile Army Surgical Hospital: A Military and Surgical Legacy', *Journal of the National Medical Association*, 97/5 (2005), 648–56

Kiple, Kenneth F. (ed.), *Cambridge Historical Dictionary of Disease*, Cambridge, Cambridge University Press, 2003

Klee, Ernst, *Euthanasie im NS-Staat: Die Vernichtung lebenswunwerten Lebens*, Frankfurt-am-Main, Fischer-Taschenbuch, 2004

Kleinkauf, H. and van Dohren, H. (ed.), *Fifty Years of Penicillin Application: History and Trends*, Prague, PUBLIC Ltd., 1980

Kogon, Eugen, Langbein, Hermann and.Ruckerl, Adalbert, *Nazi Mass Murder: A Documentary History of the Use of Poison Gas*, New Haven, Yale University Press, 1993

Koven, Seth, 'Remembering and Dismemberment: Crippled Wounded Soldiers and the Great War in Great Britain', *American Historical Review*, 99/4 (1994), 1167–1202

Laffin, John, *Combat Surgeons*, Stroud, Sutton Publishing, 1999

Le Minor, Jean Marie, 'Des Dérives de la Craniologie aux Crimes Contre l'Humanité: August Hirt (1898–1945) à Strasbourg de 1941 à 1945', in B. Schnitzler (ed.), *Histoire(s) de Squelettes* (2006), pp. 291–3

Leneman, Leah, 'Medical Women at War, 1914–1918', *Medical History*, 38 (1994), 160–77

_____, *In the Service of Life: the Story of Elsie Inglis and the Scottish Women's Hospitals*, London, Mercat Press, 1994

Leval, Gaston, *L'Espagne libertaire, 1936–1939: L'oeuvre constructive de la révolution espagnole*, Paris, Editions de Cercle, 1971

Lozano, Miguel, and Cid, Joan, 'Frederic Duran-Jorda: A Transfusion Medicine Pioneer', *Transfusion Medicine Reviews*, 21/1 (2007), 75–81

Lewis, John, *The Politics of Motherhood: Child and Maternal Welfare in England 1900–1939*, London, Croom Helm, 1980

Lindsay, Oliver and Harris, John R., *The Battle for Hong Kong 1941–1945: Hostage to Fortune*, Staplehurst, Spellmount, 2005

Longman, Jere, *Among the Heroes: The Story of United Flight 93 and the Passengers and Crew who Fought Back*, London, Simon and Schuster, 2002

Lloyd, Mark, *The London Scottish in the Great War*, Barnsley, Leo Cooper, 2001

Longden, Sean, *To the Victor the Spoils: D-Day to VE Day, the Reality Behind the Heroism*, Moreton in Marsh, Arris Books, 2004

Loudon, Irvine 'On Maternal and Infant Mortality 1900–1960', *Social History of Medicine*, 4 (1991), 29–73

Low-Beer, Daniel, Smallman-Raynor, Matthew and Cliff, Andrew, 'Disease and Death in the South African War: Changing Disease Patterns from Soldiers to Refugees', *Social History of Medicine*, 17/2 (2004), 223–45

MacArthur, Brian, *Surviving the Sword: Prisoners of the Japanese, 1942–45*, London, Abacus, 2006

McLaughlin, Redmond, *The Royal Army Medical Corps*, London, Leo Cooper, 1972

Macnichol, John, 'The Effects of the Evacuation of Schoolchildren on Official Attitudes to State Evacuation' in H.L. Smith (ed.), *War and Social Change in British Society in the Second World War* (1996), pp. 3–31

Macpherson, W.G., Herringham, W.P., Elliot, T.R. and Balfour A. (ed.), *History of the Great War: Medical Services*, London, HMSO, 1922

Martinez, Lluis, 'Perque la sang és vida', *Avui* (22 May 2005), 28–33

Marwick, Arthur, *The Deluge: British Society and the First World War*, London, Macmillan, 1973

Mayhew, E.R., *The Reconstruction of Warriors: Archibald McIndoe, the Royal Air Force and the Guinea Pig Club*, London, Greenhill Books, 2004

Mayou, Roger (ed.)., *International Red Cross and Red Crescent Museum*, Geneva, International Red Cross, 2000

Mellor, W. Franklin (ed.), *Casualties and Medical Statistics: History of the Second World War: United Kingdom Medical Services*, London, HMSO, 1972

Merridale, Catherine, *Ivan's War: The Red Army 1939–45*, London, Faber and Faber, 2005

Mines, Samuel, *Pfizer: an Informal History*, New York, Pfizer, 1978

Moorehead, C., *Martha Gellhorn: A Life*, London, Chatto and Windus, 2003

Mortimer, Philip P., 'Arsphenamine Jaundice and the Recognition of Instrument-Borne Virus Infection', *Genitourinary Medicine*, 71 (1995), 109–119

Neushul, Peter, 'Science, Government and the Mass Production of Penicillin', *Journal of the History of Medicine and the Allied Sciences*, 48 (1993), 371–95

Noble, W.C., Coli: *Great Healer of Men, the Biography of Dr Leonard Colebrook*, London, William Heinemann, 1974

O'Brien, T.H., *History of the Second World War: Civil Defence*, London, HMSO, 1955

Oram, Gerard, *Worthless Men: Race, Eugenics and the Death Penalty in the British Army During the First World War*, London, Francis Boutle, 1998

Packenham, Thomas, *The Boer War*, London, Abacus, 1992

Pairault, François, *Images de Poilus: La Grande Guerre en Cartes Postales*, Paris, Tallandier, 2005

Parascandola, John (ed.), *The History of Antibiotics: A Symposium*, Madison, Illinois, American Institute of the History of Pharmacy, 1980

Patterson, James T., *Grand Expectations: The United States 1945–1975*, Oxford, Oxford University Press, 1996

_____, Restless Giant: *The United States from Watergate to Bush v. Gore,* Oxford, Oxford University Press, 2005

Patterson, K. David, 'Typhus and its Control in Russia, 1870–1940', *Medical History,* 37 (1993), 361–81

Paul, Christa, *Zwangs Prostitution: Staatlich Erricht Bordelle im Nationalsozialismus,* Berlin, Hentrich, 1994

Pieroth, I., 'Penicillin: A Survey from Discovery to Industrial Production', in H. Kleinkauf and H. van Dohren (ed.), *Fifty Years of Penicillin Application* (1980), pp. 33–6

Porritt, Arthur, *History of the Second World War: United Kingdom Medical Services,* Surgery, London, HMSO, 1953

Porter, Roy, *The Greatest Benefit to Mankind: A Medical History of Humanity from Antiquity to the Present,* London, Harper Collins, 1997

Pressel, David M., 'Nuremberg and Tuskegee: Lessons for Contemporary American Medicine, *Journal of the National Medical Association,* 95/12 (2003), 1216–25

Preston, Paul, *Doves of War: Four Women of Spain,* London, Harper Collins, 2002

Prochaska, Frank, *Royal Bounty: The Making of a Welfare Monarchy,* New Haven, Yale University Press, 1995

Proctor, Robert, *The Nazi War on Cancer,* Princeton, Princeton University Press, 1999

Powell, Allan, *The Metropolitan Asylums Board and its Work, 1867–1930,* London, Metropolitan Asylums Board, 1930

Rafferty, Anne Marie, Robinson, Jane and Elkan, Ruth (ed.), *Nursing History and the Politics of Welfare,* London, Routledge, 1997

Rees, Laurence, *Auschwitz: the Nazis and the Final Solution,* London, BBC Books, 2005

Reznick, Jeffrey S., 'Work Therapy and the Disabled British Soldier in the First World War: the Case of Shepherd's Bush Military Hospital, London' in D.A. Gerber (ed.), *Disabled Veterans in History* (2000), pp. 185–203

Richter, Donald, 'The Experience of the British Special Brigade in Gas Warfare' in H. Cecil and P.H. Liddle (ed.), *Facing Armageddon* (1996), pp. 353–64

Roemer, M.I., 'Internationalism in Medicine' in W.F. Bynum and R. Porter (ed.), *Companion Encyclopaedia of the History of Medicine* (1993), pp. 1408–26

Rollet, Catherine, 'The Other War: Setbacks in Public Health', in J. Winter and J.L. Robert (ed.), *Capital Cities at War* (1999), pp. 456–86

Rose, Kenneth, *King George V,* London, Phoenix Press, 2000

Rosen, Irving B., 'Dr Norman Bethune as a Surgeon', *Canadian Journal of Surgery,* 39 (1996), 72–7

Ryder, R., *Edith Cavell,* London, Hamish Hamilton, 1975

Sacharski, Susan M., *To Be a Nurse,* Chicago, Northwestern Memorial Hospital, 1990

St Dunstan's Association for Blind Ex-Servicemen and Women, *The Spirit of St Dunstan's*, London, St Dunstan's Association for Blind Ex-Servicemen and Women, 2006

Saint, Andrew, (ed.), *Politics and the People of London: the London County Council, 1889–1965*, London, Hambledon Press, 1989

Seidelman, William E., 'Nuremberg: Lamentation for the Forgotten Victims of Medical Science', *British Medical Journal*, 313 (1996), 1463–7

Schneider, William H., 'Blood Transfusion in Peace and War, 1900–1918', *Social History of Medicine*, 10/1 (1997), 105–26

———, 'Blood Transfusion Between the Wars', *Journal of the History of Medicine and the Allied Sciences*, 58 (2003), 187–224

Schnitzler, Bernadette (ed.), *Histoire(s) de Squelettes: Archéologie, Médecine et Anthropologie en Alsace,* Strasbourg, Musées de Strasbourg, 2006

Schwartz, Michael, 'Euthanasie: Debatten in Deutschland 1895–1945', *Vierteljahreshefte fur Zeitgeschichte, 46* (1998), 629

Scott, Helen G. and Wise, Elizabeth A. (ed.)., *Centenary Book of the Newcastle upon Tyne Church High School 1885–1985*, Newcastle, Newcastle upon Tyne Church High School, 1985

Searle, G.R., *Quest for National Efficiency*, Oxford, Oxford University Press, 1971

———, *A New England? Peace and War 1886–1918*, Oxford, Oxford University Press, 2004

Shama, Gilbert and Reinarz, Jonathan, 'Allied Intelligence Reports on Wartime German Penicillin Research and Production', *Historical Studies in the Physical and Biological Sciences*, 32/2 (2002), 347–68

Sheldrake, J., 'The L.C.C. Hospital Service', in A. Saint (ed.), *Politics and the People of London: the London County Council, 1889–1965* (1989), pp. 187–98.

Shephard, Ben, *A War of Nerves: Soldiers and Psychiatrists 1914–1994*, London, Pimlico, 2002

Shepherd, Mary P., *Heart of Harefield: The Story of the Hospital*, London, Quiller Press, 1990

Silbey, David, 'Bodies and Cultures Collide: Enlistment, the Medical Exam and the British Working Class, 1914–1916', *Social History of Medicine*, 17/1 (2004), 61–76

Slinn, Judy, 'The Development of the Pharmaceutical Industry' in S. Anderson (ed.), *Making Medicines* (2005), pp. 155–74

Stainton, Leslie, *Lorca: A Dream of Life*, London, Bloomsbury Publishing, 1998

Starns, Penny, *March of the Matrons: Military Influence on the British Civilian Nursing Profession, 1939–1969*, Peterborough, DSM, 2000

Strachan, Hew, *The First World War*, London, Simon and Schuster, 2003

Smith, F.B., *The Retreat of Tuberculosis, 1850–1950*, London, Croom Helm, 1988

Smith, Harold L. (ed.), *War and Social Change in British Society in the Second World War*, Manchester, Manchester University Press, 1996

Steppe, Hilde, 'Nursing under Totalitarian Regimes: The Case of Nazi Germany' in A.M. Rafferty, J. Robinson and R. Elkan (ed.), *Nursing History and the Politics of Welfare* (1997), pp. 10–27

Summers, Anne, *Angels into Citizens*, London, Routledge and Kegan-Paul, 1988

Sun, Sue, '*Where the Girls Are*: the Management of Venereal Disease by United States Military Forces in Vietnam', *Literature and Medicine*, 23/1 (2004), 66–87

Sutphen, Molly, 'Striving to be Separate? Civilian and Military Doctors in Cape Town during the Anglo-Boer War' in R. Cooter, M. Harrison and S. Sturdy (ed.), *War, Medicine and Modernity* (1998), pp. 48–64

Taylor, A.J.P., *English History 1914–1945*, Oxford, Oxford University Press, 1965

Taylor, Frederick, *Dresden: Tuesday 13 February 1945*, London, Bloomsbury, 2004

Thébaud, Françoise, *La Femme au Temps de la Guerre de 14*, Paris, Éditions Stock, 1994

Thomas, Hugh, *The Spanish Civil War*, Harmondsworth, Penguin, 1977

Titmuss, Richard M., *History of the Second World War: Problems of Social Policy*, London, HMSO, 1950

Tognotti, Eugenia, 'Scientific Triumphalism and Learning from the Facts: Bacteriology and the Spanish Flu Challenge of 1918', *Journal of the Society for the Social History of Medicine*, 16 (2003), 97–110

Tomkins, S.M., 'The failure of Expertise: Public Health Policy in Britain During the 1918–1919 Influenza Epidemic', *Social History of Medicine*, 5 (1992), 435–54

Townsend, Kim, *Manhood at Harvard: William James and Others*, Cambridge, Massachusetts, Harvard University Press, 1996

Venus, Nigel and Willis, Patsy. *The Home on the Hill: the Story of the Royal Star and Garter Home, Richmond for Disabled Ex-Servicemen and Women*, Richmond, Royal Star and Garter Home, 2006

Villarroya, Joan and Juliana Enric, 'El bombardeo de Barcelona en 1938: Y Mussolini decidió experimentar', *La Vanguardia* (12 March 2003), 3–5

Weindling, Paul, *The Rise of Medical Internationalism*, Oxford, Oxford University Press, 1996

Whitehead, Ian R., 'Not a Doctor's War? The Role of the British Regimental Medical Officer in the Field' in H. Cecil and P.H. Liddle (ed.), *Facing Armageddon* (1996), pp. 466–74

_____, Doctors *in the Great War*, Barnsley, Leo Cooper, 1999

Wilensky, Robert J., 'The Medical Civic Action Program in Vietnam: Success or Failure', *Military Medicine*, 166/9 (2001), 815–9

Willcox, Philip A., *The Detective Physician: The Life and Work of Sir William Willcox*, London, Heinemann, 1970

Winkler, Allan, *Life Under a Cloud: American Anxiety About the Atom*, New York and Oxford, Oxford University Press, 1993

Winter, Jay M., *The Great War and the British People*, London, Macmillan, 1985

_____, and Robert, Jean Louis, (ed.), *Capital Cities at War: Paris, London and Berlin, 1914–1919*, Cambridge, Cambridge University Press, 1999

Woodward, Scott C., 'The Story of the Mobile Army Surgical Hospital', *Military Medicine*, 168/7 (2003), 503–13

Worboys, Michael, 'Almroth Wright at Netley: Modern Medicine and the Military in Britain, 1892–1902' in R. Cooter, M. Harrison and S. Sturdy (ed.) *Medicine and Modern Warfare* (1999), pp. 77–97

Yagisawa, Y., 'Early History of Antibiotics in Japan' in J. Parascandola (ed.), *The History of Antibiotics* (1980), pp. 69–81

Ziegler, Philip, *London at War, 1939–1945*, London, Sinclair-Stevenson, 1995

Index

Abbott Laboratories, 133
accident and emergency medicine,
    200–1
advanced dressing station, 42
Afghanistan War, 10, 209
Agent Orange, 202–3
air medical evacuation, 195–7
air raid shelters, 156–7
air raids, 150–3, 155–8
Airborne Medical Division, 113
Albert I, king of the Belgians, 74
alcohol controls, 80–1
Alexander, General, 126
Alexandra, Princess Arthur of
    Connaught, 75
Alexandra, queen of Great Britain,
    29, 75
All Quiet on the Western Front, 46–7
Allbutt, Thomas Clifford, 64
Allen, Chesney, 121
Allyson, June, 198
Al-Qaeda, 213
Altman, Robert, 201
Ambrose, Paul, 212
ambulance train, 42–3,
American Psychological Association, 40
anaesthesia, 46, 93
Anderson, Sergeant, 178
Andrews, Dana, 161
antibiotics, 129–38, 198
Apel, Otto, 198
Apollinaire, Guillaume, 87
Appelt, August, 71
Army Blood Transfusion Service,
    117–9
Army Medical Department, 21, 27
Army Nursing Service, 28
Army Transport Command, 133
Arthur of Connaught, Prince, 75
(see also Alexandra, Princess Arthur
    of Connaught)

aspirin, 86
atom bomb, 191–4
Auctioneers and Estate Agents Institute,
    78
Auschwitz Concentration Camp, 172–7
aviation medicine, 111–2, 114–5, 174–5

Bacinol, 137
bacterial warfare, 185–6, 192–3, 208,
    214
bacteriology, 49, 115–7
Bailey, Second Lieutenant, 114
Baker, F.M., 140
Baker, Newton D., 82
Balfour, Arthur, 49
Balilla, 167–8
Bannon, Dorothy, 147
barbed wire disease, 83–4
Barcelona Blood Transfusion Service,
    103–5
Barnes, John Gray, 132
Basingstoke Hospital, 160
Bataan Death March, 178
Battle Circus, 198
Bayer, 175
Begg, Mrs, 178
Belgrade Hospital, 37
Belsen Concentration Camp, 164–5
Berwick and Alba, Duke of, 93
Best Years of Our Lives, 160–1
Bethune, Norman, 105
Beveridge Report, 162
Biafran War, 212
Bier, Professor, 46
Bikini Atoll, 193
Binding, Karl, 166
Binet, Alfred, 40
Bishop, Dr, 146
Black, George, 178
blackout, 148–9
Blake, Edgar, 155

blitz, 150–3, 156–8
Blood Protection Law, 167
blood transfusion, 44–5, 103–4,
    117–9, 155, 198–9, 203
Boer War, 13–26
Bogart, Humphrey, 198
Bolton Act of Congress, 154
Boots the Chemist, 86
Borbón, Ataúlfo de, 94
Borkenau, Franz, 96, 105–6
Boston, Kenneth, 93
Boulogne 14th General Hospital
    (Casino), 48
Bowlby, Arthur, 43, 111
Boy Scouts, 33
Boys Brigade, 33
Brand, Karl, 170
Brierley, Henry, 150
Brighton Board of Guardians, 68
Brighton Pavilion, 68
Bristol Blood Supply depot, 118
British Medical Aid Unit, 92
British Women's Hospital
    Committee, 78
Brittain, Vera, 75–6
Brock, Arthur, 63
Broderick, John, 29
Broggi, Moises, 101–2
Broyles, William, 206
Brompton Hospital, 79
Brown, Sidney Hamilton, 94
Bruce, David, 23, 53
brucellosis, *see* Malta Fever
bubonic plague, 52–3
Buchan, John, 63
Bull, John, 73
Bullock, Arthur, 33, 41
Burckhardt, Carl, 188
Burdett-Coutts, William, 16, 20, 26
Burgess, Alice, 150
Burma Railway, 184

burns, 115–7, 202–3, 207
Burroughs Wellcome, 86
Buttle, G.E., 118
Byng, Douglas, 121

Cadet Nurse Corps, 154
Cairns, Hugh, 128, 135
Calder, Ritchie, 156
Calmette, Albert, 79
Cambridge Military Hospital,
   Aldershot, 59–60
Care of Mothers and Young
   Children Act, 86
Carrel, Alexis, 44–5
casualty clearing station, 42–3
Catel, Werner, 152
Cavell, Edith, 76
Chailey Heritage Hospital, 77
Chain, Ernst, 130–1
Chamberlain, Neville, 139
Changi balls, 181
Changi Camp, Singapore, 180
Charing Cross Hospital Medical
   School, 72
Charité hospital, Berlin, 85
Charleson, Miss, 18–19
Charters, David, 121
Chavasse, Noel, 41
Chelmno Concentration Camp, 173
chemical warfare, 208
child welfare, 100, 135, 147–8, 209
cholera, 184
Christie, Agatha, 74
Church Lads Brigade, 33
Churchill, Winston, 115, 122, 126,
   129, 191
Ciano, Galeazzo, 167–8
CIBA, 137
civil defence, 193
civilian internees, 83–4, 179–83
Civilian War Casualty Program, 204
Clauberg, Carl, 174
Clayponds Hospital, 150
Clemenceau, Georges, 82
clothes rationing, 158
Cockburn, Henry D. ('Cocky'), 112
Coghill, Robert, 137
Cold War, 191–4
Colebrook, Leonard, 116
combat support hospitals, 200–1
Commission on Training Camp
   Activities, 81–2
Conan Doyle, Arthur, 20
concentration camps, 24–6, 164–5,
   172–7, 188–9
Copeman, Frank, 109
Corlette, Ewan, 184
Craig, Chris, 208
Craiglockhart Hospital, 63–4
Crile, George, 44–5
Curie, Marie, 73
Cushing, Harvey, 45–6
Cutting, Irving S., 155

CWCP, *see* Civilian War Casualty
   Program

Dakin, Henry, 44–5
Dawson, Lord, 86, 161
Day, Frances, 121
DDT, 125
Defence of Realm Act, 82
Derby, Lord, 49
Diana, princess of Wales, 211
Digging for Victory, 158
Dimitrijevitch, Djurdge, 70–1
Domagk, Gerhard, 102–3
Donald, Ian, 10
Donald, James, 145
Dooley, Tom, 204
drug addiction, 205
Duhamel, Georges, 65, 74
Dunant, Henri, 186
Dunant, Paul, 189
Dunlop, Edward ('Weary'), 184–5
Duran i Jordà, Frederic, 103–5, 108

Eberth, Carl, 17
Egerton, Commander, 18
Egle, Edward, 187
Ehrlich, Paul, 86–7
Elisabeth, queen of the Belgians, 74
Elizabeth, queen of Great Britain,
   150, 157–8
Elosegui, Carlos, 103
Emergency Blood Transfusion
   Service, 155
Emergency Medical Service, 139–45,
   161
Ena, queen of Spain, 91
Endell Street Military Hospital, 73
ENSA, 128
enteric fever, *see* typhoid
Epidemic Prevention and Water
   Supply Unit, 185
Ethiopian War, 94
eugenics, 30–1, 165–7, 169
euthanasia, 169–71
evacuation, 142–3, 146–8
Exham, Commander, 19–20

Fabian Society, 31
Falklands War, 206–7
Fantus, Bernard, 104
Faramus, Anthony, 176
Fat Man, 191
Fawcett Commission, 26
Fawcett, Millicent, 25–6
field ambulance, 16, 28, 43
Fielding, Garrison, 64
Fields, Gracie, 128
Fildes, Paul, 186
first aid post, 42
First Gulf War, 207–9
First London General Hospital, 75
First World War, 37–87
Fisher, H.A.L., 67

Fitzgerald, Scott, 61
Flanagan, Bud, 121
Fleming, Alexander, 56–7, 130, 131,
   137
Florey, Howard, 128, 130–2, 135, 137
food rationing, 107, 158–9
forensic pathology, 213–4
Formby, George, 149
Fosdick, Raymond B., 81–2
Foulkes, Howard, 57
Fragner, Jiri, 137
Franco, Carmen, 88
Franco, Francisco, 88, 98
Frankland, Bill, 180–1
Franz Ferdinand, archduke of
   Austria, 37
Frewer, H.E., 151
Fuyschott, Cornelius, 136

Gable, Clark, 121
Galen, Clemens August von, 171
Gallipoli, 52
Galsworthy, John, 76
Gandhi, Mohandras K., 16–17
Garcia Lorca, Federico, 90
Garvin, J.L., 73
gas masks, 58, 148–9, 194
gas poisoning, 119–20, 194
Gedroitz, Vera, 35
Geigy Corporation, 125
Gellhorn, Martha, 97
General Mola Military Hospital, 93
General Penicillin Committee, 134
General Service Selection Scheme,
   122
Geneva Convention, 186, 188, 189
George V, king of Great Britain,
   67, 81
George VI, king of Great Britain,
   126, 150, 157
Gillies, Harold, 59–61
Gillies, Harold, 119
Gioventi Fascisti, 168
Glasgow Burns Unit, 116
Glass, Al, 200
Glasser, Ronald, 202
Goebbels, Joseph, 166, 167
Gosse, Philip, 52
Gould, Elliot, 201
Graefeneck Asylum, 171
Grande Covián, Dr, 107–8
Grau Blanc, Josep Maria, 91
Graves, Robert, 47
Great Ormond Street Children's
   Hospital, 85
Greenmantle, 63
Grenfell, Joyce, 121
Guernica, bombing of, 99
Guillan, Georges, 62
Guinea Pig Club, 121
Gulf War Syndrome, 208
Gurney, Louisa, 67
Guy's Hospital, 70, 146

Haber, Fritz, 57
Hachiya, Michihiko, 191
Haefliger, Louis, 189
Haffkine, Waldemar, 22
Hailie Selassie, emperor of Ethiopia, 94
Haldane, J.G., 114
Haldane, Lord, 28–9
Hammersmith Hospital, 77
Harcourt Got, Joaquin d', 102
Harefield County Sanatorium, 140, 143
Harstad General Hospital, 118
Heatley, Norman, 131–3
Hecking, Henri, 185
Heilbron, 25
Heinebach, Otto, 46
Heller, Joseph, 124
Helm, Bill, 110
Herling, Gustav, 177
Herrington, E.W., 27
Heydrich, Reinhard, 175
Higgins, Eric, 83
Hill, Charles, 159, 163
Hillary, Richard, 116, 120–1
Himmler, Heinrich, 172, 176
Hirohito, emperor of Japan, 165
Hiroshima, 191–2
Hirschfeldt, Magnus, 84
Hirt, August, 176
Hitler Youth, 168
Hitler, Adolph, 165, 167, 170
Hobhouse, Emily, 25–6
Hoche, Alfred, 166
Hodgson Lobley, J., 66
Hofmeyr, John, 136
Holladay, Michael, 203
Holmes, Gordon, 62
Holocaust, 164–5, 172–7
Home Guard medical services, 109
homosexuality, 83–4, 123
Hooker, Richard, *see* Hornberger, Richard
Hornberger, Richard, 201
Horwitz, Mel, 197, 198
Hospital de la Sant Creu i Sant Paul, 100
Hospital de Nuestra Señora de la Mar, *See* Hospital Marítim d'Infecciosos
Hospital Field Service, 18, 20
Hospital Marítim d'Infecciosos, 89–91
Howard Commission on Medical Services, 49
Howards of Ilford, 86
humanitarian aid, 210–13

ICI, 132
IG Farbenindustrie, 57, 102, 137, 175
In Which We Serve, 145
Inagaki, Katsuhiko, 137–8
Indian Nursing Services, 29

industrial welfare, 84–5
infant welfare, 31, 85–6
influenza, 87, 145, 158
Inglis, Elsie, 73
Institute of Aviation Medicine, 115
Institute of Professional Adaptation for Women, 106
Interdepartmental Committee on Physical Deterioration, 30–1
International Brigade, 91–3, 97
International Committee of the Red Cross, 186–9, 211
internment, 83–4, 108, 179–83, 187–8
Intombi Spruit, 19
Ishii, Shiro, 185

Jeanbreau, Emile, 45
Jenner, Edward, 22
Johanstadt Hospital, 152
Johns, Rosamund, 153
Johore, Sultan of, 180
Joint War Committee of Red Cross and Order of St John, 76
Jones, Private, 184–5
Jones, Robert, 77
Joubert, Piet, 19
Journey's End, 62
Junod, Marcel, 94–5, 187

Kamill, Mustapha, 150
Kanthack, Emilia, 31
Kaufmann, D., 64
Keith, Agnes, 183
Kemball Bishop, 132, 134
Keogh, Alfred, 28, 55
Kharsivan, 86
King George V Sanatorium, 151
King, Norman, 92
Kitchener, Lord, 24, 38, 42, 81
Klebs, Edwin, 17
Kobouky, Val, 181–2
Koch, Robert, 51
Korean War, 194–201
Kosovan War, 213
Kouchner, Bernard, 212–13
Kremer, Paul, 172
Kreysigg, Lothar, 171

Ladysmith, 18, 20–1
Lamp Still Burns, 153
land mines, 211
Landsteiner, Karl, 44–5
Lang, Slobodan, 211
Lauder, Harry, 62
Law for the Prevention of Genetically Diseased Offspring, 169
Lawrence, D.H., 39
Lawrence, Thomas E., 52
League of German Maidens, 168
League of Nations Health Organisation, 210

Leary, Timothy, 87
Leath, Norman, 178
Lebensborn homes, 171–2
Lee, Arthur, 42–3
Leforestier, Roger, 189
Leishman, William, 24, 53
Lest We Forget Association, 78
Levi, Primo, 177
lice, 53–5
Lickint, Fritz, 169
Lister, Joseph, 56
Little Boy, 191
Lloyd George, David, 49, 80–1
Logan, Daniel Crawford, 150
London Ambulance Service, 141–2
London bombings (2005), 214
London County Council Nursing Service, 147
London Hospital, Whitechapel, 150–1
London School of Medicine for Women, 71
London, Bishop of, 85
Loy, Myrna, 160
Lundy, John S., 104

Macintosh, Robert, 93
Madrid Blood Transfusion Service, 105
Mafeking, 25
Maidstone Lunatic Asylum, 22
malaria, 125–6, 203
Malayan Emergency, 196
Maldonado, Francisco, 88
Maling, P.B., 151
Malta Fever, 22
Manoel II, king of Portugal, 76–7
March, Frederic, 160
Marcus, Robert Otto, 71
Marital Health Law, 167
Martin, Arthur A., 48, 50
Martínez Alonso, Eduardo, 91, 129
Mary, queen of Great Britain, 67, 75, 78
MASH, *see* mobile army surgical unit
MASH , 200
maternity, 80, 100, 148
Maternity and Child Welfare Act, 86
Matthews, Bryan, 115
Mattowitz, Leo, 112
Maurice, John Frederick, 29
May and Baker, 86
McCorquodale Committee, 154
McIndoe, Archibald, 116–7, 119–21
McMillan, Margaret, 32
McRae, Peter, 145
MEDCAP, *see* Medical Civil Action Program
Médecins Sans Frontières, 212–13
Medical Civil Action Program, 203–4
medical experimentation, 173–6, 185–6, 189–90

Medical Staff Corps, 27
medical students, 70–3, 142–5
medical unit self–contained
 transportable hospitals, 201
Megías Manzano, José , 90
Mengele, Josef, 173–4
Mepacrine, 126
Merck, 133
Mesopotamia, 52
Metropolitan Asylums Board, 68
Mid and East Lothian Miners'
 Association, 79
Middleton, Captain, 47
Midwives Act (1902), 31
Milá Nolla, Mercedes, 98
MILHAP, *see* Military Provincial
 Health Assistance Program
Military Provincial Health Assistance
 Program, 204
Millán Astray, José, 88
Miller, Lee, 119, 135–6
Military Blood Programme Agency,
 203
Milne, Mary, 152–3
Milner, Alfred, 25
Ministry of Health, 86
Mira i López, Emili, 105–6, 108
Mitchell, Alexander, 183
mobile army surgical unit, 196–201
Moffat, Alex, 47
Montesinos, Manuel, 90
Montgomery, Bernard, 124–5
Moon, Arthur, 184
Moran, Lord, *see* Wilson, Charles
 McMoran
Moyer, Andrew, 133
Müller, Paul, 125, 169
munitions factories, 84
MUST, *see* medical unit self–
 contained transportable hospitals
Myers, Charles, 61–2
Mysterious Affair at Styles, 74

Naauwpoort, 6ᵗʰ General Hospital,
 20
Nagasaki, 191–2
National Blood Transfusion Service,
 155
National Filling Factory, Chittening,
 84–5
National Health Service, 161–3
National Hospital for the Paralysed
 and Epileptic, 64
National Institute for the Blind, 77
National Service, 196, 199
National Socialism, 165–7
naval surgeons, 145–6
Negrin, Dr, 107
Netley Military Hospital, 21–3, 28
New South Wales Ambulance, 16
Newcastle Church High School for
 Girls, 68
Newman, George, 87

Nigerian Civil War, 212
Nixon, Lewis, 10
Nixon, Richard, 205
Nonne, Max, 64
Norman, H.R.B., 151
Norman, Montagu, 159
North Point Camp, Hong Kong,
 179–80
North, Thomas Stanley, 70
Northern Regional Research
 Laboratory, Peoria, 132–4
Not Forgotten Association, 78
Not Yet Diagnosed Nervous
 Centres, 62
Nuremberg Code, 190
Nurses' Act (1943), 153–4
nursing, 9–10, 18–19, 28–9, 74–6,
 92–4, 96–7, 98–9, 147, 152–5,
 170–1
nursing cadets, 154
nutrition, 80, 107–8, 158–9, 181–2
Nyiszli, Myklos, 174

Office of Scientific Research and
 Development, 132
Ogston, Alexander, 28
Operation Golden Flow, 205
ophthalmology, 59
Order of St John, 67, 76
orthopaedic surgery, 42, 77, 101
Orwell, George, 96–7
Osler, William, 8–9, 18, 34, 64
ta ,Y ko, 191
Ottawa Treaty, 211
Owen, Wilfred, 58, 63–4

Paddington Green Children's
 Hospital, 85
Park Prewett Hospital, 119, 143–4
Passavant Memorial Hospital, 155
Pearson, Arthur, 77
Pearson, Karl, 24, 31
penicillin, 128–38, 159–60, 198
Perlasca, Giorgio, 189
Perry, Colin, 156, 157
Pfizer, 133–4
Phelps, Penny, 92
Philipps, Wogan, 92
Phillips, Dudley Vaughan, 144
physical training, 32–3, 199
Picasso, Pablo, 99
plastic surgery, 59–61, 119–21
poison gas, 57–8, 148–9
Portland Hospital, 21
Porton Down, 186, 194
post traumatic stress disorder, 206,
 209
Poulenc Frères, 86
Priestley, J.S., 114
Princess Christian's Army Nursing
 Service Reserve, 28–9
Princess Mary's Patriotic Union for
 Girls, 67

prisoners of war, 55, 83, 120, 177–85
psychiatry, 61–4, 105–7, 121–4, 149–
 50, 157–8, 200, 206, 208, 213
Pulvertaft, R.J., 135

Queen Alexandra's Imperial Military
 Nursing Service, 29, 74
Queen Mary's Hospital, Sidcup, 60
Queen Victoria Hospital East
 Grinstead, 119–21
quinine, 125–6

racial deterioration, 30–1
racial hygiene, 165–7, 169
Rascher, Sigmund, 175
rats, 52–3
recruitment medical inspections,
 38–9, 122–3
Red Army Military Sanitary
 Department, 113
Red Cross, 47, 67, 76, 94–5, 154,
 186–90, 211–12
rehabilitation, 77, 160–1
Reich Central Office for
 Combating Homosexuaity and
 Abortion, 176
Remarque, Eric Maria, 46–7
Retrosi, Virgilio, 9
Ricci, Renato, 167–8
Rion, Don, 202
Rivers, W.H.R., 62–3
Roberts, General, 20
Robson, Corporal, 43
Rockefeller Foundation, 79, 130
Romer, Robert, 26
Roosevelt, Eleanor, 159
Rosenberg, Isaac, 53
Rostock, Professor, 137
Royal Army Medical College,
 21–4, 28
Royal Army Medical Corps, 21,
 26–8, 47, 49
Royal Commission on the Poor
 Laws (1909), 33
Royal Commission on Venereal
 Diseases, 83
Royal Edinburgh Infirmary, 79
Royal Victoria Hospital, Netley,
 21–3, 28
Royal Warwickshire Hospital, 151–2
Royaumont Hospital, 73
Rudolph Hess Clinic, 153
Ruhleben Internment Camp, 83–4
Rushcliffe Committee, 154
Russell, Audrey, 108
Russell, Harold, 160
Russo-Japanese War, 34–6

Saddam Hussein, 207, 208
Sadí de Buen, Dr, 90
St Clair, Mabel, 54
St Dunstan's Association, 77–8, 160
St George's Hospital, 117, 152

St Mary's Hospital Medical School, 71–2
St Mary's Hospital, Paddington, 48, 68–9, 75,146, 152–3, 157–8
St Pancras School for Mothers, 31
St Stephen's College, Hong Kong, 178
St Thomas's Hospital, 151
salvarsan , 86
Salvation Army, 42
San Pablo Hospital, 90
Sanders, Gordon, 131
sanitation, 51, 125
Sarajevo State Hospital, 211
Sargant, William, 149–50
Sargent, John Singer, 58
Sassoon, Siegfried, 63–4
Saxton, Reginald, 105
Schering, 137
school medical services, 32
Scott–Ellis, Priscilla, 94
Scottish Women's Hospitals, 73
Second Gulf War, 10–11, 209
Second World War, 110–192
Selwyn-Clarke, P.S., 182–3
Semple, David, 22
Shaukiwan Medical Store, 178
shell shock, 61–4
Shepherd's Bush Military Hospital, 77
Sherriff, R.C., 62
Sinclair-Loutit, Kenneth, 95
Sino-Japanese War, 105, 185
Sir William Dunn School of Pathology, Oxford, 130–1
Slim, William, 126
Sloggett, Arthur, 49
Smith, Dean, 182
smoking, 168–9, 205
social medicine, 100
Social Security and the Allied Services, 162
Soldiers and Sailors Help Socxiety, 67
Sollenberger, Randall, 92
Sorley, Charles, 41
Souttar, Henry, 38
Spanish American War, 17
Spanish Civil War, 88–109
Spanish Medical Aid Committee, 91–2
Speake, Hilda, 76
Squibb, 133
Stanford–Binet Test, 40
Stanley Internment Camp, 182
Star and Garter Home, 78, 160
Steer, George, 99
Steevens, George, 19
Stephen Westman, 46, 85

sterile dressings, 14–15
Stokes, Adrian, 53
sulphonamides, 102–3, 136–7, 175
surgeon probationer, 70
surgery, 15, 28, 43–8, 100–2, 202
Sutherland, Donald, 201

T-4, 170–2
Taylor, Gordon, 117
Taylor, William, 30
Tender is the Night, 61
Terman, Lewis, 40
Territorial Army Nursing Service, 29
tetanus, 50–1
Thomas splint, 42, 101
Thomas, Lieutenant, 178
Thomas, Wade, 156
Thomson, Andrew, 214
Tobruk splint, 101
Tolomay, Jim, 206
Tonks, Henry, 59–60
Traill, Henry, 184
transport of wounded, 16–17, 42–3, 95–6, 111–14, 195–7, 201–2
Treblinka Concentration Camp, 172–3
trench fever, 53
trench foot, 54
Treves, Frederick, 15, 28
Trias de Bes, Lluis, 91
Trinder, Tommy, 121
Trueta Raspall, Josep, 100–2, 108
Truman, Harry S., 194–5
tuberculosis, 79
typhoid, 17–24, 50–1
typhus, 54–5

Udaeta, Dr, 90
ultrasound, 10
Unamuno, Miguel de, 88
UNICEF, *see* United Nations International Children's Emergency Fund
Unit 73, 185
United Airlines Flight 93, 213
United Nations International Children's Emergency Fund, 210
United Nations Relief and Rehabilitation Administration, 210
Usach, Juliet, 189

vaccination, 21–3, 50–1, 100
Valadier, Charles, 59
Vaughan, Janet, 108, 164
venereal disease, 81–3, 123, 126–9, 165, 204–5
Victory Volunteers, 155

Vietnam War, 201–6
Vincenzi, Roberto, 92
Vives Ma e, Josep, 105
Voluntary Aid Detachments (VADs), 75–6
Vukovar Hospital, 211

Wallace, William, 59
Wallenberg, Raoul, 189
War Cabinet Scientific Advisory Committee, 115
war memorials, 41
War on Terror, 10, 212, 213–14
Ward, V.J., 132
Warrack, Captain, 181
Warren Low, Vincent, 14
Waters, Doris , 158
Waters, Elsie, 158
Watson Cheyne, William, 57
Watts, J.C., 110, 118
Weil's Disease, 52–3
Wellcome Laboratories, 131
Wermacht medical services, 112–13
Wesley Memorial Hospital, 154–5
West, R., 113–4
Weston, Simon, 207
Whitby, Leonard, 117
Where the Girls Are, 204
White Paper on Health (1944), 163
White, Arnold, 29–30
White, Sir George, 18
Whitney, John, 178
Widal, Ferdinand, 18
Wilhelm II, Kaiser of Germany, 165
Wilson Committee, 141
Wilson, Charles McMoran, 62–3, 126, 140–1, 144, 199
Wilson, Woodrow, 82
Wimborne Cottage Hospital, 68
Wingate, Lieutenant, 15
Wingate, Orde, 125
Winthrop, 133
Women's Hospital Corps, 73
Wooster, Reginald, 41
World Health Organization, 210–11
World Trade Center, 213–4
wound infections, 55–7, 100–1
Wright, Almroth, 21–4, 48–51, 53, 55–7
Wright, Teresa, 161

Yaron, Barna, 189
Yealland, Lewis, 64
Yudin, Serge, 104
Yugoslavian Wars, 210–11, 214

Ziegler, Benno, 38, 40
Zindel, Rudolf, 187–8